theclinics.com

EMERGENCY MEDICINE CLINICS OF NORTH AMERICA

Pediatric Emergencies in the First Year of Life

GUEST EDITORS
Ghazala Q. Sharieff, MD and
James E. Colletti, MD

CONSULTING EDITOR
Amal Mattu, MD

November 2007 • Volume 25 • Number 4

SAUNDERS

An Imprint of Elsevier, Inc.
PHILADELPHIA   LONDON   TORONTO   MONTREAL   SYDNEY   TOKYO

W.B. SAUNDERS COMPANY
A Division of Elsevier Inc.

1600 John F. Kennedy Boulevard, Suite 1800 • Philadelphia, Pennsylvania 19103-2899

http://www.theclinics.com

EMERGENCY MEDICINE CLINICS   **Volume 25, Number 4**
OF NORTH AMERICA   **ISSN 0733-8627**
November 2007   **ISBN-13: 978-1-4160-5561-7**
Editor: Patrick Manley   **ISBN-10: 1-4160-5561-4**

The ideas and opinions expressed in *Emergency Medicine Clinics of North America* do not necessarily reflect those of the Publisher. The Publisher does not assume any responsibility for any injury and/or damage to persons or property arising out of or related to any use of the material contained in this periodical. The reader is advised to check the appropriate medical literature and the product information currently provided by the manufacturer of each drug to be administered to verify the dosage, the method and duration of administration, or contraindications. It is the responsibility of the treating physician or other health care professional, relying on independent experience and knowledge of the patient, to determine drug dosages and the best treatment for the patient. Mention of any product in this issue should not be construed as endorsement by the contributors, editors, or the Publisher of the product or manufacturers' claims.

Emergency Medicine Clinics of North America (ISSN 0733-8627) is published quarterly by Elsevier Inc., 360 Park Avenue South, New York, NY, 10010-1710. Months of issue are February, May, August, and November. Business and Editorial Offices: 1600 John F. Kennedy Boulevard, Suite 1800, Philadelphia, PA 19103-2899. Customer Service Office: 6277 Sea Harbor Drive, Orlando, FL 32887-4800. Periodicals postage paid at New York, NY, and additional mailing offices. Subscription prices are $109.00 per year (US students), $212.00 per year (US individuals), $339.00 per year (US institutions), $145.00 per year (international students), $285.00 per year (international individuals), $400.00 per year (international institutions), $145.00 per year (Canadian students), $261.00 per year (Canadian individuals), and $400.00 per year (Canadian institutions). International air speed delivery is included in all *Clinics'* subscription prices. All prices are subject to change without notice. POSTMASTER: Send address changes to *Emergency Medicine Clinics of North America*, Elsevier Periodicals Customer Service, 6277 Sea Harbor Drive, Orlando, FL 32887-4800. **Customer Service: 1-800-654-2452 (US). From outside of the US, call 1-407-345-4000. E-mail: hhspcs@harcourt.com.**

Emergency Medicine Clinics of North America is covered in *Index Medicus, Current Contents/Clinical Medicine, EMBASE/Excerpta Medica, BIOSIS, SciSearch, CINAHL, ISI/BIOMED,* and *Research Alert.*

Printed in the United States of America.

CONSULTING EDITOR

AMAL MATTU, MD, Program Director, Emergency Medicine Residency; and Associate Professor, Department of Emergency Medicine, University of Maryland School of Medicine, Baltimore, Maryland

GUEST EDITORS

GHAZALA Q. SHARIEFF, MD, FACEP, FAAEM, FAAP, Director of Pediatric Emergency Medicine, Palomar-Pomerado Health System/California Emergency Physicians; Medical Director, Division of Emergency Medicine, Rady Children's Hospital, San Diego, California

JAMES E. COLLETTI, MD, FAAEM, FAAP, Associate Residency Director, Department of Emergency Medicine, Mayo Clinic College of Medicine, Rochester, Minnesota

CONTRIBUTORS

KELLY BARRINGER, MD, Department of Emergency Medicine, Regions Hospital, St. Paul, Minnesota

MICHELLE D. BLUMSTEIN, MD, Pediatric Emergency Medicine Fellow, Division of Emergency Medicine, Miami Children's Hospital, Miami, Florida

JAMES E. COLLETTI, MD, FAAEM, FAAP, Associate Residency Director, Department of Emergency Medicine, Mayo Clinic College of Medicine, Rochester, Minnesota

STEPHANIE J. DONIGER, MD, FAAP, Attending Physician, Pediatric Emergency Medicine; and Emergency Ultrasound Fellow, St. Luke's-Roosevelt Hospital Center, New York, New York

MARLA J. FRIEDMAN, DO, Attending Physician, Division of Emergency Medicine, Miami Children's Hospital, Miami, Florida

MARTIN HERMAN, MD, Professor of Medicine, University of Tennessee Health Sciences Center, College of Medicine; Pediatric Emergency Medical Staff, Division of Pediatric Emergency Medicine, LeBonheur Children's Medical Center, Memphis, Tennessee

PAUL ISHIMINE, MD, Associate Clinical Professor, Departments of Medicine and Pediatrics, University of California, San Diego School of Medicine; Director, Pediatric Emergency Medicine, Department of Emergency Medicine, University of California, San Diego Medical Center; and Attending Physician, Division of Emergency Medicine, Rady Children's Hospital and Health Center, San Diego, California

DANIELLE M. JACKSON, MD, Department of Emergency Medicine, Regions Hospital, St. Paul, Minnesota

KEVIN P. KILGORE, MD, Department of Emergency Medicine, Regions Hospital, St. Paul, Minnesota

SAMIP KOTHORI, MD, Department of Pediatrics, University of Arizona, Tucson, Arizona

KENNETH T. KWON, MD, RDMS, FACEP, FAAP, Associate Clinical Professor, Department of Emergency Medicine, University of California, Irvine School of Medicine; Director of Pediatric Emergency Medicine, University of California Irvine Medical Center, Orange, California; Co-Director, Pediatric Emergency Services, Mission Regional Medical Center/Children's Hospital of Orange County at Mission, Mission Viejo, California

AUDREY LE, MD, Pediatric Emergency Medicine Fellow, University of Tennessee Health Sciences Center, College of Medicine, Memphis, Tennessee

JEFFREY P. LOUIE MD, Staff Physician, Department of Emergency Medicine, Children's Hospitals and Clinics of Minnesota; Adjunct Instructor, Department of Pediatrics, University of Minnesota, Minneapolis, Minnesota

MERLIN C. LOWE, Jr, MD, FAAP, Assistant Professor of Clinical Pediatrics, Department of Pediatrics, The University of Arizona, Tucson, Arizona

SEEMA SHAH, MD, Pediatric Emergency Medicine Fellow, Division of Emergency Medicine, Rady Children's Hospital, University of California, San Diego, San Diego, California

GHAZALA Q. SHARIEFF, MD, FACEP, FAAEM, FAAP, Director of Pediatric Emergency Medicine, Palomar-Pomerado Health System/California Emergency Physicians; Medical Director, Division of Emergency Medicine, Rady Children's Hospital, San Diego, California

VIRGINIA W. TSAI, MD, Resident in Emergency Medicine, Department of Emergency Medicine, University of California, Irvine School of Medicine, Orange, California

DALE P. WOOLRIDGE, MD, PhD, FAAEM, FAAP, FACEP, Assistant Professor, Department of Emergency Medicine and Pediatrics, The University of Arizona, Tucson, Arizona

LINTON YEE, MD, Associate Professor, Department of Pediatrics, Division of Hospital and Emergency Medicine; and Department of Surgery, Division of Emergency Medicine, Duke University School of Medicine, Durham, North Carolina

CONTENTS

The Normal Newborn Exam, or Is It?   921
Merlin C. Lowe Jr and Dale P. Woolridge

> Despite the broad technologic advancements of medicine, screen-
> ing for illness in infants is highly reliant on a complete physical
> exam. For this reason it is critical that the examining physician not
> only have a thorough understanding of abnormal findings but also
> the normal findings and their variants. The vast majority of infants
> are healthy and findings predictive of future health problems are
> subtle and infrequent. Yet, outcomes can be devastating. Therefore
> it is critical the physician remain diligent when screening for these.
> It is our hope that this article will assist you in this task and allow
> for more accurate and timely diagnosis that prevents or minimizes
> long-term health problems in children.

Pediatric Resuscitation Update   947
Stephanie J. Doniger and Ghazala Q. Sharieff

> In 2005, the American Heart Association updated the guidelines for
> newborn and pediatric resuscitation. These changes are now being

taught in the current Basic Life Support and Pediatric Advanced Life Support classes. This article reviews the pertinent new changes in caring for the critically ill child.

Pediatric Respiratory Infections

Seema Shah and Ghazala Q. Sharieff

Pediatric respiratory infections are a common presenting complaint to the emergency department. This article discusses the presentation and management of infectious conditions, including bacterial tracheitis, bronchiolitis, croup, epiglottitis, pertussis, pneumonia, and retropharyngeal abscess.

Cardiac Emergencies in the First Year of Life

Linton Yee

Cardiac emergencies in the first year of life can be anxiety provoking for the health care provider. An understanding of the pathophysiology involved in the most common emergency department presentations is crucial to the development of appropriate treatment plans. This article discusses the most common causes of cyanotic and acyanotic heart disease in infants.

Essential Diagnosis of Abdominal Emergencies in the First Year of Life

Jeffrey P. Louie

There are a myriad of abdominal emergencies in the first year of life. Some are more common than others, but each very serious. Any delay in determining the diagnosis can lead to significant morbidity and even mortality. This article discusses neonatal and infant medical and surgical abdominal emergencies often encountered in the emergency department.

Metabolic Emergencies

Kenneth T. Kwon and Virginia W. Tsai

Metabolic diseases can vary as much in clinical presentation as they can in classification, and neonates and infants frequently present with symptoms similar to those seen with other emergencies. Vomiting, alterations in neurologic status, and feeding difficulties are the most prominent features of metabolic emergencies. This article discusses the recognition and management of specific disorders, including diabetic ketoacidosis, congenital adrenal hyperplasia, inborn errors of metabolism, and thyrotoxicosis. Also highlighted are specific laboratory entities, including hypoglycemia, hyponatremia, and metabolic acidosis.

FORTHCOMING ISSUES

RECENT ISSUES

GOAL STATEMENT
The goal of *Emergency Medicine Clinics of North America* is to keep practicing physicians up to date with current clinical practice in emergency medicine by providing timely articles reviewing the state of the art in patient care.

ACCREDITATION
The *Emergency Medical Clinics of North America* is planned and implemented in accordance with the Essential Areas and Policies of the Accreditation Council for Continuing Medical Education (ACCME) through the joint sponsorship of the University of Virginia School of Medicine and Elsevier. The University of Virginia School of Medicine is accredited by the ACCME to provide continuing medical education for physicians.

The University of Virginia School of Medicine designates this educational activity for a maximum of *15 AMA PRA Category 1 Credits™*. Physicians should only claim credit commensurate with the extent of their participation in the activity.

The Emergency Medicine Clinics of North America CME program is approved by the American College of Emergency Physicians for 60 hours of ACEP Category I Credit per year.

The American Medical Association has determined that physicians not licensed in the US who participate in this CME activity are eligible for *15 AMA PRA Category 1 Credits™*.

Credit can be earned by reading the text material, taking the CME examination online at http://www.theclinics.com/home/cme, and completing the evaluation. After taking the test, you will be required to review any and all incorrect answers. Following completion of the test and evaluation, your credit will be awarded and you may print your certificate.

FACULTY DISCLOSURE/CONFLICT OF INTEREST
The University of Virginia School of Medicine, as an ACCME accredited provider, endorses and strives to comply with the Accreditation Council for Continuing Medical Education (ACCME) Standards of Commercial Support, Commonwealth of Virginia statutes, University of Virginia policies and procedures, and associated federal and private regulations and guidelines on the need for disclosure and monitoring of proprietary and financial interests that may affect the scientific integrity and balance of content delivered in continuing medical education activities under our auspices.

The University of Virginia School of Medicine requires that all CME activities accredited through this institution be developed independently and be scientifically rigorous, balanced and objective in the presentation/discussion of its content, theories and practices.

All authors/editors participating in an accredited CME activity are expected to disclose to the readers relevant financial relationships with commercial entities occurring within the past 12 months (such as grants or research support, employee, consultant, stock holder, member of speakers bureau, etc.). The University of Virginia School of Medicine will employ appropriate mechanisms to resolve potential conflicts of interest to maintain the standards of fair and balanced education to the reader. Questions about specific strategies can be directed to the Office of Continuing Medical Education, University of Virginia School of Medicine, Charlottesville, Virginia.

The authors/editors listed below have identified no professional or financial affiliations for themselves or their spouse/partner:
Kelly Barringer, MD; Michelle D. Blumstein, MD; James E. Colletti, MD, FAAEM, FAAP (Guest Editor); Stephanie Doniger, MD, FAAP; Marla J. Friedman, DO; Martin Herman, MD; Paul Ishimine, MD; Danielle M. Jackson, MD; Kevin Kilgore, MD; Samip Kothori, MD; Kenneth T. Kwon, MD, RDMS, FACEP, FAAP; Audrey Le, MD; Jeffrey P. Louie, MD; Merlin C. Lowe, MD, FAAP; Patrick Manley (Acquisitions Editor); Amal Mattu, MD (Consulting Editor); Seema Shah, MD; Ghazala Q. Sharieff, MD, FACEP, FAAEM, FAAP (Guest Editor); Virginia W. Tsai, MD; Dale P. Woolridge, MD, PhD, FAAEM, FAAP, FACEP; and, Linton L. Yee, MD.

Disclosure of Discussion of non-FDA approved uses for pharmaceutical products and/or medical devices:
The University of Virginia School of Medicine, as an ACCME provider, requires that all faculty presenters identify and disclose any "off label" uses for pharmaceutical and medical device products. The University of Virginia School of Medicine recommends that each physician fully review all the available data on new products or procedures prior to instituting them with patients.

TO ENROLL
To enroll in the Emergency Medicine Clinics of North America Continuing Medical Education program, call customer service at 1-800-654-2452 or visit us online at www.theclinics.com/home/cme. The CME program is available to subscribers for an additional fee of $190.00.

ELSEVIER
SAUNDERS

Emerg Med Clin N Am
25 (2007) xi

EMERGENCY
MEDICINE
CLINICS OF
NORTH AMERICA

Erratum

Airway Management in Trauma: An Update

John McGill, MD[a,b]

[a]Department of Emergency Medicine, Hennepin County Medical Center, 701 Park Avenue North,
Minneapolis, MN 55415, USA
[b]Department of Emergency Medicine, University of Minnesota, Minneapolis, MN, USA

The above article, which appeared in the August 2007 issue "Current Concepts in the Management of the Trauma Patient," contained an unfortunate error in Fig. 2C. The correct representation of this figure appears below.

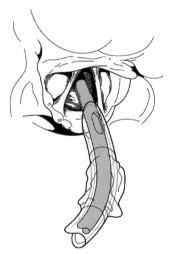

Fig. 2. (*C*) The bevel of the ET tube is facing posteriorly and allows for smooth passage through the glottis.

ELSEVIER
SAUNDERS

Emerg Med Clin N Am
25 (2007) xiii

EMERGENCY
MEDICINE
CLINICS OF
NORTH AMERICA

Erratum

Acute Complications of Extremity Trauma

Edward J. Newton, MD, John Love, MD

Department of Emergency Medicine, Keck School of Medicine, LAC+USC Medical Center,
Building GNH 1011, 1200 North State Street, Los Angeles, CA 90033, USA

In the above article, which appeared in the August 2007 issue "Current Concepts in the Management of the Trauma Patient," Dr. John Love's name did not appear on the title page. We sincerely apologize for this grave error, and fully recognize his important contributions to this article.

0733-8627/07/$ - see front matter © 2007 Elsevier Inc. All rights reserved.
doi:10.1016/j.emc.2007.09.003   *emed.theclinics.com*

ELSEVIER
SAUNDERS

Emerg Med Clin N Am
25 (2007) xv

EMERGENCY
MEDICINE
CLINICS OF
NORTH AMERICA

Erratum

Pediatric Major Trauma: An Approach to Evaluation and Management

Jahn T. Avarello, MD, FAAP[a],
Richard M. Cantor, MD, FAAP, FACEP[a,b]

[a]*Department of Emergency Medicine, SUNY Upstate Medical University,
750 East Adams Street, Syracuse, NY 13210, USA*
[b]*Central New York Poison Center, 750 East Adams Street, Syracuse, NY 13210, USA*

In the above article, which appeared in the August 2007 issue "Current Concepts in the Management of the Trauma Patient," Tables 5 and 6 and Boxes 8 and 9 should have contained the following credit line:

From Marx JA, Holberger RS. Rosen's emergency medicine: concepts and clinical practice. 5th edition. Mosby; 2002. p. 267–81; with permission.

0733-8627/07/$ - see front matter © 2007 Elsevier Inc. All rights reserved.
doi:10.1016/j.emc.2007.09.001   *emed.theclinics.com*

ELSEVIER
SAUNDERS

Emerg Med Clin N Am
25 (2007) xvii–xviii

EMERGENCY
MEDICINE
CLINICS OF
NORTH AMERICA

Foreword

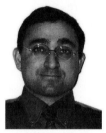

Amal Mattu, MD
Consulting Editor

"Children are not just little adults." This simple phrase likely could be considered the unofficial motto of pediatric emergency physicians around the world. The phrase has been uttered countless times by those who are involved in teaching pediatrics and pediatric emergency medicine, and it is hard to imagine that any medical student has graduated in the past several decades without hearing the phrase. There is wisdom within the meaning of the phrase: children are well known to present with atypical presentations of common diseases, their size and physiology warrant alterations in drug dosages, and there are certain diseases that occur almost exclusively in youth. Children, therefore, must not be approached, worked up, or treated like adults.

But just as children are not little adults, neonates and newborns are not just little children! Children in the first months and first year of life represent the extreme in terms of their atypical presentations, altered physiology, and distinctive diseases. Certain unique endocrine, metabolic, and cardiac emergencies occur in the newborn period. The approach to hyperbilirubinemia in neonates is far different than the approach to hyperbilirubinemia at any other time of life. Abdominal emergencies such as pyloric stenosis and midgut volvulus occur almost exclusively in the first months of life. Resuscitation issues are distinctive in the first month of life as well, so much so that neonatal resuscitation and Neonatal Advanced Life Support courses are taught at many institutions based on the model of the American Heart Association's Pediatric Advanced Life Support course.

0733-8627/07/$ - see front matter © 2007 Elsevier Inc. All rights reserved.
doi:10.1016/j.emc.2007.08.002
emed.theclinics.com

In this issue of *Emergency Medicine Clinics of North America*, Drs. Sharieff and Colletti have assembled an outstanding group of experts in pediatric emergency medicine to address acute care of children in the first year of life. The editors and authors have addressed high risk conditions of the major organ systems and common presentations that may harbor catastrophic illnesses. The reader will undoubtedly find the articles chock-full of pearls to improve practice and pitfalls to avoid. Kudos go to the editors and authors for providing us an outstanding resource to improve our practice and the care of this often perplexing patient population.

Amal Mattu, MD
Program Director
Emergency Medicine Residency, and
Associate Professor
Department of Emergency Medicine
University of Maryland School of Medicine
110 S. Paca Street, 6th Floor
Suite 100, Baltimore
Maryland 21201, USA

E-mail address: amattu@smail.umaryland.edu

ELSEVIER
SAUNDERS

Emerg Med Clin N Am
25 (2007) xix–xx

EMERGENCY
MEDICINE
CLINICS OF
NORTH AMERICA

Preface

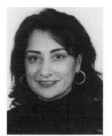 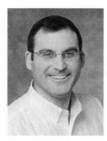

Ghazala Q. Sharieff, MD,   James E. Colletti, MD,
FACEP, FAAEM, FAAP   FAAEM, FAAP
Guest Editors

During the first year of life, children progress from a neonate, progress to an infant, and approach the toddler stage. They develop from individuals whose main functions are to smile spontaneously, feed, void and defecate to individuals who cruise, walk, speak (a few words), and have a pincer grasp. Not only do they develop through motor, language, and social skills, but also their physiologies and disease processes develop as well. Such assessment of a child in the first year of life can be challenging to even the most experienced clinician. This issue is dedicated to state of the art information regarding the emergency care of the child during his or her first year of life. Current areas of interest, clinical practice, and controversy are addressed.

Hyperbilirubinemia is a common occurrence in the newborn period. Neonatal jaundice has shifted from an inpatient issue to an outpatient issue, and management of hyperbilirubinemia is one of the most common reasons for newborn readmission. Kernicterus, the feared complication of hyperbilirubinemia, was considered to be almost extinct but has reemerged recently. Because of this, a review targeted to the emergency department presentation, evaluation, and management of the jaundiced newborn is included. Abdominal concerns are a common complaint in the emergency department. Children under a year of age may present with abdominal catastrophies with subtle presentations. In the article on abdominal emergencies, an approach to the emergent pediatric abdomen during the neonatal and infant periods is discussed. Seizures are a common neurologic problem in childhood. In this

doi:10.1016/j.emc.2007.08.003   *emed.theclinics.com*

issue of *Emergency Medicine Clinics of North America*, one article will differentiate seizures from other childhood disorders and focus on emergency treatment, patient stabilization, termination of seizure activity, and determination of seizure cause. Metabolic diseases can vary as much in clinical presentation as it can in classifications. Neonates and infants who have metabolic diseases frequently present with subtle symptoms that are similar to other emergencies. The article on metabolic illness discusses recognition and management of specific disorders and specific laboratory entities including hypoglycemia, hyponatremia, and metabolic acidosis. The crying infant can present a sense of anxiety and a diagnostic dilemma to the clinician; a discussion of differential diagnosis and management of the crying infant is included. In 2005, the American Heart Association updated the guidelines for newborn and pediatric resuscitation. These changes currently are being taught in Pediatric Advanced Life Support classes. One article reviews the pertinent changes in the care for the critically ill child. A detailed discussion of the newborn exam for background information complements all of these articles.

We thank all of our authors for their time and effort in preparing the articles. We also thank our loving spouses (Jeahan, and Javaid) and our wonderful children (Jimmy, Mariyah, Aleena, and Grace) for their support, patience, and understanding during this endeavor.

Ghazala Q. Sharieff, MD, FACEP, FAAEM, FAAP
Palomar-Pomerado Health System/California Emergency Physicians
San Diego, CA, USA
and
Division of Emergency Medicine
Rady Children's Hospital
3020 Children's Way
San Diego, CA 92123, USA

James E. Colletti, MD, FAAEM, FAAP
Department of Emergency Medicine
Mayo Clinic College of Medicine
200 First St. SW
Rochester, MN 55905, USA

E-mail address: jamesecolletti@gmail.com (J.E. Colletti)

ELSEVIER
SAUNDERS

Emerg Med Clin N Am
25 (2007) 921–946

EMERGENCY
MEDICINE
CLINICS OF
NORTH AMERICA

The Normal Newborn Exam, or Is It?

Merlin C. Lowe, Jr, MD, FAAP[a],
Dale P. Woolridge, MD, PhD, FAAEM,
FAAP, FACEP[b],*

[a]Department of Pediatrics, The University of Arizona, 1501 North Campbell Avenue,
PO Box 245073, Tucson, AZ 85724-5073, USA
[b]Department of Emergency Medicine and Pediatrics, The University of Arizona,
1515 North Campbell Avenue, Tucson, AZ 85724-5057, USA

In today's modern world of high technology imaging and sophisticated laboratory examinations, medicine has come to rely on technology much more than in the past. So much so that at times we forget about the power of a thorough physical exam in detecting medical issues. In this article we will explore the normal newborn examination, discuss the importance of knowing normal versus abnormal findings and discuss some common and not so common findings on the newborn examination. In healthy babies, 15% to 20% will have at least one minor anomaly with an associated 3% chance of having a major anomaly. Two, three, or more minor anomalies are found in 0.8% and 0.5% of healthy babies, respectively. In these cases the chances of major anomalies rises to 10% and 20%, respectively [1].

Newborn infants may present to the emergency department for a variety of reasons. Almost all of these derive from the parent's perception that something is wrong. In each of these cases, the role of the emergency physician is to recognize abnormality and, if no abnormality exists, to alleviate concerns of the parent. Mostly, parental concern stems from conditions that are self-limited or are variants without physiologic consequence. Less common are that these concerns are the presentation of a medical condition that has the potential to worsen or represents underlying illness. Detection of the latter can be life saving. Unfortunately, illness in the newborn is often subtle and difficult to detect. The primary difficulty lies in that the daily activities of a newborn and the newborn's interaction with the environment are extremely limited. It is therefore imperative that the emergency physician becomes familiar and comfortable with performing a newborn exam.

* Corresponding author.
E-mail address: dwoolridge@aemrc.arizona.edu (D.P. Woolridge).

Performing a complete and thorough exam on an infant can sometimes be monotonous where elements of the exam can be missed. Therefore, for the benefit of the reader, Box 1 contains a checklist that can be used as a guide while performing such an exam. A complete physical examination may not be possible in the emergency department because of time constraints. However, a systematic approach can allow a thorough examination in a matter of minutes. Focus should be placed on the heart, lungs, and abdomen as well as a general sense of the wellness of the baby. The neurological examination, in particular, is involved and often a complete neurological examination is not necessary. Generally, testing two to three of the primitive reflexes (such as the moro and sucking reflexes) and observing for spontaneous movement of the limbs will give a good sense of the neurological status of the child.

General evaluation

One of the greatest indicators of the wellness of a newborn is the general observation or gestalt that a clinician obtains by simply watching a baby before the start of a physical exam. This can be done while observing the baby in the basinet or in a parent's arms. Signs of distress such as labored breathing, persistent crying, and so forth are often the first indicators of an impending problem. The newborn infant will often be soundly asleep at the start of the examination and should be sleeping peacefully. Infants who are moaning or grunting during sleep may have underlying illness that should be sought out.

When awakened, it is important that the baby be vigorous and alert. Crying should be energetic and strong. Watch for signs of listlessness and weak cries as harbingers of problems. A baby who does not appear vigorous can have any number of reasons; all of which should raise concern.

Watch the movement and positioning of a child. A newborn, full-term child will lie with his or her upper and lower extremities flexed inward thus showing good tone. A premature or impaired child is more likely to lie at rest with his or her extremities extended from the body showing decreased tone. In addition, examine the movement of the extremities. Each limb should show spontaneous movement. Disuse of an extremity may be the first indication of an underlying pathologic problem.

Vital signs

One of the most difficult parts of pediatrics is recognizing normal versus abnormal because of the great degree of variability in the "normal" ranges of values. This particularly holds true for vital signs. A list of normal ranges can be seen in Table 1. Other clinical indicators should be correlated with the vital signs to aid in determination of significant abnormalities. For

Box 1. The normal newborn exam: a head-to-toe approach

A. Head
  - Shape
  - Fontanelle
  - Lesions/swelling
B. Eyes
  - Red reflex
  - Extraocular movement
  - Pupillary shape/size
C. Ears
  - Positioning
  - Tags
D. Nose
  - Nasal patency
E. Mouth
  - Palate
  - Dentition
  - Oral lesions
F. Neck
  - Swelling/cysts
G. Chest
  - Asymmetric chest rise with respirations
  - Retractions
  - Accessory respiratory muscle use
H. Lungs
  - Symetric aeration
  - Breath sounds
I. Heart
  - Murmur
J. Abdomen
  - Hepatosplenomegaly
  - Cord vessels at birth
K. Genital
  - Inguinal masses
  - Testicular/scrotal asymmetry
  - Genital hypertrophy/lesions
  - Rectal patency
L. Extremities
  - Tenderness
  - Extremity use/range of motion
  - Additional digits/tags
  - Hip click
M. Neurology
  - Tone
  - Suckling
  - Palmar/pantar
  - Moro

Table 1
Normal vital signs in the infant: normal ranges for specified vital signs are listed

Age	Heart rate	Respiratory rate	Systolic blood pressure
Newborn	90–180	40–60	60–90
1 mo	110–180	30–50	70–104
3 mo	110–180	30–45	70–104
6 mo	110–180	20–35	72–110

Data from Gausche-Hill M, Fuchs S, Yamamoto L. The pediatric emergency medicine resource, revised. 4th edition. Sudbury (MA): Jones & Bartlett; 2006. p. 108.

example, a respiratory rate of 50 in a newborn who is sleeping comfortably and showing no signs of retractions, and so forth, is likely ok; however, a respiratory rate of 50 associated with retractions, grunting, and nasal flaring indicates a neonate in respiratory distress.

Temperature should always be included in the vital signs of newborns. It has been well documented that temperatures higher than 38°C are associated with increased risk of serious bacterial illness in infants less than 2 months of age. These include infections such as sepsis, meningitis, urinary tract infection, enterocolitis, and osteomyelitis. The latter two often have symptoms that can lead one to suspect them. The first three can be more insidious. As a result, countless infants are hospitalized each year for a "rule out sepsis" work-up to look for these infections.

While a fever is a flag for infection work-up, one must always remember that newborns are just as likely to develop low temperatures or temperature instability in response to infections as well. Our newborn nursery uses temperature ranges from 36.5 to 37.5°C as a "normal" temperature for newborns in the first several days of life. Swings above or below normal should be a signal to evaluate the child closely for the possibility of an underlying infection or other problem.

Hypothermia and hyperthermia may be indicators of sepsis; however, infection is not the only cause that should be pursued. Hypoglycemia, hypothyroidism, and hypoxia can also present with low temperatures. Hyperthermia may be a manifestation of drug withdrawal, intracranial hemorrhage, or adrenal hemorrhage [2].

While fevers/hypothermia are indicators of illness, one must remember that infants are extremely susceptible to outside influence on temperature. A neonate may easily become hyperthermic as a result of an overly warm incubator, or may become hypothermic if left unwrapped in a cool room. After these issues are corrected, continued swings in temperature should yield an infection work-up. It should be noted that bundling an infant will not produce an elevation in the core body temperature [3]. If bundling is suspected as the source of a fever, a rectal temperature should be checked. A rectal temperature higher than 38°C should prompt a sepsis evaluation.

Height, weight, and head circumference (Occipital Frontal Circumference or OFC) are critical to evaluate in the newborn. They can often give clues about other potential problems or abnormalities. In particular, weight is important to evaluate. The average weight of a term neonate at birth is 3.4 kg. Standardized growth charts that can be used when making determinations about small or large for gestational age (SGA or LGA, respectively) infants are available for download from http://www.cdc.gov/growthcharts. Infants are considered appropriate for gestational age (AGA) if they are within 2 standard deviations from the mean. It is important to know the gestational age as accurately as possible, as 1 or 2 weeks' difference can have significant effects on SGA or LGA determinations. Gestational age can be estimated based on physical characteristics of the neonate including skin creases, external genitalia, ears, breasts, and neuromuscular development [2]. One should also remember to adjust for prematurity when plotting weights of infants during an evaluation. This correction typically continues until the child is 2 years of age. LGA or SGA status should alert the practitioner to evaluate the child carefully for other possible anomalies. Twenty percent of infants with serious congenital anomalies are SGA [2].

LGA infants may be large simply due to familial inheritance. Simply stated, large parents will often have large infants. Additionally, increased maternal weight gain during pregnancy may translate into an LGA infant. Of all causes of LGA, diabetes in the mother is most common. Infants are at particularly increased risk if the mother's blood sugars are poorly controlled during the last trimester. (Of note, diabetes mellitus types 1 and 2 are linked to significantly increased risk of perinatal mortality and morbidity [4]. Associated conditions include postnatal hypoglycemia, cardiac septal hypertrophy, small left colon syndrome, and meconium plug, as well as others.)

While being an infant of a diabetic mother is the most common cause of LGA, there are several genetic syndromes that can cause babies to be LGA. Among them are cerebral gigantism (Soto's syndrome), Beckwith-Wiedemann syndrome, Simpson-Golabi-Behmel syndrome, and 11p trisomy. These syndromes all have their own characteristics and discussing them is beyond the scope of this paper; however, it is important to consider such syndromes when assessing an LGA baby. For a more thorough discussion of syndromes and their associated clinical findings, one can refer to *Smith's Recognizable Patterns of Human Malformation* [5].

OFC should be examined to assess for microcephaly or macrocephaly. The OFC can be particularly helpful when there is concern for hydrocephalus. Macrocephaly can be an isolated finding or associated with other anomalies. As an isolated finding, it is often familial with an autosomal dominant inheritance. When this is in question, the OFC of the parents can be determined and plotted on nomograms. Nomograms for head circumferences of 18 year olds can be used to extrapolate to the parents' OFC percentile. Head growth for infants with familial macrocephaly should follow standard growth. While familial macrocephaly may be the cause, one should not assign this diagnosis without ensuring that other causes are not present. In particular, hydrocephalus is the most common cause of macrocephaly and should therefore trigger an evaluation [6]. Hydrocephalus often presents with widening sutures, full feeling, possibly bulging fontanelles, and a rapidly expanding OFC. Macrocephaly can also be associated with intracranial hemorrhage (eg, subdural or epidural bleeds), enlarged brain tissue (macrencephaly), or thickening of the skull bones [6]. Daily examination while the neonate is in the hospital can identify widening suture lines or a fontanelle that is becoming more full and tense. These can be earlier indicators of a quickly enlarging head and thus an underlying pathologic problem.

Head

The newborn head shows a great degree of variability in the "normal" examination, as well as a large number of findings that are due to molding in the vaginal canal and birth trauma. These normal variants and benign birth trauma findings can make it difficult to find true pathological lesions.

A brief review of anatomy reveals that the newborn skull is composed of many bones. The "neurocranium" (the portion of the skull that encompasses the brain) is composed of eight bones. The facial skull is composed of 14 irregular bones. Most of these bones are not fused together at birth and are separated by fibrous webs, known as suture lines. Most physicians are aware of the anterior and posterior fontanelles; however, there are a total of six fontanelles. In addition to the two previously mentioned fontanelles, there are two pairs of lateral fontanelles known as the sphenoidal or anterolateral fontanelles and the mastoid or posterolateral fontanelles. The four lateral fontanelles generally fuse in infancy and are less clinically significant. The posterior fontanelle begins to close after the first few months and is generally not appreciable by 1 year of age. The anterior fontanelle is generally no longer palpable by 18 months of age [7]. Sutures are generally closed by age 12, but complete fusion continues until into the third decade [8].

Often, most commonly following vaginal birth, the newborn skull will show a significant degree of molding. While this can be distressing to new parents, reassurance is the rule, as molding will resolve relatively rapidly, often over the course of 3 to 5 days. The suture lines allow the bones to shift during the birth process. Often, they are molded into a cone shape allowing for an easier passage of the head through the birth canal. Molding can be significantly more pronounced after a long labor and delivery course. It is important to recognize molding as the OFC can increase by up to 1 cm as the head shape resolves [2].

Localized edema of the scalp can occur following birth and is referred to as caput succedaneum. This is the most common scalp injury due to birth trauma [9]. Caput succedaneum is particularly common after vaginal delivery, but can occur following cesarean section delivery as well. This edema is generally serosanguinous, and occurs due to pressure on the head after being constricted against the uterus, cervix, or vaginal vault [2]. Vacuum-extracted delivery commonly results in large caput areas because of the addition of negative pressure in the area of the vacuum attachment.

Typical caput succedaneum size is only a few centimeters in diameter; however, they can be significantly larger. Spontaneous resolution is the rule for caput succedaneum and, regardless of size, edema generally resolves within 48 hours [2]. Examination of the scalp will show a boggy, somewhat ill-defined area that may cross suture lines. This feature helps distinguish caput succedaneum from another commonly found head lesion following birth, a cephalhematoma.

Cephalhematomas result from injury to the blood vessel found in the subperiosteal area. They can be distinguished from caput succedaneum in that they do not cross suture lines. Cephalhematomas occur in 1.5% to 2.5% of all deliveries. Extraction deliveries are at a greater risk of developing a cephalhematoma with the incidence in forceps deliveries at 4.1% and vacuum extraction ranging from 9.8% to 14.8% [9,10]. Overly large hematomas or those that persist may be the first indication of an underlying bleeding disorder and should prompt evaluation.

While caput succedaneum usually resolves in 48 hours, cephalhematomas may take several days to weeks to fully resolve (further allowing them to be distinguished from a caput). Cephalhematomas will resolve without intervention. Aspiration of the cephalhematoma is generally not indicated, as it leads to an increased risk of infection within the cephalhematoma [11]. The exception to this is a cephalhematoma that is expanding, showing overlying erythema, or having other signs of infection. While infection is rare, it can occur, occasionally in association with scalp electrode placement. Here, aspiration may be required for diagnostic purposes.

Less common, but important to consider, is a subgaleal bleed. Clinical presentation of subgaleal bleeds is generally described as the cranium having a diffusely boggy or soft swelling of the scalp. While subgaleal bleeds may occur following difficult deliveries without extraction assistance, they most commonly will occur following vacuum extraction. Occurrence with vacuum extraction has been shown to be 59 (0.59%) in 10,000 births, compared with 4 (0.04%) in 10,000 births via spontaneous vaginal deliveries without instrumentation [12]. Infants delivered with vacuum extraction should be monitored with serial scalp exams for the development of a subgaleal bleed. These bleeds can be life threatening as large amounts of blood can fill the potential space that lies between the galea aponeurosis and the periosteum. This space extends from the orbital ridges to the superior aspect of the neck and laterally to the ears. Mortality from these bleeds approaches 22% [13]. Infants may require intravenous fluid support, blood transfusions, or antibiotic management of infections that may establish themselves in the bleed area. Additionally, because of the increased red cell breakdown, these infants are at risk of hyperbilirubinemia.

Normally, the bones of the head are separated by suture lines to allow for molding of the skull during birth as well as head growth. Head growth is primarily driven by brain growth. As the brain grows, the neurocranium expands to allow more room. Brain growth is at a tremendous rate in utero and continues to rapidly grow during the first 3 years of life. At birth, the infant brain is about 40% of adult volume. By age 3, it has reached nearly 80% and by age 7 it is at 90% of adult size [8]. When a suture line is prematurely fused, termed craniosynostosis, the growth capacity of the skull in that plane is significantly reduced, but continues in the plane perpendicular to the fused suture.

Craniosynostosis can occur in nonsyndromic and syndromic patterns. Its incidence is 1 in 1700 to 2500 births and 1 in 25,000 births, respectively [14]. Simple craniosynostosis involves a single suture, and compound craniosynostosis involves two or more suture lines. Most commonly involved is the sagittal suture that is affected 40% to 60% of the time, followed by the coronal (20% to 30%), metopic (less than 10%) and finally the lambdoid suture. Isolated lambdoid synostosis occurs in approximately 3 of every 100,000 births [8,14].

The major forms of hereditary craniosynostosis exhibit autosomal dominance, but can have a significant degree of variability in penetrance and expressivity. Fibroblast growth factor receptors (FGFRs) have been shown to be associated with suture formation and mutations in these genes have been implicated in several diseases. For example, mutations in the *FGFR2* gene cause Apert's syndrome and Crouzon's disease [15].

Much more common than craniosynostosis is positional plagiocephaly (simple cranial shaping). At first glance, lambdoid synostosis and occipital plagiocephaly can look almost identical to each other. However, a thorough physical exam can readily distinguish between the two entities. The variance in head shape is best appreciated from above. With positional plagiocephaly, the affected side will show forward positioning of the ear in response to the bones being pushed forward by repeated positioning on the affected side. In craniosynostosis, the affected side will have a posteriorly displaced ear, because of failure of bone growth to move the ear forward to its normal position. Mild plagiocephaly often can be treated with simple alternating of the baby's sleep position such that the head is in a different position from night to night. More severe plagiocephaly may require a specially fitted helmet to correct the misshapen skull. The helmet molds the skull bones back into place as the skull grows by gently putting pressure on the areas that are misshapen to move them back to correct alignment. After the initial fitting period the helmet is worn for 23 hours a day. For this to be effective, it should be done before the sutures begin to fuse, ideally by age 4 to 6 months. Rarely, these devices may fail and surgical correction may be needed. If so, the optimal time to do so is before 1 year of age [16].

Fontanelle size is often not appreciated, but can be an indicator of underlying pathology. Anterior fontanelle size is measured by averaging the anteroposterior and transverse lengths. Fontanelle size is influenced by brain growth due to its stimulation of skull bone growth, suture development, and subsequent osteogenesis [17]. On the first day of life, the average infant fontanelle size is varied from 0.6 cm to 3.6 cm [18]. A large number of disorders are associated with an abnormally large fontanelle. Most commonly, a large fontanelle is found in congenital hypothyroidism, achondroplasia, Down syndrome, and increased intracranial pressure.

Small fontanelles can be a sign of normal early closure, as 1% of fontanelles will close by age 3 months. Additionally, molding can make it difficult to appreciate a truly open fontanelle. However, a small fontanelle can be the harbinger of a pathologic problem and should be investigated. Typically, a small fontanelle is associated with microcephaly. It can be associated with craniosynostosis as previously discussed, but can also be seen with abnormal brain development, fetal alcohol syndrome, congenital infections, and many genetic syndromes [17]. Conversely, soft tissues within the fontanelle may shift depending on intracranial pressure such that bulging of soft tissue within the fontanelle implies increased pressure within the cranium and sunken soft tissues implies dehydration.

Eyes

A pediatrician often examines the red reflexes of the eye at nearly every well-child visit in search of the all elusive retinoblastoma. However, the red reflex can give much more information than simply screening for tumors. A white reflex, known as leukocoria, from the eye can be associated with many other conditions including cataracts, retinal detachment or dysplasia, papillary membranes, and vitreous opacities. The differential expands much beyond this, and as such, findings of leukocoria require referral to an ophthalmologist for further evaluation. Bear in mind that babies with darker skin tones can have reflexes that do not look bright red; however, they should not be white. In addition to examining for leukocoria, the clinician can look for colobomas, examine the pupillary reflex, and look for strabismus using the ophthalmoscope.

Retinoblastoma does, indeed, present with leukocoria. It is the most common malignant intraocular tumor in childhood, with an incidence of 1 in 17,000 [19]. It may present unilaterally or bilaterally, with 30% of cases being bilateral. It is associated with mutations or deletions of the q14 band of chromosome 13 [20].

Congenital cataracts are present from birth, by definition; however, they may not be picked up until later in the first years of life. This is often because some cataracts are progressive and become larger with time. Congenital cataracts occur in 0.44% of live births, and account for 11.50% of blindness in preschool [21]. Of these, 23% are inherited (most commonly autosomal dominant with complete penetrance) and as many as 60% of bilateral cataracts are associated with metabolic (as in galactosemia) and systemic disease. Associated systemic diseases include congenital infections (rubella, toxoplasma, cytomegalovirus, and herpes simplex virus in particular), trisomies (13, 18, and 21), hypoglycemia, and prematurity [22]. On physical exam, one may see leukocoria, strabismus, nystagmus, light sensitivity or decreased visual acuity (particularly later in life). Smaller cataracts may appear as black spots in the red reflex.

When examining the eyes for red reflexes, one may notice a dysconjugate gaze. Gaze can be assessed by visualizing the papillary light reflex (using the ophthalmoscope, but not looking through its lens). At birth, dysconjugate gaze is not particularly concerning. Eyes may often be crossed or divergent. These findings generally correct without intervention by 2 months of age [23]. Dysconjugate gaze beyond this time frame may be an indication of an underlying defect in the function of one or both eyes. Dysconjugate gaze as a function of eye tracking is termed strabismus. In this condition, the weaker of the two eyes is typically patched to allow for appropriate development. In cases where strabismus is not corrected, visual acuity will be lost in the weaker eye. This condition of lost vision is termed amblyopia.

Following birth, subconjunctival hemorrhages are common. They represent a burst blood vessel and do not present a danger to the infant. They typically reabsorb in 1 to 2 weeks. After birth, they can be caused by increasing intraocular pressure, such as through coughing or sneezing, or they may occur spontaneously. One should be aware that a subconjunctival hemorrhage may be a sign of trauma that a parent may not have witnessed or may not be forthcoming so the eye should be examined thoroughly for other signs of injury.

Blue sclera is often one of the telltale signs of osteogenesis imperfecta. While this is the most commonly thought of diagnosis, blue sclera can appear in many different syndromes, including Ehlers-Danlos syndrome and Hallermann-Streiff syndrome. In addition, healthy infants may have a bluish tint to the sclera since the sclera is thinner than in adulthood [21].

While examining the eye, it is important to examine the iris as well as the sclera and pupil. The normal iris of neonates is typically blue or bluish-gray in light-skinned babies and can be darker gray or brown in infants with darker skin [21]. The iris should be examined for colobomas, which appear as a break in the continuity of the iris. Colobomas may be an isolated finding; however, they often are associated with other congenital anomalies, so their presence should prompt a full examination and workup for other findings [21]. Brushfield spots are areas of stromal hyperplasia surrounded by areas of hypoplasia giving a speckled look to the iris. These can be seen in healthy patients, but are much more common in those affected by Down syndrome. Upwards of 90% of Down syndrome patients will have Brushfield spots [24], which can be seen in Zellweger's syndrome as well.

Nystagmus is repetitive, involuntary, rhythmic movements of the eye in a particular direction. Several types of nystagmus exist, including horizontal, vertical, and rotary nystagmus. Nystagmus in neonates may be benign or may represent a pathological process. It can be secondary to retinopathy of prematurity, prematurity itself, or normal physiologic reflexes. An entity known as transient neonatal nystagmus typically develops before age 10 months (mean 2.7 months) and resolves spontaneously by age 12 months. The cause is not yet determined [25].

When examining the eyes, one should be on the look out for opsoclonus in neonates. Opsoclonus is rapid, irregular, and nonrhythmic movements of the eyes. It should not be confused for nystagmus, which is a rhythmic beating of the eyes. Opsoclonus shows beating in horizontal and vertical directions. It may be seen in association with an acute febrile illness, especially those caused by Epstein-Barr virus, varicella, Coxsackie viruses, and West Nile virus [21,26]. When seen in conjunction with myoclonus, so called opsoclonus-myoclonus syndrome, it has been associated with neuroblastoma in 2% to 3% percent of cases [26]. Opsoclonus-myoclonus is often referred to as "Dancing Eyes–Dancing Feet Syndrome" because of its clinical presentation.

Ears

Cranial molding from birth can move the ears into various positions, so molding should be taken into account when examining the ears. One should examine the ears for their position, noting low-set ears, as this has been associated with several syndromes, and malformation of the auricle. Preauricular pits or skin tags are common, and often are hereditary. These are generally inconsequential and no further work-up is needed when they are seen unless there is indication of other anomalies that are present. Hereditary preauricular pits can be associated with deafness and this should be followed as the infant grows [2]. Additionally, ear anomalies can be associated with genitourinary anomalies. As such a renal ultrasound is generally indicated in these patients.

Mouth

Several variations of a normal exam present themselves in the mouth. These include natal teeth and Epstein's pearls. In addition, one may see a cleft lip or palate. Natal teeth are defined as teeth that erupt at any point before 30 days of life. These occur in about 1 in every 3000 births and almost always involve the mandibular central incisors [27]. Structurally, they are similar to normal teeth; however, they generally lack a substantial root system. As such, they often fall out on their own at some point. There is no need to have them removed unless there is concern for aspiration of the tooth should it come loose on its own, or if the tooth prevents proper feeding [28].

Epstein's pearls and Bohn nodules are common findings in neonates. They are often yellowish or white and slightly raised, giving the appearance of a pearl. Bohn nodules are located on the alveolar ridges, and Epstein pearls are those located near the midpalatal raphe at the junction of the hard and soft palates [28]. They are remnants of embryonic development of the dental lamina and will resolve without treatment.

Cleft lip and palate represent the most common anomaly of the head and neck in newborns. Individually and their various combinations are second only to club feet in regard to neonatal birth defects [29]. Cleft lip and palate are two distinct findings; however, the combination of the two is found more commonly than isolated cleft lip or palate with 46% representing combined cases, 21% isolated cleft lip, and 33% isolated cleft palate. Cleft lip carries an incidence that varies with ethnicity ranging from 0.41 per 1000 in African Americans to 2.1 per 1000 in Asians. White ethnicities show an incidence of 1:1000 [30]. The left lip is most commonly involved, followed by the right, then bilateral clefts. Surgical correction often produces very good cosmetic results and should be considered early in cases of poor nutritional intake and abnormal speech development.

While most clefts are quite obvious upon examination, mucosal and sub-mucosal clefts can be less easy to identify visually. Generally, the clinician is able to palpate the cleft using a finger to examine the upper palate of the infant.

Neck

Congenital muscular torticollis is the third most common musculoskeletal anomaly of infants. It follows behind club foot and dysplasia of the hip and can have an incidence upwards of 1 in 250 live births [31]. The exact cause is unknown; however, it is known to be found more commonly in breech and forceps deliveries. In approximately two thirds of cases, a mass can be felt in the affected sternocleidomastoid muscle. It presents with the infant having its head flexed and the chin facing the direction opposite the affected muscle [32]. Occasionally, this contracture of the muscle can lead to plagiocephaly with abnormal placement of the eye and ear on the affected side. Physical therapy is generally therapeutic. Rarely, surgical release of the sternocleidomastoid muscle is needed [33]. If the torticollis is not corrected by age 1, plagiocephaly tends to be persistent [32].

The neck should be examined for any pits or other anomalies. These may represent branchial cleft anomalies, cysts, or sinuses. These branchial arch remnants will be found in the pinna of the ear, the preauricular area, or the lateral neck When present, these anomalies may be associated with systemic syndromes such as Goldenhar syndrome, Pierre-Robin Association, Treacher-Collins syndrome, and Hallerman-Streiff syndrome [14]. A midline neck lesion may represent a thyroglossal duct cyst or cervical cleft.

Chest

Clavicle fractures are one of the most common chest birth injuries, with an incidence of 0.2% to 3.5% [34]. They are identified by palpating crepitus in the clavicular region. Fractures can be confirmed by radiograph if necessary. No treatment is needed for clavicular fractures as they heal well, even in the presence of significant angulation.

When examining the lungs of a newborn, one should assess for symmetry and equal chest excursion as well as adequacy of air exchange. Examination of the lungs includes assessment of the respiratory rate and other indicators of respiratory distress including nasal flaring, grunting, or retractions.

Newborns will frequently exhibit transient tachypnea of the newborn (TTN), especially following cesarean section deliveries. It affects approximately 0.3% to 0.5% of newborns and presents with tachypnea, increased oxygen requirements, and a lack of hypercapnia on blood gas [35]. It is thought to represent delayed absorption of fluid in the lungs. Recovery is the rule, although infants may need ventilatory assistance for a time period. Respiratory distress typically will present a few hours after birth and resolves in 24 to 72 hours [35].

Cardiovascular

The cardiovascular exam can be difficult in a newborn because of their often rapid heart rate. To briefly review neonatal physiology of the heart, one must have a basic understanding of fetal cardiac physiology. Before birth, the infant does not use the lungs for oxygenation. As such, pulmonary pressures are high and blood is preferentially shunted through the foramen ovale and the ductus arteriosus to return to the systemic side of blood circulation. At the time of birth, many transitions must be completed, including closure of the foramen ovale and a decrease in pulmonary pressures to allow blood to flow through the lungs. The ductus arteriosus typically closes 10 to 15 hours after birth. Full permanent fusion may take up to 3 weeks [36].

Auscultation of the heart sounds of a neonate typically reveals a single S1 and a single, or very slightly split, S2 because of the continued relatively high pulmonary pressures. It can take up to 4 to 6 weeks for pulmonary pressures to fully drop to their baseline [37]. As this occurs, the S2 becomes more physiologically split. Typically, S1 is louder near the apex of the heart and S2 is louder near the base. An S3 may be heard near the apex and is considered normal. S4 is never normal in a newborn. Because of rapid heart rates, it can be difficult to truly distinguish the location of a gallop sound. As such, they are often referred to as a summation gallop.

Palpation of peripheral pulses is important to perform in newborns. Weak femoral pulses in comparison with brachial pulses (especially of the right arm) can be an indicator of coarctation of the aorta.

Several murmurs can be heard at birth. These may or may not be innocent in nature. As the pressures in the pulmonary vasculature drop, a ductus that remains patent (PDA) may begin to shunt left to right, creating a murmur often heard best just below the left clavicle near the mid clavicular line [36]. This murmur is typically not heard at birth, as the pulmonary pressures have not yet dropped sufficiently to allow enough shunting to create a murmur.

An innocent flow murmur, termed a newborn murmur, is commonly heard at birth. It is characterized as a systolic ejection murmur located in the left lower sternal border area that is vibratory in nature. This murmur is likely to represent rapid blood flow and is not considered pathologic. Innocent flow murmurs typically do not radiate to other areas and are graded as a I–II/VI in strength.

One may hear a murmur from peripheral pulmonic stenosis (PPS) equally in the left upper sternal border area, back, and axilla [37]. Typically this murmur will be a soft, I–II/VI high-pitched systolic ejection murmur. PPS murmurs typically resolve by age 2 as the sharp turns in the pulmonary vasculature resolve.

Other commonly described innocent murmurs include Still's murmurs, pulmonary ejection murmurs, and venous hums. These murmurs, in contrast to those previously described, are not typically heard in the newborn period.

Innocent murmurs tend to have a vibratory sound. More harsh-sounding murmurs should be evaluated to determine their etiology. Such harsh-sounding murmurs may represent valvular stenosis or regurgitation among other pathological causes.

Holosystolic murmurs are never innocent. Most commonly they represent ventricular septal defects (VSD). They may also represent mitral or tricuspid regurgitation or more complex variations of VSDs, such as atrioventricular septal defects (AVSD). VSDs are the second most common congenital cardiac anomaly (falling only behind bicuspid aortic valves). They represent 15% to 20% of congenital cardiac defects [38]. A VSD murmur typically will be a harsh-sounding holosystolic murmur at the left lower sternal border. Smaller VSDs typically will have a louder sound as blood is forced across with a higher velocity. Importantly, VSD murmurs may not be present at birth because of elevated pulmonary pressures. As the pressures drop, the murmur becomes more pronounced.

Certain anomalies associated with murmurs are also associated with systemic syndromes. For example, approximately 30% of patients with a complete atrioventricular septal defect will have Down syndrome [38]. Noonan syndrome is associated with a rare cardiac defect—supravalvular pulmonic stenosis. The murmur of this anomaly is essentially identical to pulmonic stenosis, except that it is located slightly higher on the chest and an ejection click is not heard [37]. If a murmur is detected in the emergency department that is concerning for pathology, evaluation is warranted. This should include a chest x-ray and an EKG. If abnormalities are found, the neonate should be admitted for further evaluation. If no abnormalities are detected and the child appears well, follow-up with a pediatric cardiologist as an outpatient is reasonable.

Abdomen

In examining the abdomen, the clinician should assess for typical abdominal components. This includes assessing for hepatomegaly, splenomegaly, and palpable enlarged kidneys. Abdominal palpation is best accomplished using the flats of the fingers rather than the tips, as they are more sensitive to masses and so forth. The liver is often felt approximately 1 cm below the costal margin. This degree of extrusion is considered normal.

In general unless it is enlarged the spleen should not be detected by palpation. An enlarged spleen in the setting of prolonged or severe jaundice should alert the clinician to the possibility of a hemolyzing state, as may be found in Rh or ABO incompatibility or other red cell morphological defects such as spherocytosis or elliptocytosis.

While attempting to palpate for an enlarged spleen, one can also palpate for enlarged or cystic-feeling kidneys. Autosomal recessive polycystic kidney disease can present with enlarged kidneys at birth [39]. Rarely, one can see congenital absence of the abdominal muscles in combination with cryptorchidism and urinary tract anomalies, termed Prune Belly Syndrome or the Eagle-Barrett triad [39]. Prune Belly syndrome has an incidence of 1 in 40,000 births, and 95% of cases are in males [40].

The umbilical cord should be inspected to ensure the presence of a single umbilical vein and two umbilical arteries. A single umbilical artery (SUA) is found in approximately 0.2% to 1% of newborns [41]. Studies have shown that infants with an SUA have a threefold higher incidence of severe renal anomalies and a sixfold higher incidence of any renal malformation when compared with the general population [42].

A scaphoid abdomen and respiratory distress at birth should raise concern for a congenital diaphragmatic hernia (CDH). When the possibility of CDH exists, the infant should be intubated in an effort to prevent the swallowing of air that occurs with spontaneous breathing or with bag-valve mask ventilation [2]. Air in the intestines will lead to worsening respiratory distress as the expanding intestines further compress the lungs and mediastinum. It should be noted that absence of a scaphoid abdomen does not rule out CDH.

The differential diagnosis for hepatomegaly in a neonate is quite extensive. First, it is important to recognize true hepatomegaly. Hepatic size can be assessed by various means, including percussion of liver span and palpation of the liver edge. When one palpates for the liver edge, it is recommended to start palpating in the lower quadrants to ensure that extreme hepatomegaly is not missed. In general, a liver edge palpable beyond 3.5 cm below the costal margin is considered enlarged. At 1 week of age, a normal liver span is 4.5 to 5.0 cm [43]. An enlarged edge below the costal margin in the presence of a normal liver span may be caused by depression of the liver downward due to lung hyperinflation or other anatomical causes.

Once hepatomegaly has been ascertained, other important factors to note are the presence or absence of jaundice, splenomegaly, and other physical anomalies or systemic symptoms. These will help guide the examiner's work-up to determine underlying causes.

Genitourinary tract

Several anomalies can be found when evaluating the genitourinary tract. As such, a thorough examination is important to identify any such findings that may exist. Neither girls nor boys are exempt from anomalies.

Newborn boys should be examined for inguinal hernias, hydroceles, varicoceles, undescended testes, or signs of hypospadias and other urethral anomalies. Inguinal hernias have an incidence of 0.8% to 4.4% in boys, representing one of the most common surgical issues for newborns [44]. They can present as a bulge in the inguinal area or may have palpable bowel in the scrotum [45]. Inguinal hernias develop when the processus vaginalis fails to close, allowing enough of an opening to let bowel pass through. Approximately 60% involve the left side, 30% the right, and 10% will be bilateral [44]. When an inguinal hernia is identified, light, constant pressure should be applied to the herniated bowel to reduce the bowel back into the abdomen. Occasionally, the bowel may become trapped and nonreducible. This represents an incarcerated hernia and is a surgical emergency. Incarceration of an inguinal hernia may compromise blood flow to the intestines or the scrotal contents resulting in damage to the end-organ. Girls are susceptible to inguinal hernias as well, although the male:female ratio is 6:1 [44]. Physical examination generally reveals a lump in the inguinal area.

When the processus vaginalis fails to fully close but allows only fluid to pass into the scrotum a hydrocele results. Hydroceles are most commonly present at birth, although they rarely can arise later. Transillumination can be used to aid in the diagnosis of a hydrocele as they tend to easily and uniformly light up, although bowel can occasionally transilluminate as well, making the distinguishing of the two difficult at times. Hydroceles do not extend into the inguinal canal. Typically they resolve within 12 to 28 months, so surgical repair is generally deferred [44].

Varicoceles result from dilation of the pampiniform plexus and internal spermatic vein. Almost always, they occur on the left, and are often described as feeling like a "bag of worms." Varicoceles are typically more easily seen with the patient upright, as this increases the hydrostatic pressure on the venous plexus. They should reduce easily or spontaneously with supine positioning. Any varicocele that does not reduce or is located on the right side should be evaluated by ultrasound, as failure to reduce is an indication of a possible blockage in venous drainage. This may be the result of an abdominal mass [45]. With typical varicoceles, surgical correction can be undertaken but such a need is debated as most are asymptomatic [39]. If correction is desired, it typically is not done in the neonatal period.

At birth, full-term boys will experience an undescended testis (cryptorchidism) about 3% to 4% of the time. By age 1, only 0.3% persist [39]. If one fails to locate a testis in the scrotum, examination of the inguinal canal area should be performed. Often, testes are not truly undescended but are retractile. These testes can be brought fully into the scrotum, although it may be difficult. Retractile testes are the result of a hyperactive cremasteric reflex and will ultimately settle into the scrotum without intervention [45].

True undescended testes cannot be manually drawn into the scrotum on examination. These will require intervention to draw the testes down into the scrotum if they have not descended by 6 months of age. Typically this is achieved by surgical orchiopexy but treatment with hCG can be attempted (success with hormonal treatment can reach approximately 30% to 40% but more often failure results) [39]. Undescended testes should be brought into the scrotum by intervention as this allows for better examination for malignancy as they have a 4 to 10 times higher risk than descended testes. Seminomas are most commonly seen [39]. Approximately 10% of those affected with undescended testes will have bilateral involvement. When bilateral undescended tests are seen, there should be suspicion of an underlying congenital adrenal hyperplasia with virilization of a female infant. This is particularly true if hypospadias is also seen [38].

Ambiguous genitalia result from virilization of females or undermasculinization of males. The range of phenotypes can run from almost normal female to almost normal male anatomy. In boys, ambiguous genitalia commonly result from problems in androgen synthesis (such as 17 alpha-hydroxylase deficiency) or end-organ resistance to these hormones (such as in 5 alpha-reductase deficiency or androgen insensitivity). In girls, congenital adrenal hyperplasia (CAH) is the leading cause of ambiguous genitalia. CAH occurs with an incidence of 0.06 to 0.08 per 1000 live births; 90% of these cases are a result of 21-hydroxylase deficiency [46].

During examination of the genitalia, the clinician should evaluate for clitoromegaly, micropenis, bifid scrotum, or fusion of the labia resulting in a scrotum-like appearance [47]. Increased pigmentation of the skin can be seen with CAH because of increased ACTH concentrations in an attempt to stimulate cortisol production.

Extremities

When examining the extremities, one should examine all four extremities for anomalies. Both hands and both feet should be examined for absent or supranumary digits. Polydactyly frequently is an isolated finding but may be associated with other malformations. While spontaneous occurrences are frequent, a family history of polydactyly yields up to a 10-fold increase in occurrences. Polydactyly of the fingers involving the "pinky" finger side is the second most common anomaly of the hand with an incidence of 1 in 3000 [48]. Involvement can range from a simple skin tag that can be removed by tying a suture at the base to a fully formed digit including bony struc- tures. These more complex digits require surgical removal. While they rarely produce a functional deficit, cosmetic reasons often lead to removal. Surgery is generally performed between 1 and 2 years of age [48]. Polydactyly of the toes commonly occurs as well. Surgical correction, if needed, for supranu- mary toes generally occurs between 6 months and 1 year.

The palms of the hands should be examined for the presence of a single transverse palmar crease. While a single palmar crease is associated with several syndromes, most notably Down syndrome, approximately 4% of the healthy population will have a unilateral single palmar crease and 1% will have bilateral single transverse palmar creases.

Talipes equinovarus, commonly known a clubfoot, is a relatively com- mon deformity with an incidence reported at 1 in 1000 live births. Bilateral involvement occurs in 30% to 50% of cases. Male to female ratios are 2:1 [48].

Clubfoot is a complex anomaly. It is composed of four main components: (1) the forefoot is inverted and adducted, (2) the heel and hindfoot are in- verted, (3) limitation of extension at the ankle and subtalar joint, and finally (4) internal rotation of the leg [49]. Physical examination reveals inability to bring the foot fully to midline. Initial correction is attempted with serial casting. Progressive casting is successful in most patients; however, in some cases, surgery may be required [49]. If needed, surgery is generally per- formed between 6 and 9 months.

Neurological

An extensive neurological examination can be quite time consuming; however, all infants should receive at least a limited neurological examina- tion including tone, primitive reflexes, and a gross assessment of muscu- lar/sensory status and cranial nerves. A list of primitive reflexes and a short description of each can be found in Box 2. As in older children, a sys- tematic approach is helpful. Often one can begin with a general assessment, followed by cranial nerves, motor function, sensory function, and reflexes. A good assessment of neurological status can often be obtained simply by careful observation of the infant. One should observe movements of the face for symmetry. Arms and legs should be watched to assess for movement or lack thereof. At birth, full-term infants show a flexed posture of the extremities and have the ability to raise their heads in the vertical midline plane, although they may still be quite unsteady [50]. Movements of the extremities should be generally smooth without a significant amount of jerk- ing. The cry should be strong and vigorous. Often neurological problems

Box 2. Common Primitive Reflexes

Rooting Reflex
Touch newborn on either side of cheek and baby turns toward stimulus.

Walking Reflex
Hold baby up in vertical position. As feet touch ground, baby makes walking motion.

Tonic Neck (Fencing) Reflex
Rotate baby's head leftward and the left arm stretches into extension and the right arm flexes up above head (opposite reaction if head is rotated rightward).

Moro Reflex (Startle Reflex)
Hold supine infant by arms a few inches above bed and gently release infant back to elicit startle. Baby throws arms out in extension and baby grimaces.

Hand-to-Mouth (Babkin) Reflex
Stroke newborn's cheek or put finger in baby's palm and baby will bring his fist to mouth and suck a finger.

Swimmer's (Gallant) Response
Hold baby prone while supporting belly with hand. Stroke along one side of spine and baby flexes entire torso toward the stroked side.

Palmar
Stroke inner palm/sole and toes/fingers curl around ("grasp") examiner's finger.

Plantar
Stroke outer sole (Babinski) and toes spread with great toe dorsiflexion.

Doll's Eyes
Give one forefinger to each hand (baby grasps both) and pull baby to sitting with each forefinger. Eyes open on coming to sitting (like a doll's).

Protective Reflex
Soft cloth is placed over the baby's eyes and nose. Baby arches head, turns head side to side, and brings both hands to face to swipe cloth away.

Crawling Reflex
Newborn placed on abdomen and baby flexes legs under as if to crawl.

will produce an altered cry such as a weak cry or a particularly high-pitched cry.

Cranial nerve (CN) assessment can begin with the eyes. By 28 weeks an infant's neurological system has developed enough to produce a blink when a bright light is shone in the eyes (CN II and VII). Between 28 and 32 weeks the papillary reflex develops (CN II and III) [2]. CN V can be tested via corneal reflex or with light touch/pin prick to the trigeminal branch areas producing a withdrawal from the stimulus. Additionally, full-term infants can often fixate and track on large objects thus allowing for testing of CN II, III, IV, and VI. It should be noted that a dysconjugate gaze is not abnormal when a neonate is not fixing on an object [2]. Facial asymmetry may indicate a lesion involving the facial nerve. Loud noises should evoke a blink, testing CN VIII. The swallowing reflex tests CN IX and X. Fasciculations of the sternocleidomastoid muscle or tongue may represent a lesion involving CN XI or XII, respectively [2]. Detailed examination of the cranial nerves is generally not necessary unless there is suspicion of a problem.

Sensation testing is generally limited to light touch and pinprick testing. During the entire newborn exam, the clinician can be assessing the response of the baby to touch. For example, infants commonly will react to the stethoscope touching their chest.

Motor examination involves assessing spontaneous movement of the head and extremities, as well as muscular tone. Neonatal hypotonia is the most common abnormal neurological sign seen in neonates [50]. It is associated with a wide array of disorders. Hypotonia can be divided into central and peripheral origins. Central hypotonia tends to be associated with other central nervous system (CNS) findings. Failure to fixate or meet other milestones, or seizures, are associated with central hypotonia [51]. Several common syndromes are associated with hypotonia include Down Syndrome and Prader-Willi syndrome. Other important considerations are hypoglycemia, hypothyroidism, hypoxic-ischemic encephalopathy, infection, and metabolic disorders. Often, central causes of hypotonia become more classic of CNS lesions resulting in increased tone, increased reflexes, and so forth. Transection of the spinal cord should also be considered, especially when there is a report of possible neck hyperextension in utero or during delivery. These infants may present severely with respiratory failure. Lower spinal level lesions may present with hypotonia that often becomes hypertonia with hyperreflexia characteristic of central CNS lesions [51].

Peripheral hypotonia, in contrast with central causes, often will present as hypotonia without any specific central signs. Eyes are able to fix well. Infants often are responsive to sounds and stimuli. Examples of this include spinal muscular atrophy, neonatal myasthenia gravis, and infantile botulism.

Infant spinal muscular atrophy, also known as Werdnig-Hoffman syndrome or SMA type 1, can present with hypotonia at birth (in 60% of cases), weakness, poor suck, and absent reflexes. This is due to anterior horn cell degeneration. Werdnig-Hoffman typically presents between 0 and 6 months [52]. In contrast to cerebral damage hypotonia, these infants are typically alert and have facial reactions.

Neonatal myasthenia gravis occurs in 10% to 15% of infants born to mothers with myasthenia gravis. The acetylcholine receptor antibodies readily cross the placenta and can attach to the infant's receptors producing a myasthenic phenotype. Signs of bulbar weakness including a weak suck and cry, hypotonia, absence of a moro reflex, and respiratory insufficiency can develop up to 72 hours after delivery. Treatment is with acetylcholinesterase inhibitors as in adults. Symptoms generally resolve by about 12 weeks of age as the maternal antibodies are cleared.

During delivery, particularly with difficult or breech deliveries, the brachial plexus may be injured causing a spectrum of resulting outcomes. The brachial plexus is formed from the C5-T1 nerve roots. Palsies involving this plexus are divided into three main types. Erb palsy involves the C5, C6, and occasionally C7. Klumpke palsy involves C8 and T1. The third type involves the complete plexus. Erb palsies present with the affected upper extremity in the classic "waiter's tip" position. Klumpke palsies yield a paralyzed hand with full function of the elbow and shoulder. This palsy is rare, comprising only 0.5% of all brachial plexus injuries [2].

Total plexus injuries yield a complete paralysis of the upper extremity. Injuries may be transient in mild cases to permanent in more severe instances. The range of resolution relates to the actual injury to the nerve roots. Mild cases generally are the result of the brachial plexus nerve roots being stretched, termed neurapraxia. In these cases, prognosis is excellent. The most severe cases result when the nerve root is avulsed from the spinal cord, known as axonotmesis. These cases have no chance for spontaneous resolution and surgical correction often does not yield good outcomes [2]. Fortunately, 80% to 95% of cases (primarily Erb palsies) will resolve spontaneously over the course of a few weeks to months.

If, on physical examination, there is difficulty determining if the infant does not move the area because of pain (as a result of a clavicular fracture, for example) or a palsy, the Moro reflex can be used. In cases of palsies, the Moro will result in asymmetric movement.

Skin

Newborn babies exhibit a plethora of skin findings. Often, these findings can be alarming to parents and result in numerous clinic and emergency department visits. Often, visual diagnosis is quite easy and can alleviate parental concerns.

Newborns often experience some degree of vasomotor instability that can present in several ways, including cutis marmorata, harlequin color changes, and acrocyanosis. Cutis marmorata is a condition resulting from uneven distribution of capillary blood flow. It gives a mottled appearance to the skin and often can be induced by cold exposure.

Harlequin color changes are precipitated by turning the baby on the side. When this is done, the lower half of the baby becomes erythematous or dusky while the upper half becomes pale. Often there is a sharp demarcation between zones. This typically resolves within a few seconds after returning to the supine position but can persist for up to 20 minutes [53]. Harlequin color changes are more commonly seen in low-birth-weight infants and often resolve after the first few weeks of life.

Acrocyanosis results from venous blood pooling in the extremities giving a bluish color to the hands, feet, and occasionally around the lips. This condition is exaggerated with cool temperatures and resolves with warming. Acrocyanosis is not pathological and will resolve as vasomotor stability improves.

Erythema toxicum is extremely common, affecting up to 50% of full-term infants [53]. It typically presents in the first 2 to 3 days of life and typically resolves in 5 to 7 days. Lesions classically are described as having a central flesh-colored papule with surrounding erythema at the base. Numbers can range from a few lesions to over 100. With many lesions, the erythema can become confluent making the appearance less classic, but examination of the margins often reveals individual papules with the typical appearance. Biopsy is generally not needed but would show the presence of eosinophils. Its etiology is not well known at this point.

Less common is neonatal pustular melanosis, which affects approximately 5% of black infants and less than 1% of white infants [2]. The pustules are always present at birth or form within the first 24 hours of life. Following pustule formation, the pustules rupture leaving the classic collarettes of scaly skin and hyperpigmentation. It is possible for the pustules to rupture in utero leaving only the collarettes and hyperpigmentation at birth. Pustules may be present on the face, neck, hands, and feet (including the palms and soles). Atypical presentations should be evaluated very closely as some infectious processes, such as impetigo, can mimic pustular melanosis and require rapid treatment [2].

Forty percent of newborns will have milia, most commonly found on the nose [53]. They represent small cysts filled with keratinocytes and sebaceous debris. They may also be seen on other areas of the body. Generally, these papules are self-resolving over the course of a few weeks. Epstein's pearls represent the same process in the oral cavity.

Neonatal acne is occasionally seen shortly after birth but typically develops between the second and fourth week of life. It peaks around 8 to 12 weeks of life, under the influence of maternal and fetal androgens, then subsequently resolves. Lesions are characteristically comedonal or pustular in appearance. Occasionally, nodulocystic acne can occur. In these cases, medical management may be indicated to prevent scarring. Persistent acne may be an indication of excess androgen production. If there are concerns about this, growth should be followed closely and a bone age can be checked for accelerated bone growth. Normal bone growth makes excess androgen production unlikely [2].

Nevus simplex is a blanching macule that is typically pink or red in color. When located on the glabella they are commonly referred to as angel kisses, and when located on the posterior neck they are often termed stork bites. While these two sites are the most common, they may be found anywhere along the midline from the eyes to the nape of the neck. Often they fade with time, although they may not completely.

Nevus simplex should be distinguished from a nevus flammeus or "port-wine stain." Port-wine stains do not tend to resolve much spontaneously. Laser treatment can help reduce their appearance. They are important to recognize, as they are associated with some syndromes. In particular, a nevus flammeus that involves the ophthalmic and maxillary regions of the trigeminal nerve (unilaterally or bilaterally) may be associated with Sturge-Weber syndrome that can have CNS involvement and lead to seizures. Port-wine stains that involve the face and/or upper extremity with hypertrophy of the affected side may have a condition termed Klippel-Trenaunay [2].

Dermal melanoses, formerly referred to as Mongolian spots, are bluish-black areas of hyperpigmentation often found on the buttocks, back, and shoulders. They are extremely common in darker skinned babies (upwards of 90% of Native American, Asian, and African American babies will have them) [53]. These spots can be confused with bruising and have resulted in evaluation for abuse in some cases. For this reason it is important to recognize them. Typically they will fade with age but may persist into adulthood.

Another commonly seen hyperpigmented macule is the café au lait spot. Typically these macules are light brown in color. A few café au lait macules are normal; however, the presence of many macules or a very large macule may indicate the presence of a systemic disease such as neurofibromatosis type 1 or McCune-Albright syndrome, respectively. The following list summarizes the National Institutes of Health criteria for the diagnosis of neurofibromatosis type 1 [54]. Any two or more clinical features are required for diagnosis.

- Six or more café-au-lait macules over 5 mm in greatest diameter in prepubertal individuals and over 15 mm in greatest diameter in postpubertal individuals
- Two or more neurofibromas of any type or one plexiform neurofibroma
- Freckling in the axillary or inguinal regions
- Optic glioma
- Two or more Lisch nodules (iris harmartomas)
- A distinctive osseous lesion such as sphenoid dysplasia or thinning of the long bone cortex with or without pseudarthrosis
- A first-degree relative (parent, sibling, or offspring) with neurofibromatosis type 1 by the above criteria

Summary

Despite the broad technologic advancements of medicine, screening for illness in infants is highly reliant on a complete physical examination. For this reason it is critical that the examining physician not only have a thorough understanding of abnormal findings but also the normal findings and their variants. The vast majority of infants are healthy and findings predictive of future health problems are subtle and infrequent. Yet, outcomes can be devastating. Therefore it is critical for the physician to remain diligent during screening. It is our hope that this article will assist the physician in this task and allow for more accurate and timely diagnosis that prevents or minimizes long-term health problems in children.

References

[1] Thilo EH, Rosenberg AA. The newborn infant. In: Hay WW, Levin MJ, Sondheimer JM, et al, editors. Current diagnosis and treatment in pediatrics. 18th edition. New York: Lange Medical Books/McGraw-Hill; 2007.

[2] Bland RD. The newborn infant. In: Rudolph CD, Rudolph AM, Hostetter MK, et al, editors. Rudolph's pediatrics. 21st edition. New York: McGraw-Hill; 2003. p. 55–222.

[3] Grover G, Berkowitz CD, Lewis RJ, et al. The effects of bundling on infant temperature-Pediatrics 1994;94(5):669–73.

[4] Macintosh MC, Fleming KM, Bailey JA, et al. Perinatal mortality and congenital anomalies in babies of women with type 1 or type 2 diabetes in England, Wales, and Northern Ireland: population-based study. BMJ 2006;333(7560):157–8.

[5] Jones KL. Smith's recognizable patterns of human malformation. Philadelphia: Saunders; 1997.

[6] DeMyer W. Normal and abnormal development of the neuraxis. In: Rudolph CD, Rudolph AM, Hostetter MK, et al, editors. Rudolph's pediatrics. 21st edition. New York: McGraw-Hill; 2003. p. 2174–9.

[7] Moore KL, Dalley AF. Introduction to clinically oriented anatomy. In: Moore KL, Dalley AF, editors. Clinically oriented anatomy. Philadelphia: Lippincott Williams and Wilkins; 1999. p. 2–58.

[8] Kabbani H, Raghuveer T. Craniosynostosis. Am Fam Physician 2004;69(12):2863–70.

[9] Hillenbrand KM. Birth trauma. In: Perkins RM, Swift JD, Newton DA, editors. Pediatric hospital medicine. Philadelphia: Lippincott Williams and Wilkins; 2003. p. 592–6.

[10] Caughey AB, Sandberg PL, Zlatnik MG. Forceps compared with vacuum: rates of neonatal and maternal morbidity. Obstet Gynecol 2005;106(5 Part 1):908–12.

[11] Blom NA, Vreede WB. Infected cephalhaematomas associated with osteomyelitis, sepsis and meningitits. Pediatr Infect Dis J 1993;12:1015–7.

[12] Plauche WC. Subgaleal haematoma: a complication of instrumental delivery. JAMA 1980; 244:1597–8.

[13] Chadwick LM, Pemberton PJ, Kurinczuk JJ. Neonatal subgaleal haematoma: associated risk factors, complications and outcome. J Paediatr Child Health 1996;32:228–32.

[14] Carey JC, Bamshad MJ, et al. Clinical genetics and dysmorphology. In: Rudolph CD, Rudolph AM, Hostetter MK, et al, editors. Rudolph's pediatrics. 21st edition. New York: McGraw-Hill; 2003. p. 713–86.

[15] Wilkie AO, Slaney SF, Oldridge M, et al. Apert syndrome results from localized mutations of FGFR2 and is allelic with Crouzon syndrome. Nat Genet 1995;9:165–72.

[16] Liptak GS, Serletti JM. Consultation with the specialist: pediatric approach to craniosynostosis. Pediatr Rev 1998;19:352–9.

[17] Kiesler J, Ricer R. The abnormal fontanel. Am Fam Physician 2003;67(12):2547–52.

[18] Popich GA, Smith DW. Fontanels: range of normal size. J Pediatr 1972;80:749–52.

[19] Phillipi C, Christensen L, Samples J. Index of suspicion. Pediatr Rev 2005;26(8):295–301.

[20] Veeramachaneni V, Fielder PN. Index of suspicion. Pediatr Rev 2001;22(6):211–5.

[21] Miller KM, Apt L. The eyes. In: Rudolph CD, Rudolph AM, Hostetter MK, et al, editors. Rudolph's pediatrics. 21st edition. New York: McGraw-Hill; 2003. p. 2351–417.

[22] Bashour M, Menassa J. Congenital cataract. E-medicine. Available at: http://www.emedicine.com. Accessed August 28, 2007.

[23] Calhoun JH. Consultation with the specialist: eye examinations in infants and children. Pediatr Rev 1997;18:28–31.

[24] Izquierdo N, Townsend W. Down syndrome. E-medicine. Available at: http://www.emedicine.com. Accessed August 28, 2007.

[25] Lim SA, Siatkowski RM. Pediatric neuro-ophthalmology. Curr Opin Ophthalmol 2004; 15(5):437–43.

[26] Hsieh D, Friederich R, Pelszynski MM. Index of suspicion. Pediatr Rev 2006;27(8):307–13.

[27] Soames JV, Southam JC. Other disorders of teeth: disorders of eruption and shedding of teeth. In: Soames JV, Southam JC, editors. Oral pathology. 4th edition. Oxford (UK): Oxford University Press; 2005.

[28] Shusterman S. Pediatric dental update. Pediatr Rev 1994;15(8):311–8.

[29] Vasconez HC, Ferguson REH, Vasconez LO. Plastic and reconstructive surgery. In: Doherty GM, Way LW, editors. Current surgical diagnosis and treatment. 12th edition. New York: McGraw-Hill Companies; 2006.

[30] Shenaq SM, Kim JYS, Bienstock A. Plastic and reconstructive surgery. In: Brunicardi FC, Andersen DK, Billiar TR, et al, editors. Schwartz's priciples of surgery. 8th edition. New York: McGraw-Hill Companies; 2005.

[31] Do TT. Congenital muscular torticollis: current concepts and review of treatment. Curr Opin Pediatr 2006;18(1):26–9.

[32] Sponseller PD. Bone, joint and muscle problems. In: McMillan JA, Feigin RD, DeAngelis C, et al, editors. Oski's pediatrics. 4th edition. Philadelphia: Lippincott Williams and Wilkins; 2006.

[33] Hackam DJ, Newman K, Ford HR. Pediatric surgery. In: Brunicardi FC, Andersen DK, Billiar TR, et al, editors. Schwartz's priciples of Surgery. 8th edition. New York: McGraw-Hill Companies; 2005.

[34] Kaplan B, Rabinerson D, Avrech OM, et al. Fracture of the clavicle in the newborn following normal labor and delivery. Int J Gynaecol Obstet 1998;63(1):15–20.

[35] Subramanian KNS, Bahri M. Transient tachypnea of the newborn. E-Medicine. 2006. Available at: http://www.emedicine.com. Accessed August 28, 2007.

[36] Hoffman JIE. The circulatory system. In: Rudolph CD, Rudolph AM, Hostetter MK, et al, editors. Rudolph's pediatrics. 21st edition. New York: McGraw-Hill; 2003. p. 1745–904.

[37] Sondheimer HM, Yetman AT, Miyamoto SD. Cardiovascular diseases. In: Hay WW, Levin MJ, Sondheimer JM, et al, editors. Current diagnosis and treatment in pediatrics. 18th edition. New York: Lange Medical Books/McGraw-Hill; 2007.

[38] Bers MH, Porter RS, Jones TV, et al. Congenital cardiovascular anomalies. In: Bers MH, Porter RS, Jones TV, et al, editors. The Merck manual of diagnosis and therapy. 18th edition. Whitehouse Station (NJ): Merck Research Laboratories; 2006.

[39] Siegel NJ. Kidney and urinary tract. In: Rudolph CD, Rudolph AM, Hostetter MK, et al, editors. Rudolph's pediatrics. 21st edition. New York: McGraw-Hill; 2003. p. 1629–743.

[40] Available at: http://www.prunebelly.org/. Accessed August 28, 2007.

[41] Bourke WG, Clarke TA, Mathews TG, et al. Isolated single umbilical artery—the case for routine screening. Arch Dis Child 1993;68(5):600–1.

[42] Srinivasan R, Arora RS. Do well infants born with an isolated single umbilical artery need investigation? Arch Dis Child 2005;90(1):100–1.

[43] Wolf AD, Lavine JE. Hepatomegaly in neonates and children. Pediatr Rev 2000;21(9): 303–10.

[44] Nakayama DK, Rowe MI. Inguinal hernia and the acute srotum in infants and children. Pediatr Rev 1989;11(3):87–93.

[45] Pulsifer A. Pediatric genitourinary examination: a clinician's reference. Urol Nurs 2005; 25(3):163–8.

[46] Goodman S. Endocrine alterations. In: Potts NL, Mandleco BL, editors. Pediatric nursing: caring for children and their families. 2nd edition. Clifton Park (NY): Thompson Delmar Learning; 2002.

[47] Anhalt HE, Neely K, Hintz RL. Ambiguous genitalia. Pediatr Rev 1996;17(6):213–20.

[48] Crawford AH. Orthopedics. In: Rudolph CD, Rudolph AM, Hostetter MK, et al, editors. Rudolph's pediatrics. 21st edition. New York: McGraw-Hill; 2003. p. 2419–57.

[49] Gore AI, Spencer JP. The newborn foot. Am Fam Physician 2004;69(4):865–72.

[50] Mercuri E, Ricci D, Pane M, et al. The neurological examination of the newborn baby. Early Hum Dev 2005;81:947–56.

[51] Stiefel L. In brief: hypotonia in infants. Pediatr Rev 1985;6(9):282–6.

[52] Tsao B, Stojic AS, Armon C. Spinal muscular atrophy. E-Medicine. 2006. Available at: http://www.emedicine.com. Accessed August 28, 2007.

[53] Morelli JG, Burch JM. Skin. In: Hay WW, Levin MJ, Sondheimer JM, et al, editors. Current diagnosis and treatment in pediatrics. 18th edition. New York: Lange Medical Books/ McGraw-Hill; 2007.

[54] Stumpf DA, Alksne JF, Annegers JF. Neurofibromatosis: conference statement. Arch Neurol 1988;45:575–8.

ELSEVIER
SAUNDERS

Emerg Med Clin N Am
25 (2007) 947–960

EMERGENCY
MEDICINE
CLINICS OF
NORTH AMERICA

Pediatric Resuscitation Update

Stephanie J. Doniger, MD, FAAP[a],*, Ghazala Q. Sharieff, MD, FACEP, FAAEM, FAAP[b,c]

[a]Pediatric Emergency Medicine, St. Luke's-Roosevelt Hospital Center,
1111 Amsterdam Avenue, New York, NY 10025, USA
[b]Palomar-Pomerado Health System/California Emergency Physicians, University
of California, San Diego, 3020 Children's Way, San Diego, CA 92123, USA
[c]Division of Emergency Medicine, Rady Children's Hospital, 3020 Children's Way,
San Diego, CA 92123, USA

The majority of cardiac arrest in children results from a progression of shock and respiratory failure to cardiac arrest. The goal for resuscitation is to urgently reestablish substrate delivery to meet the metabolic demands of vital organs [1]. It is important to recognize that successfully applied techniques of basic and advanced life support are crucial to reducing neonatal and childhood mortality. Currently there are no data on the incidence of pediatric resuscitations performed in the United States each year; however, it can be estimated by extrapolating data from childhood mortality rates (Fig. 1A, B).

In 2005, the American Heart Association (AHA) set forth updated guidelines for Basic Life Support, Neonatal Advanced Life Support (NALS), and Pediatric Advanced Life Support (PALS). Overall, the updated guidelines simplify resuscitation for prehospital as well as for advanced providers. The pediatric age group is now defined to include those children from 1 year of age to the onset of puberty. This is determined by the presence of secondary sexual characteristics that usually occur between 12 and 14 years of age. For the lay rescuer, pediatric guidelines are applied to children between 1 and 8 years old, with adult ACLS guidelines applied to those patients older than 8.

Once it is recognized that a child needs resuscitation, it is important to approach the evaluation and management in a stepwise manner. First, the airway is assessed, then breathing, and finally circulation. If there is an abnormality at any step of this A-B-C assessment, intervention must be

---

* Corresponding author.
E-mail address: sjdoniger@hotmail.com (S.J. Doniger).

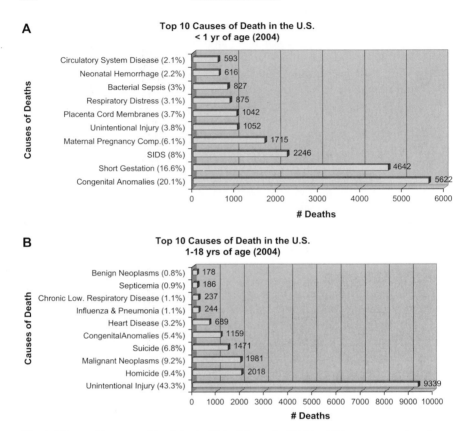

Fig. 1. The top 10 causes of death in the United States in 2005 in children younger than 1 year (*A*), and 1 to 18 years of age (*B*). (*Data from* Centers for Disease Control and Prevention/NCHS. 2004 National Vital Statistics System, mortality. Available at: http://www.cdc.gov/nchs.)

initiated to stabilize the patient. The goal of early, high-quality cardiopulmonary resuscitation (CPR) and defibrillation is to improve overall survival from arrest. Only one third of out-of-hospital cardiac arrest victims receive CPR before emergency medical service (EMS) arrival [2]. Those who actually receive CPR do not receive enough effective CPR. When CPR is performed, suboptimal CPR is often performed with too few, too shallow (37%), and too weak chest compressions. Ventilations (61%) are often excessive, with too many interruptions in chest compressions [3].

Airway

Evaluation

The first priority in basic and advanced life support is evaluating the airway. To assess upper airway patency, the provider should look, listen, and feel whether there is adequate breathing. The provider should look for chest rise, listen for breath sounds and air movement, and feel the movement of air at the nose and mouth. Clinical signs of an airway obstruction include breathing difficulty, the inability to speak or breathe, poor air exchange, a silent cough, or poor air exchange. It is crucial to determine whether the airway is maintainable by simple maneuvers, or not maintainable, necessitating advanced interventions [4].

Management

Simple measures to restore airway patency include positioning, suctioning, relieving a foreign-body airway obstruction, and the use of airway adjuncts. More advanced interventions, include endotracheal intubation.

Rather than waiting for respiratory arrest, those who do not exhibit adequate breathing should receive rescue breaths. It is recommended to try "a couple of times" to deliver two effective rescue breaths [5]. In those who are not breathing, but have a pulse, only respirations should be delivered, without compressions. The health care provider should administer 12 to 20 breaths per minute (1 breath every 3 to 5 seconds) for infants and children, and 10 to 12 breaths per minute (1 breath every 5 to 6 seconds) for adults. Rescue breaths should be given over 1 second, with enough volume to create visible chest rise. There are no indications stating specific tidal volumes, since it is difficult to estimate tidal volumes delivered during rescue breaths. In fact, much less tidal volume is required during resuscitation than in normal healthy individuals. During CPR, there is 24% to 33% less blood flow to the lungs. Therefore, fewer breaths with smaller volumes are needed for oxygenation and ventilation [5].

The preferred method of opening the airway for the lay rescuer is the head tilt–chin lift maneuver for both injured and noninjured victims. It is also recommended for the health care provider in nontrauma settings. In trauma situations in which a cervical spine injury is suspected, a jaw thrust maneuver without a head tilt is recommended to open the airway and maintain manual stabilization of the head and neck. The jaw thrust is no longer recommended for lay rescuers because it is difficult to learn and perform, may be ineffective, and may cause spinal movement [6].

In situations of airway foreign bodies, action must be taken in those cases of severe airway obstruction. If the individual is unresponsive, it is recommended to activate EMS and perform CPR. It is unadvisable to perform blind finger sweeps, and it is not recommended to perform the "jaw thrust" maneuver. This technique is difficult, especially for inexperienced providers. The preferred method of opening the airway for the lay rescuer is the head tilt–chin lift maneuver. The recommendation is to perform five back blows and five chest thrusts for infants, and to perform the Heimlich maneuver in older children.

In addition, suctioning may be required to further open the airway. Airway adjuncts such as oropharyngeal and nasopharyngeal airways may assist in opening the airway, and facilitate in delivering oxygen by bag-valve mask.

The method of maintaining a proper airway depends on the skill level of the provider. For those untrained in advanced airway, one must focus on effective bag-valve mask technique. However, for those trained in endotracheal tube placement, it is the preferred route of securing an airway. Because insertion of an advanced airway may cause a prolonged interruption in compressions, one must weigh the risks and benefits. The use of a cuffed endotracheal tube may be used in all ages except neonates. A cuffed endotracheal tube is especially useful for those with poor lung compliance, increased airway resistance, or in those with a large glottic air leak [7]. Attention must be paid to tube size, position, and pressures. For children 1 to 10 years of age, the endotracheal size can be calculated by the following formulas [8].

The size of a cuffed endotracheal tube is determined by:

$$\text{Size(mm internal diameter)} = (\text{age in years}/4) + 3$$

The size of an uncuffed endotracheal tube is determined by:

$$\text{Size(mm internal diameter)} = (\text{age in years}/4) + 4$$

Once placed, the endotracheal tube cuff pressure should be maintained at less than 20 cm H_2O [9]. When endotracheal intubation is not possible, a reasonable alternative is the placement of a laryngeal mask airway (LMA). However, the placement of LMAs is associated with a higher incidence of complications in children [10].

Confirmation of tube placement should include clinical assessment and auscultation of breath sounds. New recommendations include measuring exhaled CO_2, which can be measured by a calorimetric detector or by capnography. However, their use is limited to those patients exhibiting a perfusing rhythm [11]. In those patients weighing more than 20 kg, one may consider esophageal detector devices for confirmation of tube placement [12]. It is important to repeatedly verify endotracheal tube placement after the tube is inserted, during transport, and after the movement of the patient.

Breathing

Evaluation

The assessment of breathing includes an evaluation of the respiratory rate and effort, lung sounds, and pulse oximetry. Normal respiratory rates depend on the age of the patient (Table 1). Tachypnea is defined as a rate that is more raid than normal for age, whereas bradypnea is a rate that is slower than normal for age. Apnea is defined as a complete cessation of breathing for 20 seconds or more.

Table 1
Expected respiratory rates, according to age [4]

Age, y	Breaths, per min
<1	30–60
1–3	24–40
4–5	22–34
6–12	18–30
13–18+	12–16

With regard to increased respiratory effort, a child may exhibit nasal flaring, retractions or accessory muscle use, or irregular respirations. Further factors to assess are adequate and equal chest wall excursion, and the auscultation of air movement. Abnormal lung sounds include stridor, grunting, gurgling, wheezing, and crackles.

Management

Once an advanced airway is in place, respirations should be administered simultaneously with chest compressions, at a rate of 8 to 10 per minute. Note that this rate is markedly lower than previous recommendations. Hyperventilation is not recommended, as it can actually be harmful. Increased respiratory rates cause an increased intrathoracic pressure, thereby decreasing venous return and coronary perfusion pressure. This has been shown to decrease survival rates [13].

Neonates

In the situation of neonates, it is often necessary to provide positive-pressure ventilation. This can be achieved with the use of a self-inflating bag, a flow-initiating bag, or a T-piece device. The T-piece is a valved device in which regulated pressure and limits flow [14]. The best indicator of successful ventilation is in an increase in the heart rate.

Whenever positive pressure is indicated for resuscitation, supplemental oxygen is recommended. For those babies who are breathing but have central cyanosis, free-flow oxygen is indicated. The standard is to use 100% F_iO_2; however, it is reasonable to begin with an oxygen concentration less than 100% or room air. If there is no improvement after 90 seconds, oxygen should be administered. This updated recommendation reflects the possible adverse effects that high-concentration oxygen has on the respiratory physiology and cerebral circulation of newborns [15]. On the same token, oxygen deprivation and asphyxia cause further tissue damage. Therefore, the goal is to provide adequate oxygenation, which is a balance between oxygen delivery and tissue demand.

In a vigorous infant, it is no longer recommended to perform oropharyngeal and nasopharyngeal suctioning of meconium-stained amniotic fluid at the perineum. A large multicenter trial showed that suctioning is ineffective in preventing meconium aspiration [16]. Those infants who are not vigorous warrant endotracheal suctioning immediately after birth.

Circulation

Evaluation

The assessment of cardiovascular function includes heart rate and rhythm, blood pressure, peripheral and central pulses, capillary refill time, and skin color and temperature.

Heart rate varies according to the child's age, and includes a wide range (Table 2). Typically the rate will be much slower in a sleeping or athletic child. Tachycardia is a heart rate faster than expected for a child's age, whereas bradycardia is slower than normal.

Similarly, blood pressures vary according to age (Table 3). Hypotension is defined as below the fifth percentile of expected blood pressures for age. Hypotension represents a state of shock, either due to hemorrhage, sepsis, or cardiac failure.

The heart rhythm can initially be determined as being regular or irregular. To determine the specific rhythm, one must attach at least a three-lead ECG. Various rhythm disturbances, or arrhythmias, can be recognized to initiate appropriate interventions. The important dysrhythmias to recognize are ventricular fibrillation (Fig. 2), ventricular tachycardia (Fig. 3), pulseless electrical activity (PEA), asystole, and supraventricular tachycardia (Fig. 4).

Further factors in the cardiac assessment include central and peripheral pulses. In addition, the capillary refill time reflects skin perfusion. A delayed capillary refill time, greater than 2 seconds, may be a result of dehydration, shock, or hypothermia.

Management

The management recommendations for cardiovascular function include obtaining IV access, performing cardiac compressions, defibrillation, and the administration of drugs for rhythm disturbances.

Table 2
Expected heart rates, according to age

Age	Rate (mean)
0–3 mo	80–205 (140)
3 mo–2 y	75–190 (130)
2–10 y	60–140 (80)
>10 y	50–100 (75)

Data from Ralston M, Hazinski M, Zaritsky A, et al. Pediatric assessment. Pediatric advanced life support, provider manual. American Heart Association; 2006. p. 1–32.

Table 3
Expected systolic and diastolic blood pressures according to age

Age	Systolic BP (mm Hg)	Diastolic BP (mm Hg)
0 d	60–76	30–45
1–4 d	67–84	35–53
1 mo	73–94	36–56
3 mo	78–103	44–65
6 mo	82–105	46–68
1 y	67–104	20–60
2 y	70–106	25–65
7 y	79–115	38–78
15 y	93–131	45–85

Of note, females have slightly lower systolic blood pressures, and slightly higher diastolic blood pressures when compared with males of the same age [4].

Intravenous access

Intravenous or intraosseous routes are preferred for vascular access and for the administration of all drugs. Drug administration via the endotracheal tube is not recommended since drug delivery is unpredictable. In addition to lower drug concentrations in the blood, some drugs can cause detrimental b-adrenergic effects [17]. However, if vascular access is unavailable, lipophilic drugs may be administered at higher doses through the endotracheal tube. These drugs include "LEAN": lidocaine, epinephrine, atropine, and narcan [18].

Compressions

Effective chest compressions are crucial in improving survival. Compressions provide blood flow to vital organs, such as the heart and brain during resuscitation. The AHA now recommends "push hard and push fast." Interruptions in compressions should be limited to less than 10 seconds for interventions such as placing an advanced airway or defibrillation. Interruptions in compressions have shown to decrease the rate of return to spontaneous circulation. Rhythm checks should be performed every 2 minutes, or 5 cycles of CPR. Once an advanced airway is in place, compressions and breaths should be performed continuously without interruption.

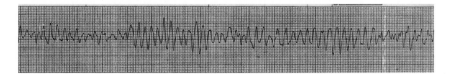

Fig. 2. Rhythm strip of ventricular fibrillation (torsades de pointes). This child had a history of dilated cardiomyopathy, and returned to sinus rhythm after defibrillation. (*Courtesy of* CDR Jonathan T. Fleenor, MD, San Diego, CA.)

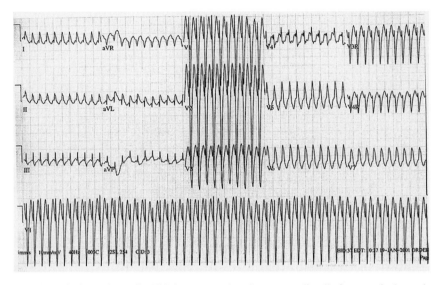

Fig. 3. Ventricular tachycardia. This is an example, of an extraordinarily fast ventricular tachycardia with a heart rate of almost 300 BPM. (*Courtesy of* CDR Jonathan T. Fleenor, MD, San Diego, CA.)

In those patients without a pulse, or newborns and children with a heart rate less than 60 beats per minute, compressions should be initiated. Since bradycardia is often a terminal rhythm in children, it is not necessary to wait for pulseless arrest to initiate compressions. Compressions should be

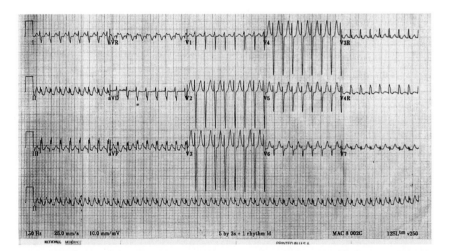

Fig. 4. Supraventricular tachycardia (SVT), with concomitant right ventricular hypertrophy. This 4-year- old male was postoperative from repair of congenital heart disease (Fontan repair). He was eventually converted to normal sinus rhythm after multiple doses of adenosine. (*Courtesy of* Stephanie Doniger, MD, San Diego, CA.)

performed at a rate of 100 per minute for all ages, except newborns, in whom compressions should occur at a rate of 120 per minute. The compression to ventilation ratio is 30:2 for single rescuers, while the ratio is 15:2 for two-rescuer health provider resuscitations in children. These universal rates simplify guidelines for providers, and are best for all victims of cardiac arrest, including hypoxic arrests. Furthermore, it allows for sufficient time for adequate chest recoil, to allow for adequate cardiac filling and venous return [19].

To perform adequate compressions for children, the heel of one or two hands can be used to compress the lower half of the sternum to a depth of one half to one third of the chest diameter [20]. For infants, the AHA now recommends that two thumbs press on sternum, with the hands encircling the chest. In addition to compressing the sternum, the hands should squeeze the thorax. This improves coronary artery perfusion pressure, and may generate higher systolic and diastolic blood pressures [21]. When performing chest compressions, rescuers should be changed after five cycles of CPR, or 2 minutes to decrease rescuer fatigue. This switch should be performed in less than 5 seconds to minimize interruptions in CPR [22].

In neonates, compressions and ventilations should be given in a 3:1 ratio of compressions to ventilations with 90 compressions and 30 breaths in 1 minute for a total of 120 events per minute. When compressions are given continuously, the rate should be 120 compressions per minute.

Defibrillation

In situations of sudden witnessed collapse, immediate defibrillation is warranted, followed by CPR, followed by drug administration. CPR provides some blood flow, delivering oxygen and substrate to the heart muscle, thereby making it more likely to abort ventricular fibrillation. A single shock should be administered at a dose of 2 J/kg, followed by immediate CPR. In at least 90% of cases, ventricular fibrillation is eliminated by the first shock [23]. In those cases in which the first shock does not terminate ventricular fibrillation, CPR is of greater value.

CPR is beneficial immediately postdefibrillation. This "primes" the heart for the next defibrillation attempt and also treats PEA. In cases of prolonged ventricular fibrillation, it has been shown that giving CPR before defibrillation increased survival rates from 4% to 22% [24].The dosages of defibrillation are now 2 J/kg followed by 4 J/kg for subsequent dosages, regardless of the type of defibrillator. It is important to note that stacked shocks are no longer recommended. A single shock is recommended followed by CPR largely because of the prolonged period of time to administer three shocks (Fig. 5). Do not interrupt CPR until after five cycles or 2 minutes for a pulse/rhythm check. In cases of asystole or PEA one should initiate immediate CPR.

More specifically, the treatment of each rhythm disturbance can be classified according to the Tachycardia Algorithm (Fig. 6). The presence or

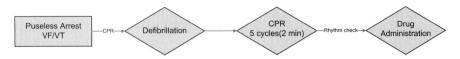

Fig. 5. Sequence of resuscitation, in pulseless arrest with ventricular fibrillation (VF) and ventricular tachycardia (VT).

absence of a pulse determines which arm of the algorithm to initiate. Of note, sinus tachycardia with adequate perfusion is no longer included in the algorithm. In addition, polymorphic ventricular tachycardia is now considered most likely to be an unstable rhythm. Therefore, it is recommended to use unsynchronized shocks rather than synchronized shocks. In contrast to previous recommendations, low-energy synchronized shocks have a high likelihood of provoking ventricular fibrillation [5].

In the community, automated external defibrillators (AEDs) have been shown to increase survival rates. There has been sufficient evidence to show that AEDs can safely be used for those older than 1 year [25]. In a sudden witnessed collapse, the AED should be used as soon as it becomes available. However, if the collapse is unwitnessed, CPR should be performed for 5 cycles or 2 minutes before the use of the AED. Pediatric AED pads and energy levels should be used in those 1 to 8 years of age. If the pediatric dose is unavailable, the adult dose is a reasonable alternative.

Drugs

For the most part, the algorithm drug dosages remain the same in the updated 2005 AHA Recommendations. Drug delivery should not interrupt CPR. The timing of drug delivery is less important than minimizing chest compressions. Amiodarone is the preferred drug for treatment for pulseless arrest, since it is more effective. Lidocaine is only recommended when amiodarone is unavailable [26]. Additionally, lidocaine is no longer listed on the stable ventricular tachycardia algorithm (see Fig. 5). It has been replaced by amiodarone and procainamide. It is important to note that amiodarone and procainamide should not be administered together as they can lead to severe hypotension and prolongation of the QT interval.

High-dose epinephrine (1:1000 concentration via IV [intravenous]) is not recommended in any age group, and is actually associated with a worse outcome, especially in cases of asphyxia [27]. Therefore, the standard recommended dose is (0.01 mg/kg IV/intraosseous) for all doses, which correlates to 0.1 mL/kg. Although the preferred routes of administration are intravenous or intraosseous, it may be given via the endotracheal tube when such access is

Fig. 6. Tachycardia algorithm. (*Adapted from* Ralston M, Hazinski M, Zaritsky A, et al. Pediatric assessment. Pediatric advanced life support, provider manual. American Heart Association; 2006. p. 1–32.)

unable to be obtained (0.1 mg/kg endotracheal tube). In exceptional cases, such as beta blocker overdoses, high-dose epinephrine may be considered.

In newborn resuscitation, drug therapy is rarely indicated [28]. However, the 2005 AHA recommendations for drug therapy in the newborn focus on the indications for the use of epinephrine and naloxone. High-dose

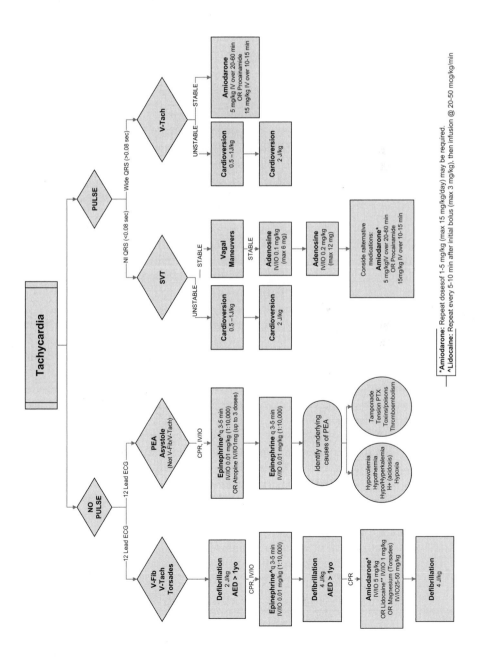

epinephrine is no longer recommended but rather at a dose of 0.01 to 0.03 mg/kg/dose. The intravenous concentration is 1:10,000 and the IV route for epinephrine administration is preferred. Although the endotracheal route for drug administration is unpredictable for drug delivery, it may be used when there is difficulty obtaining access. The endotracheal concentration of epinephrine is 1:1000. Naloxone should not be given endotracheally because of the lack of clinical data in newborns. Further, naloxone is no longer recommended in primary resuscitative efforts. Heart rate and color must first be restored through ventilatory support before its administration [6].

Postresuscitative care

In general, it is recommended to maintain a normal body temperature in postresuscitative care of neonates and children. Recent evidence is insufficient to recommend the routine use of systemic or selective cerebral hypothermia after resuscitation. However, it is important to avoid hyperthermia, especially in very-low-weight infants and hypoxic-ischemic events and very-low-weight infants. There are possible benefits of induced hypothermia (32 to 34°C) for 12 to 24 hours following successful resuscitation [29].

In addition, new recommendations recognize the probable benefits of vasoactive medications, including ionodilators (inamrinone, milrinone) to treat postresuscitation myocardial depression. However, there may be adverse effects on cerebral circulation and hyperventilation. Further studies are recommended before universal initiation of these agents [30].

New evidence suggests that the length of resuscitation is not an adequate prognostic indicator of survival. Intact survival has been reported, even in those cases with prolonged resuscitation and two doses of epinephrine have been administered [31].

Last, neonatal recommendations include guidelines regarding withholding and withdrawing resuscitative efforts. Such decisions are optimal when there are opportunities for parental agreement. It may be reasonable to withhold resuscitation in those conditions associated with an unacceptably high mortality. Such situations include extremely low birth weights (<400 g), young gestational age (<23 weeks), and certain congenital anomalies (anencephaly, trisomy 13) [6]. Alternatively, resuscitation is indicated in those cases that have a high survival rate and an acceptable mortality. In other situations, the parental desires would dictate resuscitative efforts. This occurs in babies with an uncertain prognosis, borderline survival, a relatively high morbidity rate, and a high anticipated burden to the child. Further, after 10 minutes of adequate continuous resuscitation, and there are still no signs of life (ie, no heartbeat or respiratory effort), it is reasonable to discontinue resuscitation. This is due to evidence that shows there is a high mortality rate and chance for severe neurodevelopmental disability [32].

Summary

- Emphasis on effective CPR, while limiting interruptions
- "Push hard, push fast," at 100 compressions/minute
- Universal compression: ventilation 30:2 (lone rescuer), 15:2 (2 rescuers)
- Use cuffed or uncuffed ETT, with attention to size, position, pressures
- Once advanced airway in place: simultaneous ventilations and compressions with ventilation rate: 8–10/minute
- IV/intraosseous preferable to ETT for drug administration
- Defibrillation: single shock followed by immediate resumption of CPR
- Amiodarone is preferred for pulseless arrest due to ventricular fibrillation (VF)/ventricular tachycardia (VT)

References

[1] Ludwig S, Lavelle J. Resuscitation—pediatric basic and advanced life support. In: Fleisher G, Ludwig S, Henretig F, editors. Textbook of pediatric emergency medicine. 5th edition. Philadelphia: Lippincott Williams & Wilkins; 2006. p. 3–33.

[2] Donoghue A, Nadkarni V, Berg R, et al. Out-of-hospital pediatric cardiac arrest: an epidemiologic review and assessment of current knowledge. Ann Emerg Med 2005;46(6): 512–22.

[3] Abella B, Alvarado J, Myklebust H, et al. Quality of cardiopulmonary resuscitation during in-hospital cardiac arrest. JAMA 2005;293(3):363–5.

[4] Ralston M, Hazinski M, Zaritsky A, et al. Pediatric assessment. Pediatric advanced life support, provider manual. Dallas (TX): American Heart Association; 2006. p. 1–32.

[5] ECC Committee. Highlights of the 2005 American Heart Association guidelines for cardiopulmonary resuscitation and emergency cardiovascular care. Currents in Emergency Cardiovascular Care 2006;15(4).

[6] ECC Committee SaTFotAHA. 2005 American Heart Association Guidelines for Cardiopulmonary Resuscitation and Emergency Cardiovascular Care: Part 13: Neonatal Resuscitation Guidelines. Circulation 2005;112:188–95.

[7] Newth C, Rachman B, Patel N, et al. The use of cuffed versus uncuffed endotracheal tubes in pediatric intensive care. J Pediatr 2004;144(3):333–7.

[8] Khine H, Corddry D, Kettrick R, et al. Comparison of cuffed and uncuffed endotracheal tubes in young children during general anesthesia. Anesthesiology 1997;86:627–31.

[9] Hoffman R, Parwani V, Hahn I. Experienced emergency medicine physicians cannot safely inflate or estimate endotracheal tube cuff pressure using standard techniques. Am J Emerg Med 2006;24(2):139–43.

[10] Park C, Bahk J, Ahn W, et al. The laryngeal mask airway in infants and children. Can J Anaesth 2001;48(4):413–7.

[11] Bhende M, Thompson A, Orr R. Utility of an end-tidal carbon dioxide detector during stabilization and transport of critically ill children. Pediatrics 1992;89(6 Pt 1):1042–4.

[12] Sharieff G, Rodarte A, Wilton N, et al. The self-inflating bulb as an airway adjunct: is it reliable in children weighing less than 20 kilograms? Acad Emerg Med 2003;41: 623–9.

[13] Aufderheide T, Lurie K. Death by hyperventilation: a common and life-threatening problem during cardiopulmonary resuscitation. Crit Care Med 2004;32(9 Suppl):S345–51.

[14] Allwood A, Madar R, Baumer J, et al. Changes in resuscitation practice at birth. Arch Dis Child Fetal Neonatal Ed 2003;88:F375–9.

[15] Tan A, Schulze A, O'Donnell CPF, et al. Air versus oxygen for resuscitation of infants at birth. Cochrane Database Syst Rev 2004;3:CD002273.

[16] Vain N, Szyld E, Prudent L, et al. Oropharyngeal and nasopharyngeal suctioning of meconium-stained neonates before delivery of their shoulders: multicentre, randomised controlled trial. Lancet 2004;364:597–602.

[17] Efrati O, Ben-Abraham R, Barak A, et al. Endobronchial adrenaline: should it be reconsidered? Dose response and haemodynamic effect in dogs. Resuscitation 2003;59(1):117–22.

[18] Johnston C. Endotracheal drug delivery. Pediatr Emerg Care 1992;8:94–7.

[19] Aufderheide T, Pirrallo R, Yannopoulos D, et al. Incomplete chest wall decompression: a clinical evaluation of CPR performance by EMS personnel and assessment of alternative manual chest comprssion-decompression techniques. Resuscitation 2005;64:355–62.

[20] Stevenson A, McGowan J, Evans A, et al. CPR for children: one hand or two? Resuscitation 2005;64:205–8.

[21] Ishimine P, Menegazzi J, Weinstein D. Evaluation of two-thumb chest compression with thoracic squeeze in a swine model of infant cardiac arrest. Acad Emerg Med 1998;5:397.

[22] Ashton A, McCluskey A, Gwinnutt C, et al. Effect of rescuer fatigue on performance of continuous external chest compressions over 3 min. Resuscitation 2002;55:151–5.

[23] Martens P, Russell J, Wolcke B, et al. Optimal response to cardiac arrest study: defibrillation waveform effects. Resuscitation 2001;49:233–43.

[24] Wik L, Kramer-Johansen J, Myklebust H, et al. Quality of cardiopulmonary resuscitation during out-of-hospital cardiac arrest. JAMA 2005;293:299–304.

[25] Atkinson E, Mikysa B, Conway J, et al. Specificity and sensitivity of automated external defibrillator rhythm analysis in infants and children. Ann Emerg Med 2003;42:185–96.

[26] Dorian P, Cass D, Schwartz B, et al. Amiodarone as compared with lidocaine for shock-resistant ventricular fibrillation. N Engl J Med 2002;346:884–90.

[27] Perondi M, Reis A, Paiva E, et al. A comparison of high-dose and standard-dose epinephrine in children with cardiac arrest. N Engl J Med 2004;350(17):1708–9.

[28] Perlman J, Risser R. Cardiopulmonary resuscitation in the delivery room. Associated clinical events. Arch Pediatr Adolesc Med 1995;140:20–5.

[29] Holzer M, Bernard S, Hachimi-Idrissi S, et al. Hypothermia for neuroprotection after cardiac arrest: systematic review and individual patient data meta-analysis. Crit Care Med 2005;33(2):1449–52.

[30] Abdallah I, Shawky H. A randomised controlled trial comparing milrinone and epinephrine as ionotropes in paediatric patients undergoing total correction of tetralogy of Fallot. Egyptian Journal of Anesthesiology 2003;19:323–9.

[31] Lopez-Herce J, Garcia C, Dominguez P, et al. Characteristics and outcome of cardiorespiratory arrest in children. Resuscitation 2004;63:311–20.

[32] Haddad B, Mercer B, Livingston J, et al. Outcome after successful resuscitation of babies born with apgar scores of 0 at both 1 and 5 minutes. Am J Obstet Gynecol 2000;182:1210–4.

ELSEVIER
SAUNDERS

Emerg Med Clin N Am
25 (2007) 961–979

EMERGENCY
MEDICINE
CLINICS OF
NORTH AMERICA

Pediatric Respiratory Infections

Seema Shah, MD[a],*,
Ghazala Q. Sharieff, MD, FACEP, FAAEM, FAAP[b,c]

[a]Division of Emergency Medicine, Rady Children's Hospital, University of California,
San Diego, 3020 Children's Way, San Diego, CA 92123, USA
[b]Palomar-Pomerado Health System/California Emergency Physicians,
3020 Children's Way, San Diego, CA 92123, USA
[c]Division of Emergency Medicine, Rady Children's Hospital, 3020 Children's Way,
San Diego, CA 92123, USA

Pediatric respiratory emergencies account for a large number of emergency department visits each year. Because many of these conditions may lead to life-threatening events, an appropriate understanding of the various entities that cause these emergencies will allow the provider prompt recognition and treatment. The differential diagnosis includes foreign body aspiration, allergic reaction, neoplasm, trauma, and congenital anomalies. This review discusses common infectious conditions, including bacterial tracheitis, bronchiolitis, croup, epiglottitis, pertussis, pneumonia, and retropharyngeal abscess.

Bacterial tracheitis

Epidemiology

Bacterial tracheitis, also known as laryngotracheobronchitis, pseudomembranous croup, or bacterial croup, is an entity first described in 1979 [1]. Although it is an uncommon disease, it may be life threatening. As is true for croup, the peak incidence is in the fall and winter in children with an age range between 6 months to 8 years [2]. Furthermore, Gallagher and colleagues [3] found a 2:1 male predominance. In a retrospective study of 500 patients admitted under the diagnosis of croup, 2% had bacterial tracheitis [4]. Marked subglottic edema and thick mucopurulent (membranous) secretions characterize the illness. The organisms most commonly implicated include *Staphylococcus aureus* and, to a lesser extent, alpha-hemolytic streptococcus, *Haemophilus influenzae*, *Moraxella catarrhalis*, and *Streptococcus pneumoniae* [5].

---

* Corresponding author.
  E-mail address: sshah@chsd.org (S. Shah).

0733-8627/07/$ - see front matter © 2007 Elsevier Inc. All rights reserved.
doi:10.1016/j.emc.2007.07.006 *emed.theclinics.com*

Clinical features

The clinical presentation of bacterial tracheitis has features of epiglottitis and viral croup. Typically, the child may have prodromal viral upper respiratory symptoms such as a low-grade fever, cough, and stridor, similar to patients with croup; however, the patient then experiences the rapid onset of high fever, respiratory distress, and appears toxic. Unlike patients with epiglottitis, these children typically have a cough, are comfortable lying flat, and do not drool [6].

Laboratory analysis

Radiographs are not definitive or diagnostic because the x-ray film is usually normal in appearance; however, on anteroposterior neck radiographs, bacterial tracheitis can appear similar to croup in that marked subglottic narrowing, also known as the "steeple sign," may be present. Also, a slight irregularity of the proximal tracheal mucosa or clouding of the tracheal lumen may be seen. This irregularity or clouding represents pseudomembranous detachment and varies in 20% to 82% in studies [2,7].

Routine laboratory data are not indicated. A complete blood count may show marked leukocytosis; however, Gallagher and colleagues [3] found that it varied considerably. More common was a left shift. Blood cultures are typically negative.

The diagnosis is made endoscopically by visualizing normal supraglottic structures with prominent subglottic edema, ulcerations, and copious purulent secretions. These secretions should be cultured [6]. In several studies, the majority of the patients had a positive Gram stain and culture of the tracheal secretions [1,7].

Management

If it is available, patients in severe respiratory distress are best managed in the operating suite for endoscopic diagnosis and intubation [2,3]; however, if emergency department intubation is required, a tube size smaller than the calculated size may be necessary. Copious purulent secretions can be suctioned from the endotracheal tube. These secretions should be sent for culture. Humidification of the inspired air helps prevent mucous plugging.

If endotracheal intubation is unsuccessful, a tracheostomy may be necessary but should be avoided. In the acute setting, a needle cricothyrotomy would be the next emergency intervention. Occasionally, additional endoscopy may need to be performed to remove the pseudomembranous material. Intubation is often required for 3 to 7 days until the patient is afebrile or there is an air leak present (ie, passage of air around the endotracheal tube indicating decreased edema), signifying a decrease in the quantity and viscosity of secretions. Antibiotics should be initiated with nafcillin or oxacillin (200 mg/kg/d divided every 6 h for either agent) in conjunction with a third-generation cephalosporin such as ceftriaxone (50 mg/kg daily). The addition of vancomycin should be considered if resistant organisms are present or there is multisystem involvement.

Complications of bacterial tracheitis include respiratory failure, airway obstruction, pneumothorax [1], the formation of pseudomembranes, and toxic shock syndrome. These patients frequently have concurrent sites of infection with pneumonia [8].

Bronchiolitis

Epidemiology

Bronchiolitis is the most common lower respiratory tract infection in infants that is characterized by fever, cough, coryza, expiratory wheezing, and respiratory distress [9]. The disease causes marked inflammation, edema, and necrosis of the epithelial cells of the smaller airways, increased mucous production, and bronchospasm [10]. Although it may occur in all age groups, the larger airways of older children better accommodate the mucosal edema, and severe symptoms are usually seen in children under the age of 2 years. There are approximately 125,000 hospitalizations per year with 80% of admissions occurring in children less than 1 year of age [11]. The most common cause of bronchiolitis is respiratory syncytial virus (RSV), isolated in 75% of children less than 2 years of age who are hospitalized for bronchiolitis [12] Other causes include parainfluenza virus types 1 and 3, influenza B, adenovirus types 1, 2, and 5, mycoplasma, rhinovirus, enterovirus, and herpes simplex virus. In temperate climates, RSV epidemics occur yearly beginning in winter and continue until late spring, whereas parainfluenza epidemics typically occur in the fall.

Clinical features

Patients with bronchiolitis frequently present with rhinitis, tachypnea, wheezing, cough, crackles, the use of accessory muscles, and nasal flaring [13]. The cough may be paroxysmal, and patients may also have post tussive emesis. Respiratory distress in these children manifests as tachypnea with respiratory rates as high as 80 to 100 breaths/min, nasal flaring, and intercostal and supraclavicular retractions, apnea, grunting, and cyanosis. Common caregiver complaints include poor feeding and increased fussiness, usually as a result of difficulty sleeping. Other associated findings are tachycardia and dehydration. The natural course of the illness is about 7 to 10 days but can last several weeks to a month. Unfortunately, reinfections with RSV are common throughout life [14].

Laboratory testing

Although testing for RSV may be performed, it rarely changes clinical outcomes in typical cases. The diagnosis of bronchiolitis should be a clinical one [15]. If necessary, the work-up may include a nasopharyngeal swab for a rapid ELISA to test for RSV. A chest radiograph often shows hyperinflation with flattening of the diaphragm. Although routine chest radiographs are not necessary, they are helpful in ruling out potential complications such as atelectasis, hyperinflation, or pneumonia, especially when patients are not improving at the expected rate or have acute decompensation of unclear etiology.

Infants under 3 months of age who have bronchiolitis and the presence of a fever are frequently studied to determine the risk of serious bacterial infection. Melendez and Harper showed that the risk of bacteremia or meningitis among infants aged less than 90 days with fever and bronchiolitis was low; however, the risk of urinary tract infection in febrile RSV-positive patients aged less than 60 days is significant [16,17].

Management

The mainstay of treatment of bronchiolitis is supportive care including ensuring hydration, oxygenation, nasal suction, or even endotracheal intubation and ventilation for children with respiratory failure. Many therapies have been studied, including epinephrine, beta-2 agonist bronchodilators, corticosteroids, and ribavarin, but little evidence supports a routine role in management [18]. In actual hospital practice, beta-2 agonists have been used in 53% to 73% of various studies [19,20]. Per the American Academy of Pediatrics (AAP) Subcommittee on Diagnosis and Management of Bronchiolitis, bronchodilators should not be used in the routine management of all patients with bronchiolitis; rather, inhaled bronchodilators should be used only if there is a documented positive clinical response [13] Deep airway suctioning is extremely helpful in infants who present with acute distress. Thick secretions compromise the infant's airway, and this simple therapy can provide immediate relief. The clinician should give close attention to the patient's hydration status, especially in children who present with respiratory distress, because they are often dehydrated owing to insensible losses.

Prevention

Close evaluation of children who have underlying conditions such as bronchopulmonary dysplasia, chronic lung disease, congenital heart disease, or immunodeficiencies should be completed because they are prone to apnea and respiratory failure. In a subset of children under 1 year of age, palivizumab (Synagis) has been shown to be effective in preventing severe bronchiolitis when given prophylactically. Synagis is a monoclonal antibody given intramuscularly on a monthly basis through the RSV season. The AAP has established guidelines for the administration of Synagis, but, in general, it is given to children under the age of 24 months with comorbidities such as prematurity less than 28 weeks, congenital heart disease, severe immune deficiencies, severe neuromuscular disease, or congenital airway abnormalities.

Complications include apnea, respiratory failure, or pneumonia. Sweetmann and colleagues [21] found an incidence of neurologic complications of 1.2% (0.7% seizures) in 964 patients with RSV bronchiolitis. Patients with persistent hypoxia, respiratory distress, and an inability to tolerate fluids, or patients in whom close follow-up cannot be ensured should be admitted. Admission should also be strongly considered for patients less than 2 months of age or for premature infants owing to the risk of apnea.

Croup

Epidemiology

Croup, or laryngotracheobronchitis, is the most common cause of infectious airway obstruction in children [22]. The most commonly affected group is aged 6 months to 4 years, with a peak incidence of 60 cases per 1000 children aged 1 to 2 years [23]. Croup has a peak incidence in early fall and winter, but it may be seen throughout the year. The most frequent causative organism is parainfluenza virus type I; however, other organisms such as parainfluenza types II and III, *Mycoplasma pneumoniae*, RSV, influenza A and B, and adenovirus have been implicated.

Clinical features

Initially, patients have a 1- to 2-day prodrome of nasal congestion, rhinorrhea, and cough. Often frightening to the caregiver, the patient will have the onset of a harsh barky cough often described as sounding similar to a seal or a bark. The patient may also have stridor, which is typically inspiratory, but it may also be biphasic. In addition to nasal flaring, suprasternal and intercostal retractions, and tachypnea and hypoxia, the presence of biphasic stridor indicates severe respiratory compromise [24]. Symptoms tend to be aggravated by crying and agitation; children often want to sit up or be held upright. Symptom duration is less than 1 week with a peak of 1 to 2 days.

Laboratory analysis

The diagnosis of croup is a clinical one, because complete blood counts tend to be normal. Radiographs may be helpful in differentiation of other disease entities such as epiglottitis, retropharyngeal abscess, congenital abnormalities, a foreign body, or hemangioma. The classic radiographic finding in a patient with croup is the steeple sign (Fig. 1). Distension of the hypopharynx and of the laryngeal ventricle and haziness or narrowing of the subglottic space may be seen on a lateral neck radiograph; however, the absence of this finding does not rule out croup, because almost half of patients have normal radiographs [23].

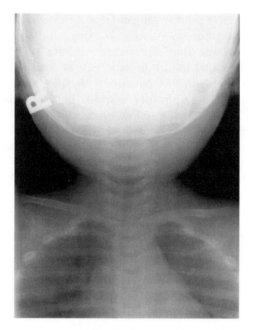

Fig. 1. Croup.

Treatment

The management of croup, usually a self-limited disease, is dependent on the severity of respiratory symptoms [22]. The most important task is airway maintenance. The administration of a mixture of helium and oxygen (heliox) can be beneficial in patients with severe croup [25].

In patients who have severe croup that is unresponsive to nebulized epinephrine, corticosteroids, and heliox, endotracheal intubation and ventilation may be necessary. If intubation is necessary, an endotracheal tube with a diameter smaller than recommended for the patient's age and size should be used.

Other therapies for mild-to-moderate croup are discussed in detail in the following sections.

Mist therapy

Traditionally, patients with croup have received humidified air to sooth the inflamed mucosa, thereby decreasing the amount of coughing due to mucosal irritation. Nevertheless, Neto and colleagues [26] described that mist therapy was not effective in improving clinical symptoms in children presenting to the emergency department with moderate croup. More recently, Scolnik and colleagues [27] found that even 100% humidity was not more effective when compared with mist therapy in the treatment of moderate croup. Because these treatments are harmless, many practitioners still use mist therapy, particularly in patients who have received racemic epinephrine and are being observed.

Glucocorticoids

The use of glucocorticoids for moderate-to-severe croup has long been recognized as a treatment modality. Both Johnson and colleagues and Klassen and colleagues showed improvement in children with severe croup treated with steroids [28,29]. Nebulized budesonide dosed at 2 and 4 mg has also shown efficacy in mild-to-moderate croup as single dose therapy [28,29].

In comparison with placebo, oral or intramuscular dexamethasone was found to decrease hospitalization rates. Donaldson and colleagues [30] found no differences in oral or intramuscular dexamethasone at doses of 0.6 mg/kg for children with moderate-to-severe croup at 24 hours or at any time in the week after treatment. Patients with mild croup have also been shown to benefit from the use of dexamethasone with faster resolution of symptoms. Although the standard dose of dexamethasone has been accepted to be 0.6 mg/kg, Geelhoed and colleagues [31,32] showed similar efficacy in patients with moderate croup using lower doses of 0.15 mg/kg and 0.3 mg/kg. Because the half-life of dexamethasone is 36 to 52 hours, it is the preferred agent for croup therapy, and it is not necessary to discharge the patient with additional doses of steroids.

Racemic epinephrine

Nebulized racemic epinephrine containing levo (L) and dextro (D) epinephrine isomers is the mainstay of treatment for moderate-to-severe croup. Although racemic epinephrine does not alter the natural course of croup, it may reduce the need for emergent airway management. The preferred dose is 0.25 to 0.5 mL with 3 mL of saline. Ledwith and Shea have recently allayed concern for the "rebound phenomenon." Patients who also received corticosteroids and experienced a sustained response to racemic epinephrine 3 hours after treatment were shown to be safe for discharge [33]. Patients who receive nebulized epinephrine should also receive dexamethasone. If racemic epinephrine is not available, epinephrine can be used in its place.

Patients who have persistent tachypnea or hypoxia, who are unable to tolerate oral fluids, or who require more than two treatments of racemic epinephrine should be admitted. Complications include potential airway obstruction, pneumonia, and respiratory arrest.

Epigottitis

Epidemiology

Epiglottitis or supraglottitis is a serious, life-threatening infection of the epiglottis and an airway emergency. Epiglottitis is an acute inflammation of the epiglottis and the structures surrounding it including the aryepiglottic folds and the arytenoid soft tissue. It is more common in the winter but can occur throughout the year. The peak incidence occurs in children between 2 and 8 years of age, but it has been increasing since the advent of *Haemophilus influenzae* type B vaccination. Before widespread vaccination against *Haemophilus influenzae* type B, the incidence was 41 cases per 100,000 children aged less than 5 years in 1987. This incidence decreased to 1.3 cases per 100,000 children in 1997 [34]. Currently, the most common identified organisms causing epiglottitis are group A beta-hemolytic streptococcus, *Streptococcus pneumoniae*, *Klebsiella*, *Pseudomonas*, and *Candida* sp.

Clinical features

Epiglottitis usually presents abruptly with a 6- to 24-hour prior duration of illness. Patients with epiglottitis classically present with a high fever, irritability, throat pain, airway obstruction, marked anxiety, and a toxic appearance. These children prefer to rest in the tripod position (ie, a sitting position with their jaws thrust forward). As the supraglottic edema worsens, it becomes difficult for the patient to swallow saliva; therefore, drooling is apparent and is a common complaint [35]. Often, a "hot potato" muffled voice may be present as well as air hunger. A temperature as high as 104°F (40.0°C) and tachycardia may be present. Blackstock and colleagues [36] described the "4 Ds" of epiglottitis: drooling, dyspnea, dysphonia, and dysphagia. Cyanosis may occur later in the illness as well as stridor, usually indicating impending airway obstruction.

Laboratory diagnosis

Airway management is of the utmost importance; routine laboratory data are not indicated, especially because agitation of the child may worsen symptoms. Only after a definitive airway has been established should cultures and sensitivities be obtained from the blood and supraglottic region. On physical examination, gentle visualization of the oropharynx may be performed but without the use of a tongue depressor because manipulation may result in complete obstruction of the airway. Occasionally, an erythematous epiglottis may be seen protruding at the base of the tongue. Radiographs are helpful in ruling out croup, retropharyngeal abscess, or a foreign body, but treatment should not be delayed to obtain radiographs. If obtained, the lateral neck radiograph is the imaging view of choice, especially with hyperextension during inspiration. The classic finding is the "thumbprint sign," indicative of a round and thick epiglottis (Fig. 2); however, this finding may be negative in up to 20% of cases [37].

Treatment

When a definitive diagnosis of epiglottitis is established, every effort should be made to avoid any anxiety provoking procedures, including

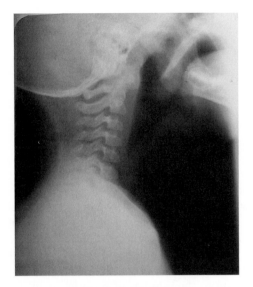

Fig. 2. Epiglottitis.

phlebotomy or intraoral examination. It is imperative to allow the patient to sit in the most comfortable position. The confirmatory diagnosis of epiglottitis is made by direct visualization with a laryngoscope; however, this should be performed under a controlled setting such as that of an operating room. The supraglottic structures, including the epiglottis, arytenoids, and aryepiglottic folds, may appear cherry red and edematous, and pooling of secretions may be present as well. Severe airway compromise requires immediate airway management by orotracheal intubation and typically requires a tube size smaller than calculated for age. When intubation is not successful, a surgical airway is necessary. If time permits, the assistance of an anesthesiologist or an ear, nose, and throat specialist is helpful. After securing the airway, the patient should be started on broad-spectrum antibiotics such as second- or third-generation cephalosporins (eg, ceftriaxone, 100 mg/kg/d intravenously; cefotaxime, 200 mg/kg/d in four divided doses; or ampicillin/sulbactam, 450 mg/kg/d in four divided doses) as an alternative until cultures return. Patients with mild symptoms may be observed in the intensive care unit. Patients who do not require immediate intervention are ideally taken to the operating room for airway control. Steroids are not routinely indicated.

Complications

While the patient is bacteremic, other sites may become involved through seeding. Patients who are not vaccinated against *Haemophilus influenzae* type B may develop meningitis, septic shock, cellulitis, and septic arthritis. Most of the complications associated with disease are centered on airway obstruction, including pulmonary edema, pneumonia, and respiratory arrest.

Pertussis

Epidemiology

Pertussis, or whooping cough, is an acute infection of the respiratory tract caused by *Bordetella pertussis,* first isolated in 1906. Other organisms may cause a similar clinical syndrome, such as *Bordetella parapertussis*, adenovirus, or *Chlamydia*. Following the introduction of immunization in the mid-1940s, the incidence of pertussis declined more than 99% by 1970 and to an all-time low of 1010 cases by 1976. Since then, a relevant increase in disease incidence has been documented, with nearly 26,000 cases reported in 2004, 40% of which were present in children aged less than 11 years [38]. The concern for the rising number of cases is that the increase in the number of reported deaths from pertussis among very young infants has paralleled the increase in the number of reported cases [39].

Clinical features

Pertussis can be divided into three phases described in the following sections.

Catarrhal phase

The first phase usually is characterized by mild cough, conjunctivitis, and coryza, and may last 1 to 2 weeks.

Paroxysmal phase

Characteristics in the second phase involve a worsening cough for 2 to 4 weeks. The classic description of the cough in this phase is that, after a spasmodic cough, the sudden inflow of air produces a "whoop." In infants, the cough usually is a staccato cough, and there is an absence of the whoop; instead, they may have an apneic episode. Vomiting frequently occurs after the episodes as well. In general, there is an absence of fever. Conjunctival hemorrhages and facial petechiae may be noted due to harsh coughing.

Convalescent phase

This third phase is typified by a chronic cough that may last several weeks.

Laboratory testing

Bordetella pertussis is a gram-negative, pleomorphic bacteria that can be cultured and is considered the gold standard for diagnosis; however, a polymerase chain reaction testing of the nasopharyngeal specimens is available.

According to Heininger and colleagues [40], 75% of unvaccinated patients with pertussis have a lymphocytosis on complete blood count. The leukocytosis may reach 20,000 to 50,000/mm^3; however, this finding is not often seen in children less than 6 months of age. A poor prognosis in infants is associated with leukocytosis with a lymphocytic predominance and the presence of pulmonary infiltrates [41]. Chest radiographs are usually normal but may infrequently show a shaggy right-sided heart border.

Treatment

Treatment is of minimum benefit by the time the paroxysmal phase has begun; however, treatment should be started within 3 to 4 weeks to prevent disease dissemination. The options are erythromycin, azithromycin, or clarithromycin. Trimethoprim-sulfamethaxazole may be used for patients with an allergy to macrolides (Table 1). Erythromycin has been associated with a risk of pyloric stenosis when used in infants less than 1 month of age [42].

Patients with pertussis should be placed in respiratory isolation to prevent further infections. Prophylaxis is recommended for all close contacts (see Table 1) regardless of age and vaccination status. Patients less than 7 years of age who are unimmunized or who have received less than four doses of the pertussis vaccine should be evaluated for vaccine initiation.

Complications

Major complications of pertussis infection include pneumonia (20%), encephalopathy and seizures (1%), failure to thrive, and death (0.3%). Pneumonia accounts for 90% of deaths from pertussis [41]. Other secondary complications as a result of severe coughing and increased intrathoracic

Table 1
Antibiotics for prophylaxis and treatment of pertussis

Antibiotic	Dosing guidelines	Commentary
First line		
Azithromycin	10 mg/kg 1st day, then 5 mg/kg for 4 days	For <6 months, use 10 mg/kg/d for 5 days
Clarithromycin	15 mg/kg div q12h for 7 days	Not recommended for use in infants <6 months of age
Erythromycin ethyl succinate	40–50 mg/kg/d div q6h for 14 days	Linked to infantile hypertrophic pyloric stenosis in infants <1 month
Macrolide allergy		
Trimethroprim-sulfamethoxazole	8 mg/kg/d div q12h for 14 days	Contraindicated in infants <2 months

pressure are intracranial hemorrhage, diaphragmatic rupture, pneumothorax, and rectal prolapse.

Pneumonia

Epidemiology

Community-acquired pneumonia is one of the most serious infections of childhood, leading to significant mortality and morbidity in the United States. The annual incidence in Europe and North America for children under 5 years of age is 34 to 40 cases per 1000 population [43–46]. Although there are several definitions for pneumonia, the most commonly accepted definition is the presence of fever, acute respiratory symptoms, or both, plus evidence of parenchymal infiltrates on a chest radiograph as defined by McIntosh and colleagues [47].

Etiology

The most causative organisms vary by age group. In neonates from birth to 3 weeks of age, group B streptococcus and gram-negative bacteria are common pathogens. This infection is from vertical transmission from the mother. In infants 3 weeks to 3 months of age, *Streptococcus pneumoniae* is usually implicated. From 3 months of age into the preschool years, viruses are the predominant causative organisms; however, the etiology of bacterial pneumonia is still predominantly *Streptococcus pneumoniae*. There are other potential bacteria, including *Mycoplasma pneumoniae, Haemophilus influenzae* type B and non-typeable strains, *Staphylococcus aureus,* and *Moraxella catarrhalis.*

Clinical features

The clinical features of pneumonia depend on various factors, such as the age of the patient, the presence of immunosuppression or comorbid diseases, and the causative organism. Bacterial pneumonia generally has an abrupt onset with fever and chills, productive cough, and chest pain. Toikka and colleagues [48] found that 93% of patients with bacterial pneumonia had a high fever ($>39.0°C$), 28% had no respiratory symptoms, and 6% presented with only gastrointestinal symptoms such as vomiting and vague abdominal pain in addition to fever. Frequently, the respiratory rate and work of breathing have been studied as predictors of pneumonia; however, Rothrock and colleagues [49] showed that tachypnea was predictive of only 24% of cases of pneumonia based on a respiratory rate of greater than 40 breaths/min. One study reviewed the predictive factors for the presence of focal infiltrates in children and found that decreased breath sounds, crackles, grunting, and retractions were clinically significant [50]. Upper lobe pneumonias may manifest as suspicion for meningitis because pain may radiate to the neck. The presence of vague abdominal pain and fever should also raise the suspicion for pneumonia. Wheezing is typically associated with viral pneumonias, *Mycoplasma*, or chlamydial infections. Patients with chlamydial pneumonia often present with a staccato-like cough and are afebrile on examination.

Laboratory testing

In an uncomplicated patient with a lower respiratory tract infection that is otherwise stable, no testing is necessary. A peripheral white blood cell count as well as a sedimentation rate and assay for C-reactive protein are not helpful in differentiating a viral from bacterial infection [51]. Conversely, Bachur and colleagues [52] showed that chest radiography should be considered a routine diagnostic test in children with a temperature of 39°C or greater and white blood cell count of $20,000/mm^3$ or greater without an alternative major source of infection. Classic characteristic radiographic findings vary by causative organism, such as lobar infiltrates with air bronchograms seen in bacterial pneumonia or perihilar infiltrates seen in atypical pneumonia. Pneumococcal pneumonia may present as a round or lobar infiltrate; however, many of these radiographic findings may be seen in both bacterial and viral infections [53]. Decubitus chest radiographs are helpful in the evaluation of pleural effusions. Children who are dehydrated might not have an infiltrate on initial radiography. Another diagnostic test is a mycoplasma IgM, which is especially helpful in children less than 3 years of age who present with pneumonias that are not responsive to amoxicillin.

Management

Once a diagnosis has been made, management is based on the presumed causative agent. For bacterial or viral pneumonia, supportive care should be initiated with hydration, maintaining oxygenation, and continuous cardiorespiratory monitoring for ill-appearing children. If a virus is suspected, supportive care should be continued. Children with a large pleural effusion who are ill appearing or in an immunocompromised state should have a thoracentesis as well as chest tube placement to relieve respiratory distress and for diagnostic purposes. In infants less than 2 months of age, blood, urine, and cerebrospinal fluid cultures should be obtained; otherwise, blood cultures are rarely positive in pneumonia [54]. Bronchodilators and steroids should be considered in patients with wheezing or a history of reactive airway disease. An arterial or venous blood gas should be obtained in ill-appearing children or infants in respiratory distress. Endotracheal intubation followed by mechanical ventilation should be initiated in children with respiratory failure. Antibiotics should be initiated based on the presumptive causative organism. For infants aged less than 28 days, one should consider empiric ampicillin, 50 mg/kg every 6 hours, and a third-generation cephalosporin such as cefotaxime at 50 mg/kg every 6 hours. For patients older than 3 months who are stable for discharge home, amoxicillin may be used at 100 to 120 mg/kg/d divided three times per day. In children older than 3 years, azithromycin may be initiated in atypical pneumonia at a dose of 10 mg/kg the first day followed by 5 mg/kg/d for the next 4 days.

Complications

Infants less than 3 months of age should be admitted for intravenous antibiotics due to the high risk for sepsis and meningitis. Patients who meet admission criteria include those who have a poor social situation for whom appropriate follow-up is difficult, and patients who have persistent hypoxia, an inability to tolerate fluids, or outpatient antibiotic failure. Complications include bacteremia, with seeding of infection causing meningitis, pericarditis, epiglottitis, and septic arthritis.

Retropharyngeal abscess

Epidemiology

A retropharyngeal abscess is an infection of one of the deep spaces of the neck and is another potential life-threatening infection in children. The retropharyngeal space is a potential space located between the anterior border of the cervical vertebrae and the posterior wall of the esophagus. The space contains connective tissues and lymph nodes that receive lymphatic drainage from adjacent structures. There are two potential ways that the space may become infected. The first is through an upper respiratory tract infection that causes inflammation of the retropharyngeal nodes. The second is infection introduced through penetrating trauma to the oropharynx, such as in children who fall with an object in their mouth.

Fifty percent of cases occur in patients between 6 months and 12 months of age and 96% of all cases occur in children less than 6 years of age because the nodes of Rouvière that drain the retropharyngeal space typically atrophy after this age [55]. There is also a slight male predominance, in some studies, up to 75% of cases [56]. The most common causative organisms are group A streptococcus, anaerobic organisms, and *Staphylococcus aureus*.

Clinical features

The clinical presentation of a retropharyngeal abscess is similar to that of other illnesses such as croup, epiglottitis, tracheitis, and peritonsillar abscess. Patients frequently present with symptoms of an upper respiratory tract infection, fever, dysphagia, odynophagia, trismus, neck stiffness, and poor intake. As the purulent material collects, a fluctuant mass may compress the pharynx or trachea. Patients may then present with drooling, stridor, and respiratory distress. On examination, visualization of the oropharynx may reveal a mass; however, this is only present in half of all children with retropharyngeal abscess [57]. Patients often present with a stiff neck and may be misdiagnosed with meningitis.

Laboratory analysis

Routine laboratory testing is not useful in the diagnosis of a retropharyngeal abscess. A lateral neck radiograph with attention to the retropharyngeal space is very useful in the initial diagnosis of retropharyngeal abscesses. In children, the normal parameters are that the soft tissue should measure no more than 7 mm at the level of the second cervical vertebrae, less than 5 mm anterior to the third and fourth cervical vertebrae (or less than 40% of the anteroposterior diameter of the vertebral body), and 14 mm at the sixth cervical vertebrae on a film done with proper neck extension (Fig. 3). In general, the anteroposterior diameter of the retropharyngeal space should not exceed that of the contiguous vertebral body. Retropharyngeal thickening is seen in 88% to 100% of cases on the lateral neck radiograph [55,56,58]. In clinically stable patients, a CT scan of the neck is helpful to delineate whether there is a retropharyngeal cellulitis rather than a true abscess [59].

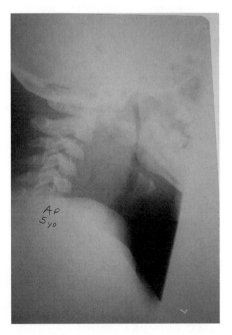

Fig. 3. Retropharyngeal abscess. (*Courtesy of* Lee Harvey, MD, San Diego, CA.)

Occasionally, there may be leukocytosis on a peripheral complete blood count, but a normal white blood cell count does not rule out retropharyngeal abscess.

Treatment

In cases of retropharyngeal abscess diagnosed by CT, antibiotics alone successfully treat 37% [59]. Antibiotic therapy should be initiated in these patients; clindamycin is an appropriate first choice (30 mg/kg/d intravenously divided four times a day), and cefazolin is an alternative (100 mg/kg/d intravenously divided four times a day). Previously, the standard of care for the management of retropharyngeal abscess had been surgical drainage. For cases in which there is a concern for airway obstruction, endotracheal intubation followed by surgical drainage by a qualified surgeon is still the treatment of choice. If endotracheal intubation needs to be performed due to airway compromise, caution should be taken when visualizing the airway owing to distortion from the mass and the possibility of inducing rupture.

Complications

Because retropharyngeal abscess is a life-threatening airway illness, all patients should be closely monitored and admitted. Complications include airway compromise, abscess rupture leading to asphyxiation or aspiration pneumonia, or spread of infection to adjacent structures in the neck, including infection of the carotid artery sheath, osteomyelitis of the cervical spine, or infection of the structures of the mediastinum. Necrotizing fasciitis is also a complication of the infection.

Summary

Respiratory track infections are common in newborns and infants. Prompt attention to the airway is essential as is the ability to recognize and manage these illnesses.

References

[1] Jones R, Santos JI, Overall JC Jr. Bacterial tracheitis. JAMA 1979;242(8):721–6.
[2] Liston SL, Gerhz RC, Siegel LG, et al. Bacterial tracheitis. Am J Dis Child 1983;137(8): 764–7.
[3] Gallagher PG, Myer CM 3rd. An approach to the diagnosis and treatment of membranous laryngotracheobronchitis in infants and children. Pediatr Emerg Care 1991;7(6):337–42.
[4] Tan AK, Manoukian JJ. Hospitalized croup (bacterial and viral): the role of rigid endoscopy. J Otolaryngol 1992;21(1):48–53.
[5] Brook I. Aerobic and anaerobic microbiology of bacterial tracheitis in children. Pediatr Emerg Care 1997;13(1):16–8.
[6] Donaldson JD, Mathby CC. Bacterial tracheitis in children. J Otolaryngol 1989;18(3):101–4.

[7] Bernstein T, Brilli R, Jacobs B. Is bacterial tracheitis changing? A 14-month experience in a pediatric intensive care unit. Clin Infect Dis 1998;27:458–62.

[8] Duncan NO, Sprecher RC. Infections of the airway. In: Cummings CW, editor. Otolaryngology-head & neck surgery. 3rd edition. St. Louis (MO): Mosby; 1998. p. 388–400.

[9] Klassen TP. Recent advances in the treatment of bronchiolitis and laryngitis. Pediatr Clin North Am 1997;44:249–61.

[10] Agency for Healthcare Research and Quality. Management of bronchiolitis in infants and children. Evidence Report/Technology Assessment No. 69. Rockville (MD): Agency for Healthcare Research and Quality; 2003. AHRQ Publication No. 03–E014.

[11] Henderson FW, Clyde WA Jr, Collier AM, et al. The etiologic and epidemiologic spectrum of bronchiolitis in pediatric practice. J Pediatr 1979;95(2):183–90.

[12] Carlsen KH, Orstavik I, Halvorsen K. Viral infections of the respiratory tract in hospitalized children: a study from Oslo during a 90 months' period. Acta Paediatr Scand 1983;72(1): 53–8.

[13] American Academy of Pediatrics Subcommittee on Diagnosis and Management of Bronchiolitis. Diagnosis and management of bronchiolitis. Pediatrics 2006;118(4):1774–93.

[14] Shay DK, Holman RC, Roosevelt GE, et al. Bronchiolitis-associated mortality and estimates of respiratory syncytial virus-associated deaths among US children, 1979–1997. J Infect Dis 2001;183:16–22.

[15] Bordley WC, Viswanathan M, King VJ, et al. Diagnosis and testing in bronchiolitis: a systematic review. Arch Pediatr Adolesc Med 2004;158(2):119–26.

[16] Melendez E, Harper MB. Utility of sepsis evaluation in infants 90 days of age or younger with fever and clinical bronchiolitis. Pediatr Infect Dis J 2003;22(12):1053–6.

[17] Zorc JJ, Levine DA, Platt SL, et al. Multicenter RSV-SBI Study Group of the Pediatric Emergency Medicine Collaborative Research Committee of the American Academy of Pediatrics. Pediatrics 2005;116(3):644–8.

[18] King VJ, Viswanathan M, Bordley WC, et al. Pharmacologic treatment of bronchiolitis in infants and children: a systematic review. Arch Pediatr Adolesc Med 2004;158(2):127–37.

[19] Mansbach JM, Edmond JA, Camargo CA. Bronchiolitis in US emergency departments 1992 to 2000: epidemiology and practice variation. Pediatr Emerg Care 2005;21:242–7.

[20] Plint AC, Johnson DW, Wiebe N. Practice variation among pediatric emergency departments in the treatment of bronchiolitis. Acad Emerg Med 2004;11:353–60.

[21] Sweetman LL, Ng YT, Butler IJ, et al. Neurologic complications associated with respiratory syncytial virus. Pediatr Neurol 2005;32(5):307–10.

[22] Denny FW, Murphy TF, Clyde WA Jr, et al. Croup: an 11-year study in a pediatric practice. Pediatrics 1983;71(6):871–6.

[23] Skolnik NS. Treatment of croup: a critical review. Am J Dis Child 1989;143(9):1045–9.

[24] Shroeder LL, Knapp JF. Recognition and emergency management of infectious causes of upper airway obstruction. Semin Respir Infect 1995;10(1):21–30.

[25] Gupta VK, Cheifitz IM. Heliox administration in the pediatric intensive care unit: an evidence-based review. Pediatr Crit Care Med 2005;6(2):204–11.

[26] Neto GM, Kentab O, Klassen TP, et al. A randomized controlled trial of mist in the acute treatment of moderate croup. Acad Emerg Med 2002;9(9):873–9.

[27] Scolnik D, Coates AL. Controlled delivery of high vs. low humidity vs. mist therapy for croup in emergency departments: a randomized controlled trial. JAMA 2006;295(11):1274–80.

[28] Klassen TP, Craig WR, Moher D, et al. Nebulized budesonide and oral dexamethasone for treatment of croup: a randomized control trial. JAMA 1998;279(20):1629–32.

[29] Johnson DW, Jacobson S, Edney PC, et al. A comparison of nebulized budesonide, intramuscular dexamethasone, and placebo for moderately severe croup. N Engl J Med 1998; 339(8):498–503.

[30] Donaldson D, Poleski D, Knipple E, et al. Intramuscular versus oral dexamethasone for the treatment of moderate-to-severe croup: a randomized, double blind trial. Acad Emerg Med 2003;10(1):16–21.

[31] Geelhoed GC, Turner J, Macdonald WB. Efficacy of a small single dose of oral dexameth-asone for outpatient croup: a double blind placebo controlled clinical trial. BMJ 1996; 313(7050):140–2.

[32] Geelhoed GC, Macdonald WB. Oral dexamethasone in the treatment of croup: 0.15 mg/kg versus 0.3 mg/kg versus 0.6 mg/kg. Pediatr Pulmonol 1995;20(6):362–8.

[33] Ledwith C, Shea L. The use of nebulized racemic epinephrine in the outpatient treatment of croup. Ann Emerg Med 1995;25(3):331–7.

[34] Progress toward eliminating *Haemophilus influenzae* type B disease among infants and chil-dren-United States, 1987–1997. MMWR Morb Mortal Wkly Rep 1998;47(46):993–8.

[35] Mauro RD, Poole SR, Lockhart CH. Differentiation of epiglottitis from laryngotracheitis in the child with stridor. Am J Dis Child 1988;142(6):679–82.

[36] Blackstock P, Adderhey RJ, Steward DJ. Epiglottitis in young infants. Anesthesiology 1987; 67:97–100.

[37] Loos GD. Pharyngitis, croup and epiglottitis. Prim Care 1990;17(2):335–45.

[38] Centers for Disease Control. Pertussis: epidemiology and prevention of vaccine-preventable diseases. (The Pink Book) course textbook. p.79–96.

[39] Vitek C, Pascual B, Murphy T. Pertussis deaths in the United States in the 1990s. In: Ab-stracts of the 40th Interscience Conference on Antimicrobial Agents and Chemotherapy, September 17–20, 2000, Toronto, Ontario, Canada. Washington (DC): American Society for Microbiology.

[40] Heininger U, Klich K, Stehr K, et al. Clinical findings in *Bordetella pertussis* infections: results of a prospective multicenter surveillance study. Pediatrics 1997;100(6):E10.

[41] Greenberg DP, von Konig CH, Heininger U. Health burden of pertussis in infants and chil-dren. Pediatr Infect Dis J 2005;24(Suppl 5):S39–43.

[42] Cooper WO, Griffin MR, Arbogast P, et al. Very early exposure to erythromycin and infan-tile hypertrophic pyloric stenosis. Arch Pediatr Adolesc Med 2002;156(7):647–50.

[43] Murphy TF, Henderson FW, Clyde WA Jr, et al. Pneumonia: an eleven-year study in a pe-diatric practice. Am J Epidemiol 1981;113:12–21.

[44] Foy HM, Cooney MK, Allan I, et al. Rates of pneumonia during influenza epidemics in Se-attle, 1964 to 1975. JAMA 1975;241:253–8.

[45] Jokinen C, Heiskanen L, Juvonen H, et al. Incidence of community-acquired pneumonia in the population of four municipalities in eastern Finland. Am J Epidemiol 1993;37:977–88.

[46] McConnochie KM, Hall CB, Barker WH. Lower respiratory tract illness in the first two years of life: epidemiologic patterns and costs in a suburban pediatric practice. Am J Public Health 1988;78:34–9.

[47] McIntosh K. Community-acquired pneumonia in children. N Engl J Med 2002;346(6): 429–37.

[48] Toikka P, Virkki R, Mertsola J, et al. Bacteremic pneumococcal pneumonia in children. Clin Infect Dis 1999;29:568–72.

[49] Rothrock SG, Green SM, Fanella JM, et al. Do published guidelines predict pneumonia in children presenting to an urban ED? Pediatr Emerg Care 2001;17(4):240–3.

[50] Lynch T, Platt R, Gouin S, et al. Can we predict which children with clinically suspected pneumonia will have the presence of focal infiltrates on chest radiographs? Pediatrics 2004;113(3 Pt 1):e186–9.

[51] Nohynek H, Valkeila E, Leinonen M, et al. Erythrocyte sedimentation rate, white blood cell count and serum C-reactive protein in assessing etiologic diagnosis of acute lower respiratory infections in children. Pediatr Infect Dis J 1995;14:484–90.

[52] Bachur R, Perry H, Harper MB. Occult pneumonias: empiric chest radiographs in febrile children with leukocytosis. Ann Emerg Med 1999;33(2):166–73.

[53] Korppi M, Kiekara O, Heiskanen-Kosma T, et al. Comparison of radiological findings and microbial aetiology of childhood pneumonia. Acta Paediatr 1993;82:360–3.

[54] Shah SS, Alpern ER, Zwering L, et al. Risk of bacteremia in young children with pneumonia treated as outpatients. Arch Pediatr Adolesc Med 2003;157(4):389–92.

[55] Coulthard M, Isaacs D. Retropharyngeal abscess. Arch Dis Child 1991;66:1227–30.
[56] Yeoh LH, Singh SD, Rogers JH. Retropharyngeal abscesses in a children's hospital. J Laryngol Otol 1985;99:555–6.
[57] Broughton RA. Nonsurgical management of deep neck infections in children. Pediatr Infect Dis J 1992;11(1):14–8.
[58] Morrison JE, Pashley NRT. Retropharyngeal abscesses in children: a 10-year review. Pediatr Emerg Care 1988;4:9–11.
[59] Craig FW, Schunk JE. Retropharyngeal abscess in children: clinical presentation, utility of imaging, and current management. Pediatrics 2003;111:1394–8.

ELSEVIER
SAUNDERS

Emerg Med Clin N Am
25 (2007) 981–1008

EMERGENCY
MEDICINE
CLINICS OF
NORTH AMERICA

Cardiac Emergencies in the First Year of Life

Linton Yee, MD[a,b,*]

[a]Department of Pediatrics, Division of Hospital and Emergency Medicine,
Duke University School of Medicine, Durham, NC 27710, USA
[b]Department of Surgery, Division of Emergency Medicine,
Duke University School of Medicine, Durham, NC 27710, USA

The presence of a distressed or obtunded infant in any adult or pediatric emergency department can prove to be a challenging process in airway management, vascular access, and decision making. Cardiac emergencies, as well as a number of other diseases, can present in this manner. It is essential to accurately diagnose and expeditiously care for these potentially complicated cardiac patients. Diagnosis can be difficult because of a number of nonspecific elements in the history and physical exam. However, by developing an effective strategy in dealing with these patients, the emergency department management of these individuals can be completed in an efficient and prompt manner.

The most challenging scenarios of cardiac emergencies in the first year of life include cyanotic episodes, congestive heart failure, cardiogenic shock or collapse, and arrhythmias. All of these emergent presentations can be the result of either the initial presentation of disease or as a known complication of an already diagnosed cardiac lesion.

In approaching cardiac emergencies, cardiac disease can be divided into structural disease, conduction abnormalities, and acquired illnesses. While recognizing that many lesions can be a combination of many defects, structural congenital heart disease can be divided into cyanotic and acyanotic categories. The cyanotic category can be further subdivided into increased and decreased pulmonary blood flow. Division of the acyanotic category is based on left-to-right shunting and left ventricular outflow obstruction. Conduction abnormalities can be congenital or the result from a new-onset illness. Acquired heart disease includes cardiomyopathies, myocarditis, pericarditis, endocarditis, and Kawasaki's disease.

* Department of Pediatrics, Division of Hospital and Emergency Medicine, Duke University School of Medicine, Durham, NC 27710.
 E-mail address: linton.yee@duke.edu

doi:10.1016/j.emc.2007.08.001

A cyanotic patient suggests that there is cyanotic congenital heart disease with shunting from the right to the left. In a patient with cardiogenic shock or collapse (the result of outflow obstruction and pump failure), the infant may appear mottled, ashen, and gray. A patient with left-to-right shunting and congestive heart failure can appear to be normal in color [1–7]. This article will discuss the cardiac emergencies that may present within the first year of life.

Basic pathophysiology

There are a number of changes that occur within the cardiovascular system in the transition from a fetus to a newborn. The placenta functions as the pulmonary system for the fetus, as oxygenated blood is transferred from the placenta to the fetus via the umbilical vein. At birth, blood then travels through a now lower resistance pulmonary system for oxygenation with closure of the shunts that were used between the pulmonary and systemic circulations (foramen ovale, ductus arteriosus, ductus venosus). Expansion of the lungs and the elimination of fluid from the lungs cause dilatation of the pulmonary vasculature, which then leads to a decrease in pulmonary resistance and increased pulmonary blood flow. Oxygenation of the blood through the pulmonary system leads to the closure of the umbilical vessels, the ductus arteriosus, and the ductus venosus. Decreased pulmonary artery resistance and subsequent increased systemic resistance changes the flow though the atria, with pressures now higher in the left atria than the right, resulting in the closure of the foramen ovale [8,9].

Cyanosis

Cyanosis is seen when desaturated blood is present in the capillary beds. Deoxygenated hemoglobin is blue and the presence of cyanosis means that there is 3 to5 mg/dL of deoxyhemoglobin in the blood. This corresponds with a room air oxygen saturation of 70% to 85% [10,11]. Because the oxygen carrying capacity is based on the amount of hemoglobin available to carry oxygen, an infant who is polycythemic and cyanotic is still able to deliver oxygen to tissues as opposed to an anemic infant who may not appear cyanotic but is not able to deliver oxygen to tissues.

It is important to differentiate between central and peripheral cyanosis as the evaluation and treatment differ based on the underlying cause. There are a number of different causes for central cyanosis. These include central nervous system (CNS) depression, pulmonary disease, and cardiac disease as well as sepsis and metabolic disease and toxic ingestions. Peripheral cyanosis is the result of acrocyanosis, exposure to cold, and decreased peripheral perfusion.

Factors to keep in mind when assessing cyanosis are the arterial oxygen saturation, the oxygen binding capacity (hemoglobin), and the arteriovenous oxygen difference [10].

Cyanotic heart disease

There are five well-known cyanotic congenital heart lesions—also known as the "Terrible Ts." They are Tetralogy of Fallot (TOF), Transposition of the Great Arteries (TGA), Tricuspid Atresia (TA), Total Anomalous Venous Return (TAPVR), and Truncus Arteriosus.

Tetralogy of Fallot

Tetralogy of Fallot is the most common form of cyanotic congenital heart disease in the post infancy period and represents up to 10% of all congenital heart disease [12,13]. Tetralogy of Fallot consists of four basic lesions. The lesions are a large ventricular septal defect (VSD), right ventricular outflow obstruction (from pulmonic stenosis), an overriding aorta, and right ventricular hypertrophy. Two of the lesions will determine the extent of the disease pathophysiology. There must be right ventricular outflow obstruction and the VSD must be large enough to equalize pressures in both of the ventricles.

The extent of obstruction of the right ventricular outflow track will determine the amount of cyanosis present in the patient. Systolic pressures are equally balanced in the right and left ventricle because of the nonrestrictive VSD. There will be a left-to-right shunt, a bidirectional shunt, or a right-to-left shunt depending on the extent of the right ventricular outflow tract obstruction. If the pulmonic stenosis is severe, there will be a right-to-left shunt with subsequent cyanosis and decreased pulmonary blood flow. If there is mild pulmonic stenosis, a left-to-right shunt will occur resulting in an acyanotic Tetralogy of Fallot.

In addition to cyanosis, the physical exam may show a systolic thrill at the lower and middle left sternal border. A loud and single S2, an aortic ejection click, and a loud grade 3 to 5/6 systolic ejection murmur in the middle to lower left sternal border will also be found. A continuous patent ductus arteriosus (PDA) murmur may also be present.

The ECG will show right axis deviation (RAD) and right ventricular hypertrophy (RVH).

A boot-shaped heart with a main pulmonary artery segment is characteristic of the cyanotic Tetralogy of Fallot. The heart size is normal with decreased pulmonary vascular markings. Acyanotic Tetralogy of Fallot will have chest x-rays similar to that of moderate VSDs.

Transposition of the great arteries

Transposition of the great arteries represents around 5% to 8% of congenital heart disease and is the most common cyanotic heart lesion in the newborn period [14]. There are many variations of the disease, with the underlying factor being that the aorta originates from the right ventricle and that the main pulmonary artery has origins in the left ventricle. Within these two distinct circulatory systems, the main pulmonary artery has a significantly higher oxygen saturation than the aorta, with hyperoxemic blood traveling through the pulmonary system and hypoxic blood traveling within the systemic system.

The presence of a VSD, atrial septal defect (ASD), or PDA is essential to survival, because the mixing of the circulations is the only way of providing oxygenated blood to the systemic system. A VSD can be found in approximately 20% to 40% of patients.

With progressive closure of the PDA, cyanosis becomes more prevalent. Hypoxia and acidosis result from the suboptimal mixing of oxygenated and deoxygenated blood.

Congestive heart failure is a common presentation in the first week of life, with dyspnea and feeding difficulties in addition to the cyanosis. If the interventricular septum is intact, these patients will be the critically ill. The severe arterial hypoxemia will not respond to the administration of oxygen. Acidosis as well as hypocalcemia and hypoglycemia are common. They will respond well to PGE1 infusion and, ultimately, a Rashkind balloon septostomy. If there is a VSD or large PDA, these patients will not be as cyanotic but will present with congestive heart failure and obstructive pulmonary disease.

There will be a loud, single S2. If there is a VSD, a systolic murmur can be heard. Otherwise, there are no specific auscultatory findings.

The ECG will show right axis deviation (RAD) and right ventricular hypertrophy (RVH).

The egg-shaped heart with a narrow mediastinum is the characteristic chest x-ray. There is cardiomegaly with increased pulmonary vascular markings (Fig. 1).

Echocardiogram will show two circular structures instead of the circle and sausage pattern of normal great arteries.

Total anomalous pulmonary venous return

TAPVR represents around 1% of congenital heart disease [15]. The pulmonary veins bring the blood from the lungs to the right atrium instead of the left atrium. TAPVR is generally divided into four groups, depending on where the pulmonary veins drain. In the supracardiac type (50%) the common pulmonary vein attaches to the superior vena cava. In the cardiac type (20%) the common pulmonary vein empties into the coronary sinus. In the infracardiac/subdiaphragmatic type (20%), the common pulmonary vein empties into the portal vein, ductus venosus, hepatic vein, or inferior vena cava. A mixed type is seen in 10% of the lesions, which is a combination of any of the types. An ASD or patent foramen ovale is necessary for mixing of the blood.

Pulmonary venous return is delivered to the right atrium, and there is mixing of the pulmonary and systemic circulations. Blood flow then travels to the left atrium through the ASD and to the right ventricle. Systemic

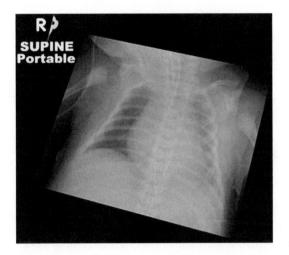

Fig. 1. Chest radiograph of TGA with cardiomegaly and increased vascular markings.

arterial desaturation occurs as the result of mixing of pulmonary and systemic blood. Pulmonary blood flow determines the amount of desaturation of systemic arterial blood. If there is no obstruction to pulmonary venous return, there is minimal desaturation of the systemic blood. If there is obstruction to pulmonary venous return, there is significant cyanosis. With the blood from both the pulmonary and systemic circulations pumped by the right ventricle, there can be volume overload, with subsequent right ventricular and atrial enlargement.

In a patient without pulmonary venous obstruction, there can be a history of frequent pneumonias and growth difficulties. Patients will frequently present with a congestive heart failure presentation with tachypnea, tachycardia, and hepatomegaly, in addition to slight cyanosis. There will be a hyperactive right ventricular impulse, with a split and fixed S2. A grade 2 to 3/6 systolic ejection murmur is at the upper left sternal border, with a mid diastolic rumble at the left lower sternal border.

The ECG will show right axis deviation, right ventricular hypertrophy, and right atrial enlargement (Fig. 2).

Chest x-ray will exhibit significant cardiomegaly with increased pulmonary vascular markings (Fig. 3). The characteristic "snowman sign" is found in infants older than 4 months.

In those patients with TAPVR and pulmonary venous obstruction, cyanosis and respiratory distress dominate the presentation. There can be minimal cardiac exam findings aside from a loud and single S2 and gallop rhythm. A murmur is usually not found.

The ECG will also show right axis deviation and right ventricular hypertrophy and the chest radiograph will have a normal heart silhouette with lung fields consistent with pulmonary edema.

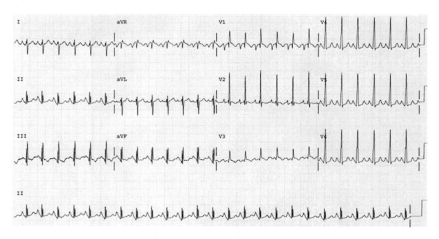

Fig. 2. ECG of TAPVR with right atrial enlargement, right ventricular hypertrophy.

Tricuspid atresia

Tricsupid atresia represents 1% to 2% of congenital heart disease in in-fancy [16]. There is no tricuspid valve and there is underdevelopment of the right ventricle and pulmonary artery. Therefore, pulmonary blood flow is decreased. With no flow across the right atrium to the right ventricle, the right atrium needs a right-to-left shunt to empty, making an ASD, VSD, or PDA essential for survival. The great arteries are transposed in 30% of the cases, with a VSD and no pulmonic stenosis. In 50% of cases there is normal artery anatomy, with a small VSD and pulmonic stenosis.

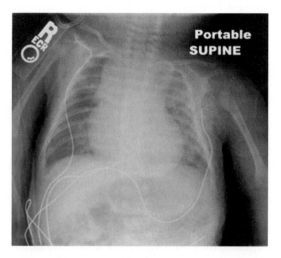

Fig. 3. Chest radiograph of TAPVR with cardiomegaly and increased vascular markings.

There will be right atrial dilatation and hypertrophy because all systemic venous return is shunted from the right atrium to the left atrium. Enlargement of the left atrium and ventricle occurs because of the work of handling both systemic and pulmonary returns.

The amount of cyanosis is inversely related to the amount of pulmonary blood flow.

Severe cyanosis, tachypnea, and poor feeding are common presentations. There is a single S2. The murmur is a grade 2 to 3/6 systolic regurgitant murmur from the VSD and is heard best at the left lower sternal border. There can also be a continuous murmur of a PDA. Hepatomegaly can be found with congestive heart failure.

The ECG has a superior QRS axis, along with right atrial hypertrophy (RAH), left atrial hypertrophy (LAH) and left ventricular hypertrophy. The chest radiograph will show a normal to slight increase in heart size along with decreased pulmonary vascular markings.

Truncus arteriosus

Truncus arteriosus is seen in less than 1% of all congenital heart disease [17]. All of the pulmonary, systemic, and coronary circulations result from a single arterial trunk. A large VSD is associated with this, as well as abnormalities of the coronary arteries.

DiGeorge syndrome (hypocalcemia, hypoparathyroidism, absence or hypoplasia of the thymus, chromosomal abnormalities) is often seen with truncus arteriosus. Pulmonary blood flow can be normal, increased, or decreased, depending on the type of truncus arteriosus.

There is a direct relationship between the amount of pulmonary blood flow and the degree of systemic arterial oxygen saturation. Cyanosis is prevalent with decreased pulmonary blood flow, and is minimal with increased pulmonary blood flow. Congestive heart failure can be seen with increased pulmonary blood flow. The left ventricle has to deal with significant volume overloads.

Usually within the first weeks of life, the patient will present with congestive heart failure and cyanosis. There will be a loud regurgitant 2 to 4/6 systolic murmur at the left sternal border, sometimes associated with a high-pitched diastolic decrescendo murmur or a diastolic rumble. The S2 will be single and accentuated.

The ECG will usually show bilateral ventricular hypertrophy and the chest radiograph will have cardiomegaly with increased pulmonary vascular markings.

Acyanotic heart disease

Left-to-right shunt lesions include ventricular septal defects, atrial septal defects, patent ductus arteriosus, and endocardial cushion defects. This group comprises almost 50% of all congenital heart disease [18]. Left-to-right shunt lesions have blood shunted from the systemic system into the pulmonary system. The high pulmonary vascular resistance in the neonate controls the amounts shunted but once pulmonary vascular resistance starts to drop in the first few weeks of life, pulmonary blood flow and pressures will increase. The extent of the lesion is directly related to the degree of pulmonary vascular blood flow. More blood flow will lead to chamber enlargement, and increased pulmonary vascular pressures and subsequent signs of congestive heart failure.

Atrial septal defects

Atrial septal defects comprise up to 10% of all congenital heart disease [19]. In infancy this connection from the left to right atria has the potential for causing problems in about 10% of patients [14]. If there is a large defect, or if there are associated defects, there will be considerable left-to-right shunting and subsequent overload of the pulmonary circulation. Some defects will close spontaneously but larger defects will require surgical intervention.

Difficulty feeding and difficulty gaining weight are common complaints.

The cardiac exam will have a widely split and fixed S2, with a grade 2 to 3/6 systolic ejection murmur at the upper left sternal border, sometimes associated with a mid-diastolic rumble.

ECG findings include right axis deviation and right ventricular hypertrophy or right bundle branch block.

Chest radiograph will have cardiomegaly with increased pulmonary vascular markings.

Ventricular septal defects

Ventricular septal defects are the most common type of congenital heart disease. Seen in approximately 25% of all congenital heart disease cases [20], ventricular septal defects allow for mixing of blood in the ventricles. The extent of the defect determines the degree of disease. Small defects will have minimal impact, as compared with large defects, which will cause pulmonary hypertension and congestive heart failure. Large VSDs have volume and pressure overload in the right ventricle as well as volume overload in the left atrium and left ventricle.

In larger VSDs, poor weight gain along with delayed development are common. Congestive heart failure and cyanosis are frequent presentations.

The exam will have a grade 2 to 5/6 systolic murmur (holosystolic) heard best at the left lower sternal border. A systolic thrill or diastolic rumble can also be present with a narrowly split S2.

ECG findings in a moderate VSD will show left atrial hypertrophy and left ventricular hypertrophy. In a larger VSD there will be left and right ventricular hypertrophy and left atrial hypertrophy. The chest radiograph can show cardiomegaly as well as increased pulmonary vascular markings.

Patent ductus arteriosus

Seen in 10% of all congenital heart disease, the ductus arteriosus remains patent and does not close as it ordinarily would [18]. The degree of the left-to-right shunting is dependent on the lesion length and diameter and pulmonary vascular resistance. The larger the left-to-right shunt, the more symptomatic the patient will be. Ordinarily, in healthy patients the ductus arteriosus will close within 15 hours after birth and then will completely seal around 3 weeks of age, becoming the ligamentum arteriosum. Hypoxia and prematurity have a tendency to keep the ductus arteriosus patent.

If the defect is large, as with all left-to-right shunts, signs of congestive heart failure will be present.

Physical exam will be remarkable for a grade 1 to 4/6 continuous machinery like murmur heard best at the left upper sternal border. A diastolic rumble can also be present as well as bounding peripheral pulses.

ECG findings can show left and right ventricular hypertrophy in large PDAs.

Chest radiograph will have cardiomegaly and increased pulmonary vascular markings.

Endocardial cushion defect

When the endocardial cushion does not develop properly, there will be defects to the atrial septum, the ventricular septum, and the atrioventricular valves. Complete defects involve the entire endocardial cushion and will have atrial and ventricular septal lesions and a common atrioventricular valve. Incomplete or partial defects have atrial involvement with an intact ventricular septum. There can also be variations of both complete and incomplete lesions. A history of failure to thrive, and multiple respiratory tract infections are common. Endocardial cushion defects represent around 3% of congenital heart disease and almost two thirds have the complete form [18]. Down's syndrome is strongly associated with the complete form of endocardial cushion defects.

Left-to-right shunting is directly dependent on the extent of the defects, with complete lesions presenting with congestive heart failure early from volume overload in both the left and right ventricles.

Cardiac exam will be remarkable for a hyperactive precordium, a systolic thrill, a loud holosystolic regurgitant murmur, and a loud and split S2.

The ECG will show a superior QRS axis with RVH, right bundle branch block (RBBB), and left ventricular hypertrophy, along with a prolonged PR interval (Fig. 4).

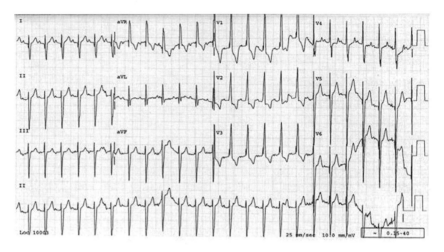

Fig. 4. ECG of CAVC (common AV canal) or endocardial cushion defect with superior QRS axis.

Coarctation of the aorta

Coarctation of the aorta represents 8% to 10% of congenital heart disease and is seen in males in a 2:1 ratio [21]. There is congenital narrowing of the aorta, in the upper thoracic aorta in the region of the ductus arteriosus. The extent of illness is a factor of the degree of narrowing, the length of the narrowing and the presence of other cardiac defects. If the right ventricle supplies the descending aorta via the PDA in fetal life, infants will be symptomatic early. Many other cardiac defects are present such as a VSD, PDA, and aortic hypoplasia and collateral circulation is underdeveloped.

The PDA is able to temporarily negate the obstructive effects of the coarctation obstruction. Additionally, the PDA can maintain blood flow to areas distal to the obstruction. When the PDA eventually closes, the development of pulmonary hypertension and subsequent pulmonary venous congestion leads to congestive heart failure.

Tachypnea, feeding difficulties, and minimal urine output along with shock and metabolic acidosis are common presentations. When presenting in congestive heart failure, there will be a loud gallop, a murmur may or not be present, and pulses will be weak.

The ECG will show RVH or RBBB. There will be significant cardiomegaly as well as pulmonary edema on chest radiograph (Fig. 5). In older children, the appearance of notching of the first rib, also known as the "3 Sign" may be present.

The presence of decreased pulses in the lower extremities is key in the diagnosis of a coarctation. Comparison of the right upper extremity blood pressures and pulse oximeter readings with the lower extremity aids in the

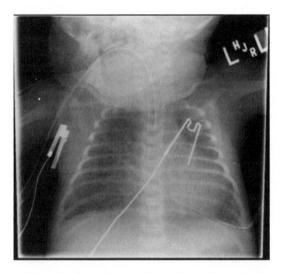

Fig. 5. Chest radiograph of coarctation with cardiomegaly and pulmonary edema.

diagnosis. If the patient is in significant shock, however, pressures can be decreased everywhere.

Hypoplastic left heart syndrome

Hypoplastic left heart syndrome (HLHS) includes hypoplasia of the left ventricle and hypoplasia of the ascending aorta and aortic arch. There can be atresia or marked stenosis of the mitral and aortic valves. The left atrium is also underdeveloped. The ultimate result is that of minimal left ventricular outflow [22].

In utero, the pulmonary vascular resistance is higher than the systemic vascular resistance. The right ventricle (through the right-to-left shunt of the ductus arteriosus) and the elevated pulmonary vascular resistance are able to keep a normal perfusion pressure to the descending aorta and systemic fetal system. The hypoplastic left ventricle does not contribute. An ASD allows the left atrium to decompress. All systemic blood flow is dependent on the ductus arteriosus. After birth, significant problems occur. Systemic vascular resistance is now greater than pulmonary vascular resistance, reversing the pressure system. The patent ductus arteriosus now begins to gradually close. With the nonfunctioning left side and increased systemic vascular resistance, cardiac output falls and aortic pressure drops. This leads to circulatory shock and metabolic acidosis. Increased pulmonary blood flow leads to an increase in left atrial pressure and subsequent pulmonary edema.

These patients appear listless, dusky with tachypnea. There is a single heart sound with a systolic ejection murmur and diminished pulses. The

ECG will show right atrial enlargement, right ventricular hypertrophy, and peaked P waves. The chest radiograph will show cardiomegaly.

Aortic stenosis

Aortic stenosis is seen in 6% of congenital heart disease, with a 4:1 ratio in males [23]. The stenosis will be at the valvular, supravalvular, or subvalvular level, with the degree of obstruction determining the severity of disease in the patient. Those with severe obstruction (approximately 10% to 15%) will present with congestive heart failure in infancy [24]. Left ventricular hypertrophy will develop with severe stenosis. The most common type of aortic stenosis is a bicuspid aortic valve. William Syndrome has supravalvular stenosis in addition to elfin facies, mental retardation, and pulmonary artery stenosis.

The physical exam will be remarkable for a systolic thrill in the region of the upper right sternal border, suprasternal notch, or carotid arteries. There can be an ejection click. The murmur will be a rough or harsh systolic murmur grade 2 to 4/6 at the right intercostal space or left intercostal space with transmission to the neck.

In cases of severe aortic stenosis, the ECG will show left ventricular hypertrophy. If there is resultant congestive heart failure, the chest radiograph will show cardiomegaly.

Anomalous origin of the left coronary artery (ALCAPA Syndrome, Bland-White-Garland Syndrome)

In anomalous origin of the left coronary artery (also known as ALCAPA or Bland-White-Garland Syndrome), the left coronary artery has origins in the pulmonary artery instead of the aorta. When pulmonary artery pressure diminishes in the second to third month of life, there will be decreased perfusion of the left ventricle, resulting in a distressed patient with cardiomegaly and congestive heart failure. There may or may not be a murmur consistent with mitral regurgitation [25,26].

The ECG will show myocardial infarction with abnormally deep and wide Q waves, inverted T waves, and ST segment changes in the precordial leads (Fig. 6). The chest radiograph will be most likely show cardiomegaly. An echocardiogram will help in the diagnosis, with an aortogram if necessary.

Acquired disease

Inflammatory diseases of the heart are grouped under carditis. Included in this group are myocarditis, pericarditis, and endocarditis (along with valvulitis).

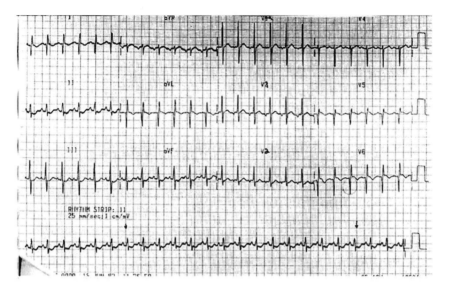

Fig. 6. ECG of anomalous origin of the left coronary artery (ALCAPA) with deep and wide Q waves, inverted T waves, and ST segment changes.

Myocarditis

There are a number of different etiologies in myocarditis. Infectious and autoimmune, as well as toxin-mediated processes can contribute to the inflammatory response in the myocardium [27,28].

Viruses, such as adenovirus, coxsackievirus, echovirus, mumps, and rubella, are the most commonly associated infectious agents. Nonviral causes such as protozoans (Chaga's Disease seen in South America) also cause myocarditis. Less frequently, bacteria, rickettsia, fungal, mycobacteria, and other parasites can be etiologic agents.

Kawasaki's disease and acute rheumatic fever as well as collagen vascular disease can also be seen with myocarditis. Toxic myocarditis is the result of drug ingestion.

Infants may present with vomiting, decreased activity, poor feeding, and congestive heart failure, with tachycardia, tachypnea, a gallop rhythm, and decreased heart tones.

There are no specific lab tests for myocarditis. Erythrocyte sedimentation rate, white blood cell count, myocardial enzymes, and cardiac troponin will be normal or elevated. Troponin levels are thought to be more sensitive than cardiac enzymes [29]. Chest radiograph will show cardiomegaly and, depending on the extent of the disease, pulmonary venous congestion.

ECG abnormalities are common but are nonspecific. There will be tachycardia, low QRS voltages, flattened or inverted T waves with ST-T wave changes, and prolongation of the QT interval. Arrhythmias such as premature contractions are also seen.

Echocardiogram studies will show dilatation of the heart chambers and decreased left ventricular function. The echocardiogram will also help to evaluate myocardial contractility and the presence of a pericardial effusion. Radionuclide scanning and endomyocardial biopsies can help in confirming the disease.

The mortality rate in symptomatic neonates with acute viral myocarditis can be significant. Management of myocarditis revolves around identifying an etiologic agent and, if identified, treating that suspected agent, treating the congestive heart failure, and controlling the arrhythmias. Rest, supplemental oxygen, rapid-acting diuretics like furosemide, and rapid-acting inotropic agents such as dopamine and dobutamine are mainstays in treatment along with the use of angiotensin-converting enzyme inhibitors like captopril. Digoxin is used cautiously because of its potential to induce arrhythmias. In Kawasaki's disease, high-dose immunoglobulins have been beneficial. Other treatment modalities, such as immunosuppressive agents and corticosteroids (except in severe rheumatic carditis) are not universally accepted.

Pericarditis

Inflammation of the pericardium is the hallmark of pericarditis. The most common cause in infancy is a viral etiology such as coxsackie, echovirus, adenovirus, or influenza. Viral pericarditis is usually associated with a viral myocarditis, with the myocarditis being the more prominent entity. Bacterial causes include *Staphylococcus aureus, Streptococcus pnuemoniae, Haemophilus influenzae, Neisseria meningitides,* and streptococci as well as tuberculosis. Acute rheumatic fever, collagen vascular disease, and uremia can also cause a pericarditis. Postpericardiotomy syndrome is seen in patients who have had cardiac surgery involving interruption of the pericardium.

Since the pericardium is a fixed space, the extent of symptoms and signs of disease will be determined by the rate of accumulation of fluid and by the health of the myocardium.

If the myocardium is normal and fluid accumulation is slow, then the patient will tolerate the pericarditis better than if there was underlying myocardial injury with a slow collection of fluid or if there was a rapid collection of a large amount of fluid.

If pericardial tamponade were to occur, the heart, to improve hemodynamics would increase heart rate (improves cardiac output), increase systemic vascular resistance (offset hypotension), and improve diastolic filling by systemic and pulmonary venous constriction.

There is usually a predisposing illness in the history, with an upper respiratory infection or, in the case of a bacterial pericarditis, a pneumonia, empyema, osteomyelitis, pyelonephritis, or tonsillitis.

A pericardial friction rub is diagnostic. A murmur may not be found and the heart will be hypodynamic.

On ECG there will be a low-voltage QRS complex. Early in the disease, ST segments will be elevated everywhere except in V1 and aVR. Later in the disease, ST segments will return to normal and the T waves will flatten or invert. A chest radiograph will show cardiomegaly, with the heart in a water-bottle shape.

Echocardiogram is the key to establishing the presence of an effusion. Additionally, the echo can also evaluate for cardiac tamponade, as it will show the collapse of the right atrial wall or the right ventricular wall in diastole.

To treat pericarditis or pericardiocentesis, surgical intervention is essential, especially if an infectious etiology is suspected. Multiple blood cultures are also indicated as well as standard fluid studies. In milder cases not requiring drainage or antibiotics, antivirals, or antifungals, nonsteroidal anti-inflammatory drugs can be used to treat the discomfort.

In postpericardiotomy syndrome, which can affect as many as 30% of pediatric patients who undergo cardiovascular surgery involving the pericardium, the patients will present with fever, irritability, and a pericardial friction rub anywhere from a month to a few months postoperatively. The etiology is thought to be autoimmune [30].

In cardiac tamponade with signs of tachycardia, tachypnea is an immediate concern.

Chest radiograph will have cardiomegaly and pleural effusion. ECG will have ST segment elevation and flat or inverted T waves. The most helpful test is an echocardiogram because this will assess the amount of pericardial effusion as well as the presence of cardiac tamponade.

Endocarditis

Congenital heart disease is a significant risk factor in infective endocarditis. It is thought that turbulent flow from pressure gradients leads to endothelial damage and thrombus formation. Transient bacteremia then seeds the damaged areas. With the exception of a secundum ASD, all congenital heart diseases and valvular heart diseases are prone to endocarditis, especially if there is any artificial material within the heart (prosthetic heart valve or graft). Common bacterial causes include *S viridans*, enterococci, and *S aureus* as well as fungal and bacteria such as Eikenella, Cardiobacterium [31].

In infancy, endocarditis is rare and is associated with open-heart surgery. The usual presentation is with fulminant disease and a septic appearance. A heart murmur and fever are always present. Embolic phenomena tend to be seen more in the adult population.

Using the Duke Criteria for Infective Endocarditis, a patient must have two major criteria or one major criterion with three minor criteria or five minor criteria. Major criteria include two separately obtained positive blood cultures growing the typical microorganisms and an echocardiogram with endocardial involvement such as an intracardiac mass on a valve, abscess, partial dehiscence of a prosthetic valve, or new valvular regurgitation. Minor criteria include predisposing conditions, fever, vascular phenomena (emboli, hemorrhages, Janeway lesions), and immunologic phenomena (glomerulonephritis, Osler's nodes, Roth spots, rheumatoid factor), microbiological evidence (positive blood culture not meeting major criteria), and echocardiographic findings (not meeting major criteria).

While an echocardiogram identifying valvular vegetation is helpful in the evaluation, the echocardiogram is not 100% sensitive or specific. Because of this, a negative echocardiogram does not exclude endocarditis. A more definitive diagnosis is made by obtaining a positive blood culture. The isolation of a specific microorganism is key to determining antibiotic therapy. Treatment regimens may take place for weeks to be certain that the microorganism has been eliminated.

Kawasaki's disease

Kawasaki's disease (mucocutaneous lymph node syndrome) is a self-limiting generalized systemic vasculitis of indeterminate etiology. Fever, bilateral nonexudative conjunctivitis, erythema of the mucous membranes (lips, oral mucosa), rash, and extremity changes are the hallmarks of the disease. It is among the most common systemic vasculitic illnesses along with Henoch-Schoenlein Purpura. Kawasaki's primarily affects infants and younger children, and can occur in endemic or community-wide epidemic forms [32].

Coronary artery aneurysms or ectasia have been found in 15% to 25% of untreated children with Kawasaki's [33]. These coronary artery lesions can lead to myocardial infarction, sudden death, or ischemic heart disease [34,35].

In the acute phase of Kawasaki's, there can be involvement of all parts of the heart—the pericardium, the myocardium, the endocardium, the valves, and the coronary arteries. The cardiac exam can show a hyperdynamic precordium, tachycardia, a gallop, and a flow murmur or regurgitant pansystolic murmur. Depressed myocardial function can present as cardiogenic shock. The ECG will show nonspecific ST and T wave changes, a prolonged PR interval, or arrhythmia.

The classic Kawasaki's patient will present with fever greater than or equal to 5 days' duration, and at least four of the primary physical criteria, which include involvement of the extremities, the skin, the conjunctivae, the lips and mouth, and the cervical lymph nodes. The extremity changes include erythema to the palms and soles, with induration and desquamation to the fingers and toes. There can be an extensive erythematous rash that is usually a nonspecific diffuse maculopapular rash. Sometimes early desquamation in the perineal region can occur. Bilateral conjunctival injection involving the bulbar conjunctivae is seen around the time of the fever. There can be erythema; peeling, cracking, or bleeding from the lips and mouth; a strawberry tongue; and diffuse erythema of the mucosa of the oropharynx. The cervical lymphadenopathy is generally unilateral, and usually one node is greater than 1.5 cm in diameter.

Lab findings include thombocytosis (appears in second week, peaking in third week), leukocytosis, and anemia. Thrombocytopenia in active disease is a risk factor for coronary aneurysms. There is elevation of the C-reactive protein (CRP) and erythrocyte sedimentation rate (ESR). Serum transaminases can be moderately elevated. Gammaglutamyl transpeptidase (GGT) is elevated in a majority of patients.

In the younger patient, an incomplete or atypical presentation is common [36]. Diagnosis is often made by echocardiogram findings of coronary artery abnormalities [37].

Pharmacologic management of the acute phase of Kawasaki's includes aspirin and intravenous immunoglobulin (IVIG). High-dose aspirin at 80 to 100 mg/kg per day dosed four times a day along with IVIG have an additive anti-inflammatory effect [32]. Length of treatment with aspirin is variable. IVIG is thought to have a generalized anti-inflammatory effect and is dosed at 2 g/kg in a single infusion. Best results are seen when IVIG is started within the first 7 to 10 days of illness.

Cardiomyopathies

Cardiomyopathies affect the heart muscle and are divided into three categories. They are hypertrophic, dilated, or congestive and restrictive (Fig. 7).

In hypertrophic cardiomyopathies, there is significant ventricular muscular hypertrophy and increased ventricular contractility but these factors limit or reduce ventricular filling.

An autosomal dominant link has been documented [38]. The left ventricle is relatively stiff and affects diastolic ventricular filling. The physical exam is notable for a sharp upstroke of the arterial pulse [39]. There can be a systolic ejection murmur or holosystolic murmur.

The ECG will show left ventricular hypertrophy, ST and T wave changes, deep Q waves, and decreased R waves. The chest radiograph may show a globular heart or cardiomegaly.

Dilated or congestive cardiomyopathies have ventricular dilatation with diminished contractility. This is the most common form of cardiomyopathies and results from infectious or toxic etiologies. They will present with evidence of congestive heart failure. A significant S3 will be found on exam.

Restrictive cardiomyopathies limit diastolic filling of the ventricles. This is the least common form and results from noncompliant ventricular walls that have been subject to an infiltrative process such as a glycogen storage disease.

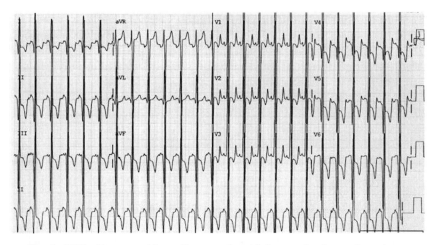

Fig. 7. ECG of hypertrophic cardiomyopathy with increased voltages throughout.

Arrhythmias

Damage, from either congenital or acquired causes, to cardiac structure will predispose the patient to arrhythmias. There can be congenital abnormalities to the conduction system, injured conduction pathways from surgery or postinflammatory changes, or irritation to the conduction system from injured myocardium. Arrhythmias have their origins in the atrial or ventricular conduction systems.

The most common arrhythmia is paroxysmal SVT [40,41]. The usual cause is idiopathic. The majority of patients with SVT have normal hearts, with 23% having congenital heart disease and 22% with Wolff-Parkinson-White (WPW) syndrome [42].

WPW is associated with congenital heart disease, such as transposition of the great arteries. WPW is a preexcitation syndrome with an accessory pathway between the atria and ventricles.

SVT is a narrow complex tachycardia with a rate ranging from 220 to 280 beats per minute in the 1-year age group. The determination of sinus tachycardia and a reentrant tachycardia must be made before the initiation of therapy. In this age group, pulse rate will linearly increase with body temperature, at a ratio of 10 beats per minute per °C increase in body temperature [43].

The ECG in SVT will show a regular rhythm with no beat-to-beat variability and a heart rate greater than 220 beats per minute in the infant. P waves can be present but are usually not. In most cases, the QRS complex is narrow. In a hemodynamically unstable SVT, immediate synchronized cardioversion with 0.5 to 1.0 J per kilogram should be done. In a hemodynamically stable SVT, vagal maneuvers can be initiated. Applying a bag of ice water to the face for 15 to 30 seconds can be used. Adenosine is the drug of choice. Adenosine acts by temporarily blocking conduction at the AV node, thereby interrupting the reentrant circuit. Because the drug is rapidly metabolized, IV access as close to the heart is ideal, with the drug delivered via a rapid intravenous injection. Constant cardiorespiratory monitoring should be in place. Initial dosing of adenosine is 0.1 mg/kg. If there is no response, the next dose should be doubled. The maximum dosing is 0.25 to 0.35 mg/kg (Fig. 8A, B). Verapamil should not be used in the patient younger than 1 year because of the potential for hypotension and cardiovascular collapse [44].

In WPW there is a ventricular preexcitation pathway because of an accessory pathway between the atria and ventricles [3]. There is a short PR interval, a prolonged QRS duration, and delta waves (Fig. 9). Slowing the conduction through the atrioventricular node can allow another pathway to become dominant.

In a WPW-induced SVT, adenosine can cause atrial fibrillation, which can then lead to ventricular fibrillation. This underscores the need for always having resuscitation material at the bedside whenever dealing with arrhythmias.

Sick Sinus Syndrome is usually the result of cardiac surgery involving the atria or can be from myocarditis. The sinus node no longer acts as the primary pacemaker of the heart or functions at a significantly slower rate. This leads to marked sinus bradycardia, sinus arrest with a junctional escape, atrial flutter, fibrillation, or SVT.

A

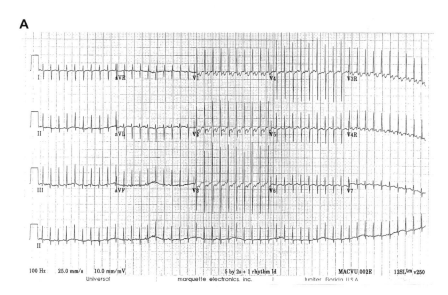

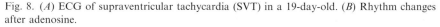

Fig. 8. (*A*) ECG of supraventricular tachycardia (SVT) in a 19-day-old. (*B*) Rhythm changes after adenosine.

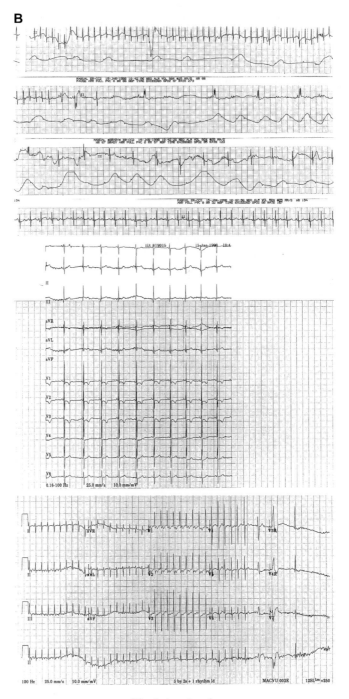

Fig. 8 *(continued)*.

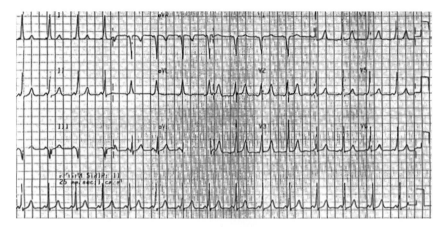

Fig. 9. ECG of WPW with delta waves.

AV block is found when there is an interruption of the conduction of the normal sinus impulse and the subsequent ventricular response. There are first-degree, second-degree, and third-degree blocks.

The first-degree block has a prolonged PR interval because of delayed conduction through the AV node. This is the result of a cardiomyopathy, congenital heart disease, postcardiac surgery, or digitalis toxicity or can be found in healthy patients.

In a second-degree block, not all of the P waves are followed by QRS complexes. The Mobitz Type I Wenckebach phenomenon has a PR interval that gets progressively longer until the QRS complex is completely dropped. The block is at the AV node level and can be attributed to myocarditis, cardiomyopathy, surgery, congenital heart disease, or digitalis toxicity. The Mobitz Type II block has similar etiologies but the block is at the Bundle of His. AV conduction is either all or none. There is potential for a complete block to develop. In two-to-one or three-to-one blocks, the block is at the level of the AV node, but can also be at the Bundle of His.

Third-degree or complete heart blocks have independent atrial and ventricular activity. There are regular P waves at a normal heart rate for age. The QRS complexes are also regular but at a slower rate than the P waves. The usual presentation in infancy is congestive heart failure. Congenital complete heart blocks have a normal QRS complex duration and can be found in patients with a structurally normal heart. A history of maternal lupus or connective tissue disease such as Sjogen's Syndrome predispose a patient to complete heart block (Fig. 10). It is thought that there is transplacental passage of autoimmune antibodies affecting the atrioventricular node [45]. Acquired complete heart blocks are the result of cardiac surgery but can also be attributed to cardiomyopathies and myocarditis and have a prolonged QRS duration.

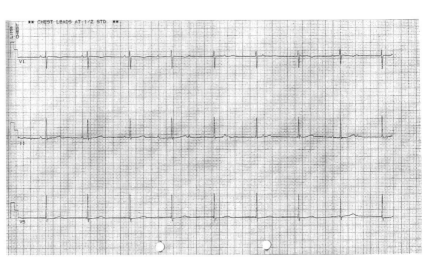

Fig. 10. ECG of complete heart block, patient's mother with lupus.

If asymptomatic, no intervention is indicated. If symptomatic, atropine, isoproterenol or temporary transvenous ventricular pacing are sometimes required.

Surgical repairs

The surgical repair of congenital heart disease continues to progress, with some lesions now repaired in the neonatal period, and most lesions repaired in the first couple of months of life. There are still patients, however, who may appear in the emergency department with no prior surgery, palliative surgery, or corrective surgery. These patients may have a less than optimal nutritional status, can be on multiple medications, or can be exhibiting post-operative complications such as a dysrhythmia or post pericardiotomy syndrome. Also a shunt could develop stenosis.

A Blalock-Taussig shunt is used in the Tetralogy of Fallot. This shunt joins the subclavian artery to the ipsilateral pulmonary artery. The modified Blalock-Taussig shunt uses a Gore-Tex shunt and requires less dissection, is not dependent on the vessel length, and has decreased shunt failure [46].

The Rastelli procedure is done in older patients, and is used in severe Tetralogy of Fallot with significant right ventricular outflow tract obstruction. There is patch closure of the VSD, with the placement of a conduit from the right ventricle to the pulmonary artery.

The Mustard and Senning operations were used in the Transposition of the Great Arteries and functioned at the atrial level. The Mustard operation was an atrial switch using prosthetic material for an intra-atrial baffle, while the Senning operation used native material for an intra-atrial baffle.

Because of atrial dysrhythmias and the inability of the right ventricle to function as a normal left ventricle in later life, these procedures were discontinued. The Arterial Switch, which has now replaced the Mustard and Senning, corrects the TGA at the great artery level. The aortic trunk is attached to the left ventricle and the pulmonic trunk is attached to the right ventricle.

The Fontan operation is done in HLHS, tricuspid atresia, and HRHS. This shunt is a cavocaval baffle to pulmonary artery anastomosis. Systemic venous return is redirected to the pulmonary artery.

The bidirectional Glenn (cavopulmonary shunt) or hemi-Fontan operation anastomoses the superior vena cava to the right pulmonary artery and is performed in patients with HLHS and HRHS. The bidirectional Glenn operation is usually done at 6 months of age, and the hemi-Fontan at 1.5 years of age.

The Norwood operation, performed in the neonatal period, is a palliative procedure in HLHS [47]. The hypoplastic aorta is reconstructed using an aortic or pulmonary artery allograft, the main pulmonary artery is divided, a Gore-Tex shunt is placed on the right to establish pulmonary blood flow, and the atrial septum is excised to provide interatrial mixing [48].

Complications that may be seen in the postoperative patient include dysrhythmias, obstruction of the surgical grafts or conduits, endocarditis, myocardial ischemia or postpericardiotomy syndrome.

Management of acute issues

Cardiac emergencies in the first couple of weeks of life will involve cyanosis and shock. The ductal-dependent lesions dominate this group and preserving ductal patency is crucial in managing these patients. While many of these patients will be diagnosed in the newborn nursery, the advent of earlier newborn discharges increases the chances that the patient will present to the emergency department for the initial diagnosis.

Cyanotic or hypoxemic episodes are seen in patients with congenital heart disease (usually Tetralogy of Fallot). They will present with hyperpnea, irritability, and increasing cyanosis along with a decreased intensity of the underlying heart murmur. A decrease in systemic vascular resistance or increased resistance to the right ventricular outflow tract increases right-to-left shunting, causing hyperpnea and, then, increased systemic venous return. This causes increased right-to-left shunting through the VSD.

To manage a "tet spell" the patient should be placed in a knee-chest position. Morphine sulfate (0.1 to 0.2 mg/kg subcutaneously [SC] or intramuscularly [IM]) will stop the hyperpnea. Oxygen may or may not help because the issue is to improve pulmonary blood flow. Sodium bicarbonate (1 mEq/kg IV) can treat the acidosis. Propanolol (0.01 to 0.2 mg/kg IV over 5 minutes) can be beneficial. Phenylephrine (0.02 mg/kg IV) can help to increase systemic vascular resistance. Ketamine (1 to 3 mg/kg IV) can also increase systemic vascular resistance and provide sedation.

Tricuspid Atresia, Transposition of the Great Arteries, Total Anomalous Pulmonary Venous Return, Truncus Arteriosus, Hypoplastic Right Heart Syndrome, and Pulmonary Atresia can all present with cyanosis or shock in the first couple of weeks of life. Cyanosis or congestive heart failure will be the usual presentation of Tetralogy of Fallot. Shock will be the initial presentation for Hypoplastic Left Heart Syndrome, Aortic Stenosis, and Coarctation of the Aorta.

The key to dealing with the ductal-dependent lesions is to start intravenous prostaglandin E1 (PGE1). Decreasing pulmonary vascular resistance will help in left-to-right shunting and increasing pulmonary blood flow. The initial dose of PGE1 is 0.05 µg/kg/min. If at all possible, consultation with pediatric cardiology as well as the critical (neonatal or pediatric) care staff is beneficial. Apnea and hypotension are potential complicating side effects of PGE1 so management of the airway is essential as well as determining that the patient is not possibly septic. Additionally, the side effect of fever can cloud the potential sepsis picture. In certain variants of TAPVR, PGE1 can actually exacerbate the symptoms. Supplemental oxygen can hasten the closure of the ductus arteriosus, so this must be used with caution.

Acyanotic lesions that are dependent on ductal flow will present with cardiogenic shock.

Those lesions with critical left heart obstruction such as HLHS, aortic stenosis, and coarctation of the aorta depend on the ductus to maintain systemic perfusion. Poor perfusion, diminished pulses, and pallor are common, and the presentation can mimic sepsis. If central cyanosis is present, a response to oxygen may not take place or the patient may become worse.

Airway management is paramount, as mechanical ventilation can increase pulmonary vascular resistance [49]. Increasing right-to-left shunting over the PDA will improve systemic perfusion. Volume assists in treating the acidosis and fluid deficits. Vasopressors can be initiated if decreased ventricular function is evident.

Patients with critical right heart obstruction such as Tetralogy of Fallot and pulmonic stenosis are also ductal dependent. Airway management is a primary concern. IV prostaglandins are also key in the management, especially with oxygen saturations less than 70%. Decreasing pulmonary vascular resistance will help in left-to-right shunting and increasing pulmonary blood flow.

Congestive heart failure in the first year of life is generally associated with congenital heart disease but can also be the result of acquired disease such as myocarditis, arrhythmias, sepsis, and respiratory and metabolic diseases. Pressure overload, volume overload, decreased inotropic function, and rhythm abnormalities can all be factors in causing congestive heart failure. Cardiac congenital abnormalities that have predisposition to presenting with congestive heart failure include left ventricular outflow obstruction (such as coarctation of the aorta and aortic stenosis) and volume overload (left-to-right shunts, VSDs, TAPVR). Endocardial cushion defects with complete involvement and AV valve insufficiency will present acutely ill in the first couple of months of life.

Difficulty feeding, tachypnea, tachycardia, cardiomegaly, hepatomegaly, and rales are all common findings. Prolonged feeding times with diaphoresis can function as a stress test for the infant. Pulmonary diseases can also present in the same fashion as cardiac disease. Supplemental oxygen may not help in differentiating between the two. Echocardiogram is much more definitive.

To treat congestive heart failure, inotropic assistance is important. Modification of preload (end diastolic volume roughly equivalent to the intravascular volume), afterload, contractility, and heart rate all play roles. Cardiac output is determined by heart rate multiplied by stroke volume. In the under 1-year-old, heart rate is the primary method of increasing cardiac output.

Airway management is important and should take precedence, as a stabilized airway and mechanical ventilation can prevent respiratory decompensation. Elevation of the head of the patient can help to decrease pulmonary blood volume. Morphine sulfate assists in treating agitation. Bicarbonate can be used in severe acidosis.

If immediate intervention is needed, dopamine and dobutamine are appropriate choices.

Dopamine is started at a continuous infusion at 5 to10 µg/kg/min. There should be a rapid response to the chronotropic effects with increases in heart rate and blood pressure and urine output. Dobutamine is also started as a continuous infusion at the same dosing. Dobutamine has less of an arrhythmic potential and chronotropic effect than dopamine and because of its vasodilatory effect, reduces afterload. Dobutamine should be used with caution in the less than 1 year of age population. Dobutamine will improve cardiac output without increasing blood pressure so if there is severe hypotension, dobutamine may be a better choice as an adjunct rather than primary agent [4,50].

Amrinone (0.5 mg/kg IV over 3 minutes) and milrinone (loading dose of 10 to 50 µg/kg IV over 10 minutes) can also be considered as potential aids in treating congestive heart failure. They do not increase the heart rate but have inotropic and vasodilator properties.

Digoxin is the inotrope of choice in the nonacute setting. Digoxin improves cardiac contractility and subsequently increases cardiac output. Care must be taken with dosing regimens. Diuretics such as furosemide promote diuresis.

Summary

The diagnosis and management of cardiac emergencies in the first year of life can be challenging and complicated. By reviewing the pathophysiology of the heart and circulation, one can be more prepared for these difficult scenarios.

Early presentations will usually be the result of ductal-dependent lesions and will appear with cyanosis and shock. Later presentations will be the result of volume overload or pump failure and will present with signs of congestive heart failure. Acquired diseases will also present as congestive heart failure or arrhythmias.

References

[1] Burton DA, Cabalka AK. Cardiac evaluation of infants. The first year of life. Pediatr Clin North Am 1994;41(5):991–1015.

[2] Flynn PA, Engle MA, Ehlers KH. Cardiac issues in the pediatric emergency department. Pediatr Clin North Am 1992;39(4):955–68.

[3] Woods WA, McCulloch MA. Cardiovascular emergencies in the pediatric patient. Emerg Med Clin North Am 2005;23(4):1233–49.

[4] Gewitz MH, Woolf PK. Cardiac emergencies. In: Fleisher GR, Ludwig S, editors. Textbook of pediatric emergency medicine. 5th edition. Philadelphia: Lippincott Williams and Wilkins; 2006. p. 717–58.

[5] Woolridge DP. Congenital heart disease in the pediatric emergency department. Part I: pathophysiology and clinical characteristics. Pediatric Emergency Medicine Reports 2002;7(7): 69–80.

[6] Woolridge DP. Congenital heart disease in the pediatric emergency medicine department. Part II: managing acute and chronic complications. Pediatric Emergency Medicine Reports 2002;7(8):81–92.

[7] Hoffman JI, Kaplan S. The incidence of congenital heart disease. J Am Coll Cardiol 2002; 39(12):1890–900.

[8] Lees MH, King DH. Cyanosis in the newborn. Pediatr Rev 1987;9(2):36–42.

[9] Friedman AH, Fahey JT. The transition from fetal to neonatal circulation: normal responses and implications for infants with heart disease. Semin Perinatol 1993;17(2):106–21.

[10] Nadas AS, Fyler DC. Hypoxemia. In: Keane JF, Lock JE, Fyler DC, editors. Nada's pediatric cardiology. 2nd edition. Philadelphia: Saunders Elsevier; 2006. p. 97–101.

[11] Martin L, Khalil H. How much reduced hemoglobin is necessary to generate cyanosis? Chest 1990;97(1):182–5.

[12] Waldman JD, Wernly JA. Cyanotic congenital heart disease with decreased pulmonary blood flow in children. Pediatr Clin North Am 1999;46(2):385–404.

[13] Breitbart RE, Fyler DC. Tetralogy of Fallot. In: Keane JF, Lock JE, Fyler DC, editors. Nada's pediatric cardiology. 2nd edition. Philadelphia: Saunders Elsevier; 2006. p. 559–79.

[14] Studer M, Blackstone E, Kirklin J, et al. Determinants of early and late results of repair of atrioventricular septal (conal) defects. J Thorac Cardiovasc Surg 1982;84(4):523–42.

[15] Keane JF, Fyler DC. Total anomalous pulmonary venous return. In: Keane JF, Lock JE, Fyler DC, editors. Nada's pediatric cardiology. 2nd edition. Philadelphia: Saunders Elsevier; 2006. p. 773–81.

[16] Keane JF, Fyler DC. Tricuspid atresia. In: Keane JF, Lock JE, Fyler DC, editors. Nada's pediatric cardiology. 2nd edition. Philadelphia: Saunders Elsevier; 2006. p. 753–9.

[17] Williams JM, de Leeuw M, Black MD, et al. Factors associated with outcomes of persistent truncus arteriosus. J Am Coll Cardiol 1999;34(2):545–53.

[18] Driscoll DJ. Left to right shunt lesions. Pediatr Clin North Am 1999;46(2):355–68.

[19] Mahoney LT, Truesdell SC, Krzmarzick TR, et al. Atrial septal defects that present in infancy. Am J Dis Child 1986;140(11):1115–8.

[20] Kidd L, Driscoll D, Gersony W, et al. Second natural history study of congenital heart defects: results of treatment of patients with ventricular septal defects. Circulation 1993; 87(Suppl 2):I38–51.

[21] Demircin M, Arsan S, Pasaoglu I, et al. Coarctation of the aorta in infants and neonates: results and assessments of prognostic variables. J Cardiovasc Surg 1995;36(5):459–64.

[22] Bailey LL, Gundry SR. Hypoplastic left heart syndrome. Pediatr Clin North Am 1990;37(1): 137–50.

[23] Fedderly RT. Left ventricular outflow obstruction. Pediatr Clin North Am 1999;46(2): 369–84.

[24] Bando K, Turrentine MW, Sun K, et al. Surgical management of hypoplastic left heart syndrome. Ann Thorac Surg 1996;62(1):70–7.

[25] Chang RKR, Allada V. Electrocardiographic and echocardiographic features that distinguish anomalous origin of the left coronary artery from pulmonary artery from idiopathic dilated cardiomyopathy. Pediatr Cardiol 2001;22(1):3–10.

[26] DeWolf D, Vercruysse T, Suys B, et al. Major coronary anomalies in childhood. Eur J Pediatr 2002;161(12):637–42.

[27] Towbin JA, et al. Myocarditis. In: Allen HD, Gutgesell HP, Clark FB, editors. Moss and Adam's heart disease in infants, children and adolescents: including the fetus and young adult. 6th edition. Baltimore (MD): Lippincott, Williams & Wilkins; 2001. p. 1197–215.

[28] Wheeler DS, Kooy NW. A formidable challenge: the diagnosis and treatment of viral myocarditis in children. Crit Care Clin 2003;19(3):365–91.

[29] Smith SC, Ladenson JH, Mason JW, et al. Elevations of cardiac troponin I associated with myocarditis. Experimental and clinical correlates. Circulation 1997;95(1):163–8.

[30] Cabalka AK, Rosenblatt HM, Towbin JA, et al. Postpericardiotomy syndrome in pediatric heart transplant recipients. Immunologic characteristics. Tex Heart Inst J 1995;22(2):170–6.

[31] Danilowicz D. Infective endocarditis. Pediatr Rev 1995;16(4):148–54.

[32] Newberger JW, Takahashi M, Gerber MA, et al. Diagnosis, treatment, and long-term management of Kawasaki disease. AHA Scientific Statement. Circulation 2004;110(17):2747–71.

[33] Genizi J, Miron D, Spiegel R, et al. Kawasaki disease in very young infants: high prevalence of atypical presentation and coronary arteritis. Clin Pediatr 2003;42(3):263–7.

[34] Dajani AS, Taubert KA, Gerber MA, et al. Diagnosis and therapy of Kawasaki disease in children. Circulation 1993;87(5):1776–80.

[35] Kato K, Koike S, Yokoyama T. Kawasaki disease. Effect of treatment on coronary artery involvement. Pediatrics 1979;63(2):175–9.

[36] Rosenfeld EA, Corydon KE, Shulman ST. Kawasaki disease in infants less than one year of age. J Pediatr 1995;126(4):524–9.

[37] Baer AZ, Rubin LG, Shapiro CA, et al. Prevalence of coronary artery lesions on the initial echocardiogram in Kawasaki syndrome. Arch Pediatr Adolesc Med 2006;160(7):686–90.

[38] Burch M, Blair E. The inheritance of hypertrophic cardiomyopathy. Pediatr Cardiol 1999; 20(5):313–6.

[39] DeLuca M, Tak T. Hypertrophic cardiomyopathy. Tools for identifying risk and alleviating symptoms. Postgrad Med 2000;107(7):127–40.

[40] Sachetti A, Moyer V, Baricella R, et al. Primary cardiac arrhythmias in children. Pediatr Emerg Care 1999;15(2):95–8.

[41] Losek J, Endom E, Dietrich A, et al. Adenosine and pediatric supraventricular tachycardia in the emergency department. Ann Emerg Med 1999;33(2):185–91.

[42] Saul PJ, Scott WA, Brown S, et al. Intravenous amiodarone for incessant tachyarrhythmias in children. A randomized, double-blind, antiarrhythmic drug trial. Circulation 2005; 112(22):3470–7.

[43] Hanna CM, Greenes DS. How much tachycardia in infants can be attributed to fever? Ann Emerg Med 2004;43(6):699–705.

[44] Epstein ML, Kiel EA, Victorica BE. Cardiac decompensation following verapamil therapy in infants with supraventricular tachycardia. Pediatrics 1985;75(4):737–40.

[45] Boutjdir M, Chen L, Zhang ZH, et al. Serum and immunoglobin G from the mother of a child with congenital heart block induce conduction abnormalities and inhibit L-type calcium channels in a rat heart model. Pediatr Res 1998;44(1):354–62.

[46] Ullom RL, Sade RM, Crawford FJ Jr, et al. The Blalock-Taussig shunt in infants: standard versus modified. Ann Thorac Surg 1987;44(5):539–43.

[47] Norwood WI, Lang P, Hansen DD. Physiologic repair of aortic atresia with hypoplastic left heart syndrome. N Engl J Med 1983;308(1):23–36.

[48] Bove EL, Lloyd TR. Stage reconstruction for hypoplastic left heart syndrome. Ann Surg 1996;224(3):387–94.

[49] Atz AM, Feinstein JA, Jonas RA. Preoperative management of pulmonary venous hypertension in hypoplastic left heart syndrome with restrictive atrial septal defect. Am J Cardiol 1999;83(8):224–8.

[50] Lee C, Mason LJ. Pediatric cardiac emergencies. Anesthesiol Clin North Am 2001;19(2): 287–308.

ELSEVIER
SAUNDERS

Emerg Med Clin N Am
25 (2007) 1009–1040

EMERGENCY
MEDICINE
CLINICS OF
NORTH AMERICA

Essential Diagnosis of Abdominal Emergencies in the First Year of Life

Jeffrey P. Louie, MD[a,b,*]

[a]Department of Emergency Medicine, Children's Hospitals and Clinics of Minnesota,
345 North Smith Avenue, St. Paul, MN 55102, USA
[b]Department of Pediatrics, University of Minnesota Medical School, 420 Delaware St. SE,
Minneapolis, MN 55455, USA

Abdominal concerns are a common emergency department (ED) complaint, representing about 10% of visits [1]. Neonates and infants only comprise a small subset of these ED visits. They, however, may present with the most devastating, life-threatening surgical and medical abdominal emergencies. This article is designed to refresh the experienced practitioner and to entice the new physician. Samuel Bard, in 1769, stated:

> "Do not therefore imagine, that from this Time [ie, on receipt of this MD degree] your studies are to cease; so far from it, you are to be considered as but just entering upon them; and unless your whole lives, are one continued series of application and improvement, you will fall short of your duty" [2].

In this article, neonates are defined as being less than 31 days of life; infants are defined as being more than 31 days of life up to 12 months of age. Based upon these definitions, the article will present and discuss abdominal emergencies as two groups: neonates and infants. This approach is more consistent with how these patients present to the ED with their surgical or medical abdominal emergencies.

General approach

With nonverbal patients, all medical information is obtained from caregivers. Clinicians must listen. Parents will know their child's condition better than clinicians upon presentation to the ED. Often, an infant will present

---

* Department of Emergency Medicine, Children's Hospitals and Clinics of Minnesota, 345 North Smith Avenue, St. Paul, MN 55102.
  E-mail address: jeffrey.louie@childrensmn.org

0733-8627/07/$ - see front matter © 2007 Elsevier Inc. All rights reserved.
doi:10.1016/j.emc.2007.07.011
emed.theclinics.com

with a distended abdomen or mass that only the parent will recognize. Obtaining an accurate history and being meticulous with the infant's signs and symptoms often will guide the astute practitioner to a child's diagnosis. For example, a parental report of bilious vomiting in an otherwise well-appearing newborn may be the only sign of malrotation with volvulus. In addition, a parental description of an 8-month-old with intermittent abdominal pain followed by lethargy is highly suggestive of intussusception.

The physical examination always should include reviewing the patient's vital signs. Abnormal vital signs must be repeated and verified. Trends and changes in heart rate and blood pressure may be evidence of shock [3,4]. Tachypnea may suggest respiratory compensation for acidosis secondary to diabetic ketoacidosis [5] or peritonitis and sepsis. Singer and Losek noted tachypnea as a clinical finding suggestive of abdominal pain [6]. Once the vital signs have been reviewed, the actual examination should proceed.

The physical examination can be difficult even for the friendliest-appearing provider. Stranger anxiety develops in the pediatric population at about 8 months of age and will not diminish, for some patients, until as late as 2 to 3 years of age [7]. Despite the best efforts of parents and the physician, an infant may not want to cooperate with an abdominal examination. Furthermore, the examination may provide little information if the child cries throughout and contracts his or her abdominal musculature. Gentle palpation during inspiration may provide some clues as to why the patient is vomiting. Many times, the infant only will allow an examination while the parent is comforting the infant. With supervision and guidance, sometimes a parent can perform an informal examination. Otherwise, the physician should try to examine the infant on the lap of the caregiver. A warm and quite examination room may allow the physician to observe an undressed infant during sleep or while in a calm moment. With luck, an inguinal hernia or a peristaltic wave suggestive of hypertrophic pyloric stenosis may be witnessed.

The age of the patient can assist greatly the physician in the differential diagnosis. Table 1 lists the age of presentation with regards to particular

Table 1
Neonatal and infant abdominal emergencies

Age	Disease	Clinical presentation
Neonate	Malrotation with volvulus	Bilious vomiting
	Necrotizing enterocolitis	Vomiting, abdominal distention
	Omphalitis	Erythema of umbilicus
	Hirschsprung's disease	Abdominal distention, diarrhea
Infant	Hypertrophic pyloric stenosis	Projectile, nonbilious vomiting
	Incarcerated inguinal hernia	Inguinal mass, vomiting
	Meckel's diverticulum	Rectal bleeding or bilious vomiting
	Intussusception	Vomiting, colicky abdominal pain, listless
	Appendicitis	Vomiting, anorexia, fussy

abdominal emergencies. Although not absolute, Table 1 is very helpful in forming an approach and diagnostic decision process. A common theme will be found in this article:

- Vomiting and abdominal distention should alert the practitioner to a life-threatening abdominal process.
- Abdominal plain films are a good screening tool.
- A thorough history and physical examination often will assist the physician in diagnosing many of the surgical and medical emergencies seen in neonates and infants.

Neonates

Malrotation with volvulus

Pathophysiology

Malrotation occurs during early fetal development and is a failure of the midgut, small bowel, right colon, and one third of the transverse colon, to undergo appropriate rotation and retroperitoneal fixation [8,9]. The superior mesenteric artery supplies vascular vessels to the midgut. If malrotation occurs during embryonic development, the midgut bowels are prone to twisting, resulting in a volvulus, and in severe cases, bowel ischemia [10,11]. Anatomically, the twisting of the midgut occurs at the distal duodenum or proximal jejunum [12]. Fibrous bands, known as Ladd's bands, may cause intestinal obstructions and are a result of anomalous fixation of the gut [13].

Epidemiology

Malrotation occurs in approximately 1 in 5000 live births [14]. About 80% of all midgut malrotation with volvulus presents in the first month of life, with most cases occurring in the first week of life [15]. Other cases will present later in childhood and rarely in adulthood [16,17]. Males have a higher incidence of malrotation by 2:1 [15].

Clinical presentation

The trademark presentation is a neonate presenting with bilious vomiting. The incidence of this single clinical finding is found in 80% to 100% of cases [18,19]. Early in the clinical course, the abdominal examination will be normal, and the neonate will appear healthy. Over time, as the midgut blood supply is compromised, hematochezia, abdominal distension or pain, and shock will present and are strongly suggestive of bowel necrosis [19–21]. Bowel necrosis can occur within 2 hours of initial presentation [22]. It should be noted that about 40% of neonatal bilious vomiting will require a surgical intervention [23]. Nevertheless, the dictum "bilious vomiting in the (neonate) should be considered as due to mechanical intestinal obstruction until proven otherwise" [23] must be followed. The midgut volvulus can present in older children and adolescents, and it should be considered in patients who have chronic intermittent vomiting or abdominal pain, feeding difficulties, or failure to thrive [17]. Other concomitant congenital anomalies are unusual in patients who have malrotation.

Differential diagnosis

Approximately 40% of neonates who have bilious emesis will have a surgical etiology [23,24]. Apart from a midgut volvulus, one should consider other surgical conditions including meconium ileus, Hirschsprung's disease, duodenal atresia, necrotizing enterocolitis, Meckel's diverticulum, intussusception, and appendicitis. Medical conditions also should be considered, including inborn errors of metabolism, nonintentional trauma, gastroesophageal reflux (GER), acute gastroenteritis (AGE), pyelonephritis, meningitis, and intracranial pathology.

Laboratory and imaging diagnostics

Generally, specific laboratory studies are not useful to diagnosing malrotation and volvulus. Plain radiographs, however, can be useful in identifying a bowel obstruction (Fig. 1) or showing a markedly dilated stomach and duodenal bulb (Fig. 2). Both radiographic findings are suggestive of malrotation with a volvulus [25]. A normal or equivocal radiograph, however, also is seen in 20% of cases [12]. An upper gastrointestinal (GI) study (UGI) is considered the gold standard and also can assist in identifying other conditions such as GER, pyloric stenosis, and duodenal atresia. Under

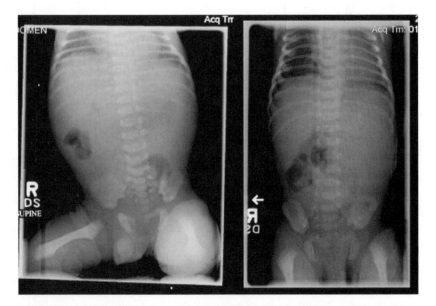

Fig. 1. Supine and decubitus radiographs showing a small bowel obstruction caused by malrotation with volvulus. (*Courtesy of* David Cox, MD, St. Paul, Minnesota.)

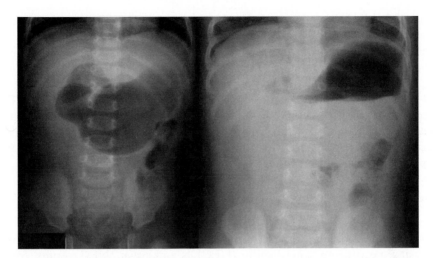

Fig. 2. Supine and upright radiographs showing a markedly dilated stomach and duodenal bulb that is highly suggestive of malrotation with volvulus. (*Courtesy of* Loren G. Yamamoto, MD, Honolulu, Hawaii.)

fluoroscopy, a spiral–corkscrew configuration of the jejunum can be found (Fig. 3), confirming a midgut malrotation with volvulus. Also, ultrasonography is becoming a valuable screening tool [26]. Orzech and colleagues [27] reported that this modality effectively ruled out intestinal malrotation by noting a normal superior mesenteric artery and vein orientation. All abnormal ultrasounds, however, should be confirmed by an UGI series.

Management

   Once the diagnosis is confirmed, consultation with a pediatric surgeon is an important pillar of management. Venous access should be obtained, and

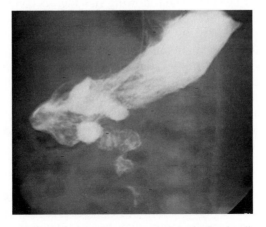

Fig. 3. The corkscrew findings during an upper gastrointestinal series diagnosing malrotation with volvulus. (*Courtesy of* David Cox, MD, St. Paul, Minnesota.)

a nasogastric (NG) tube should be placed to decompress the stomach. Other management strategies should be directed towards the overall condition of the patient, such as fluid resuscitation for volume loss, acidosis, and third spacing. Initial laboratory studies should include a complete white cell count (CBC), electrolytes with a renal panel, and type and screen. If the patient is ill-appearing, consider a venous blood gas (VBG), liver function tests (LFT), and coagulopathy laboratory tests. Finally, if intestinal necrosis is suspected, then broad-spectrum antibiotics should be given. The ED physician should provide supportive care and stabilization until the patient undergoes operative repair or is transferred to a pediatric critical care unit.

Necrotizing enterocolitis

Pathophysiology

Regarding premature and full-term infants, the precise mechanism causing necrotizing enterocolitis (NEC) is unknown. NEC results from bowel wall inflammation that leads to necrosis and bowel wall death. Pathogenic bacteria, the introduction of enteral feeds of commercial formulas, or hyperosmolar medications are some recent theories behind mucosal wall inflammation [28].

Epidemiology

NEC is not only a disease of premature infants, but also is well described in full-term infants. The overall rate of NEC in full term infants is approximately 0.7 per 1000 live births, which is almost 10% of all cases of NEC [29]. In a study by Maayan-Metzger, most of these cases were delivered by caesarian. The results of a 5-year study period show that the prevalence is increasing [30]. Age of presentation is described from birth to the first week of life [31], although case reports show NEC presenting in infants up to 6 months of age [32]. The following risk factors commonly are linked to full-term infants developing NEC: maternal eclampsia, a history of neonatal respiratory distress, congenital heart disease, neonatal asphyxia, or hypothyroidism [31]. Some infants will have no risk factors [30,31].

Term infants born at 36 weeks or more present with NEC on average at day 3 or day 4 day of life [31]. The mean presentation is 10 days of life for premature infants. This is critical, because premature infants who are discharged from the NICU earlier in life, may present to the ED with NEC. Hostetller and Schulman describe a premature NICU graduate presenting to the ED with fulminate NEC [33].

Clinical presentation

Early in the course, the most common symptom is feeding intolerance associated with emesis and abdominal distention. As the disease progresses, fevers will develop, and the infant may become irritable or lethargic. The emergency medicine practitioner may see coffee ground or bilious vomiting

[33]. The abdomen will be distended, and on physical examination, one may visualize erythema on the abdominal wall. Gentle palpation of the abdominal wall will elicit pain secondary to peritonitis. Finally, these neonates may present with fever and shock, often mimicking bacterial meningitis [29].

Differential diagnosis

Surgical conditions may include Hirschsprung's disease, malrotation with volvulus, intussusception, and appendicitis. Medical conditions such as non-accidental trauma, pyelonephritis, omphalitis, sepsis, GER, overfeeding, AGE, and meningitis also should be considered in the differential diagnosis for NEC.

Laboratory and imaging diagnostics

Abdominal radiographs are salient in the diagnosis of NEC, allowing physicians to visualize pneumatosis intestinalis, the presence of gas bubbles within the bowel wall, a characteristic of NEC (Fig. 4). Portal vein air is associated with a poor prognosis [34]. The presence of free air, especially pneumoperitoneum, also may be visualized. In addition, ultrasounds are becoming a reliable screening modality. Ultrasounds have been used to identify and predict the outcome from necrotic bowel, free peritoneal fluid, and portal air [35,36].

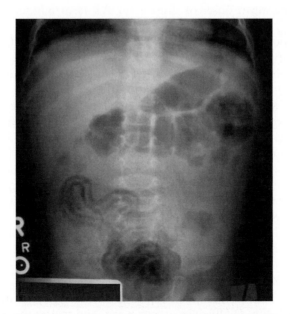

Fig. 4. An infant with pneumatosis intestinalis in the right lower quadrant. (*Courtesy of* Loren G. Yamamoto, MD, Honolulu, Hawaii.)

Management

Once the diagnosis is confirmed on radiograph, an early surgical consultation is warranted. Initial stabilization should include volume resuscitation and broad-spectrum antibiotics. Laboratory studies should include a CBC, electrolytes with a renal panel, blood culture, C-reactive protein, and blood gas analysis. An NG tube should be inserted to decompress the stomach. If the diagnosis of NEC is suspected, but not confirmed, in-patient observation and serial examinations and radiographs are warranted with early pediatric surgical and neonatology consultation.

Omphalitis

Pathophysiology

The umbilical stump is a universally acquired wound with the potential of becoming infected. Omphalitis occurs from poor hygiene or an acquired nosocomial infection [37]. As the infection intensifies, the bacteria will spread into the subcutaneous tissue causing necrotizing fasciitis [38]. Myonecrosis, an infection of the abdominal musculature and phlebitis and an infection of the portal veins also have been described [39].

Epidemiology

In developed countries, the incidence is about 7 per 1000 live births [40]. Mortality rates are over 50% if the infant develops necrotizing fasciitis [41,42]. Females are equally affected, but males have a higher rate of mortality [43]. The mean onset of disease for full-term infants is 5 to 9 days of life [43].

Umbilical cord care has changed over the last decade. Traditionally, a triple dye was applied within the first hours of birth, followed by outpatient care with alcohol [44]. Currently, the stump is left to dry, and parents are educated not to apply commercial antibacterial solutions or alcohols [44]. Research has shown autonecrosis of the umbilical cord occurs almost 2 days faster with the natural drying technique [45]. Parents, however, often complain of its appearance and foul smell [46]. Increases in infection rates have not been reported. Interestingly, in 2003, a study from Nepal showed a large reduction in omphalitis by using topical applications of chlorhexidine [47]. Obviously, controversy exists among either technique.

The most common bacterial pathogens to cause omphalitis are *Staphylococcus aureus*, *S epidermidis*, *Streptococcus pyogenes*, enterococci, and gramnegative rods [40,44,48]. The presence of community acquired-methicillin resistant *S aureus* (CA-MRSA) has yet to be reported.

Clinical presentation

Early in the infection, omphalitis presents as an erythematous rash at the umbilical cord (Fig. 5) [49]. The area is warm and tender to the touch, consistent with cellulitis. The newborn may have a fever. A malodorous smell

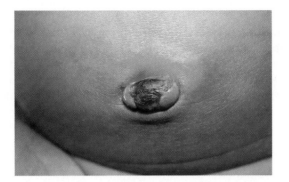

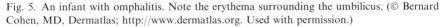

Fig. 5. An infant with omphalitis. Note the erythema surrounding the umbilicus. (© Bernard Cohen, MD, Dermatlas; http://www.dermatlas.org. Used with permission.)

may emanate from the site of infection [49]. As time progresses, the infection will spread into the subcutaneous tissue layer causing necrotizing fasciitis [39]. Palpation of the abdomen will be exquisitely tender, and crepitus also may be appreciated. An ecchymotic, violaceous discoloration may be seen around the umbilicus. Fever and lethargy signify systemic infection [48]. A thorough history and a physical examination revealing an umbilical rash will be sufficient for the astute practitioner to diagnosis this disease.

Differential diagnosis

A clear history and physical findings of an umbilical rash are almost pathognomonic for omphalitis. The clinician, however, should be aware of other medical and surgical conditions related to the umbilicus. In healthy newborns, the cord usually separates from the umbilicus at about 10 days of life. By 2 weeks of life, delayed cord separation is considered abnormal. Leukocyte adhesion deficiency (LAD) is a rare immunologic disorder resulting in a defective leukocyte function and high morbidity and mortality [50]. It often presents with delayed cord separation and omphalitis [51]. These patients require pediatric subspecialty care by immunology or infectious disease. Anatomical urachal abnormalities also can cause delayed cord separation [52,53].

Laboratory and diagnostic imaging

For afebrile and febrile neonates, obtaining surface cultures of the umbilicus may identify the causative bacteria. For afebrile neonates, a CBC and a C-reactive protein should be obtained. For febrile and ill-appearing patients, a full sepsis work-up should be performed. LFTs and coagulopathy laboratory tests also are indicated if portal vein thrombosis has occurred. An ultrasound or abdominal CT scan may show fluid accumulation between subcutaneous fat and muscle in cases with necrotizing fasciitis. Both modalities also will detect congenital umbilical anatomic abnormalities. A radiograph may demonstrate subcutaneous air.

Management

All infants will require admission for intravenous broad-spectrum antibiotics. For ill-appearing neonates, fluid resuscitation is a priority along with other supportive measures for airway, breathing, and circulation. A consultation with a neonatologist or pediatric infectious disease specialist is prudent for guidance on antimicrobial selection. A pediatric surgical consultation is warranted to remove infected tissue.

Hirschsprung's disease

Pathophysiology

From a histologic perspective, Hirschsprung's disease is caused by aganglionosis, hypoganglionosis, or dysganglionosis of the bowel [54]. The congenital agangliosis always involves the anus, and the pathology proceeds proximally for a variable length of large bowel. Both the myenteric (Auerbach) and submucosal (Meissner) plexus are absent, resulting in diminished bowel peristalsis and function. The anus will have an abnormal or absent relaxation [55]. The precise mechanism underlying the development of Hirschsprung's disease is unknown.

Epidemiology

It is estimated that 1 in 5000 newborns will have Hirschsprung's disease [56]. Three quarters of the infants will be males [57]. Familial cases have been described [30]; thus it is not surprising that after one child has the disease, subsequent offspring are at much higher risk than the general population [58]. Other congenital abnormalities have been found with Hirschsprung's disease: Trisomy 21, Smith-Lemli-Opitz syndrome, and Waardenburg's syndrome [59]. This is an abbreviated list.

Clinical presentation

In the newborn period, the most common presentation is a failure to pass meconium in the first 48 hours of life [60]. For neonates who present to the ED, there are two well-described presentations: bowel obstruction and enterocolitis. The former often will present with complaints of abdominal distention, bilious or feculent vomiting, constipation, and other signs of obstruction [15,61,62]. Older patients and adults have been diagnosed with Hirschsprung's disease. They usually complain of chronic constipation, vomiting, and failure to thrive [61]. For infants who present outside of the neonatal period, 30% will have diarrhea, which some researchers believe is a symptom of enterocolitis [63].

Enterocolitis occurs in 12% to 60% of patients with congenital agangliosis [63,64]. It is the most serious complication of Hirschsprung's disease [65]. It may occur before a diagnosis of Hirschsprung's disease is made, and it is described after corrective surgery. Mortality rates from treated Hirschsprung's disease are as high as 30% [66]. The symptoms of enterocolitis range from loose diarrhea with mild abdominal distention and no systemic manifestations to explosive diarrhea with mucosal ulceration, marked abdominal distension, and sepsis [67]. Toxic megacolon is a life-threatening complication of enterocolitis. It is associated with fever, abdominal distention, bilious vomiting, explosive diarrhea, volume depletion, and shock [63,64]. Radiographs typically will show air fluid levels and the absence of air in the distal rectosigmoid colon [68]. Pneumatosis intestinalis also may be seen on radiograph [64,68]. Spontaneous perforation is estimated to occur in about 3% of patients [66].

Differential diagnosis

For those patients who present with enterocolitis, necrotizing enterocolitis, omphalitis, appendicitis, and malrotation with volvulus should be considered. Medical conditions such as infectious colitis, congenital hypothyroidism, and meconium ileus from cystic fibrosis also should be considered for those newborns who present with abdominal distention, vomiting, and constipation.

Laboratory and imaging diagnostics

A high index of suspicion is required to diagnose Hirschsprung's disease. Abdominal radiographs may be suggestive of a toxic megacolon and may show dilated loops of bowel with mucosal changes or pneumatosis intestinalis. Free peritoneal air also can be detected. A radiograph additionally may demonstrate pathologic air–fluid levels without rectal air, which is suggestive of Hirschsprung's disease (Fig. 6). A contrast enema may show the

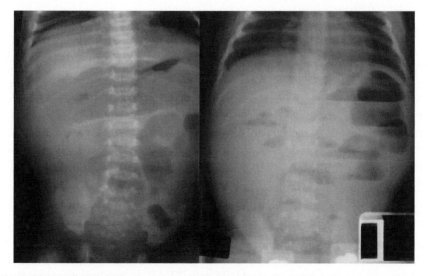

Fig. 6. Plain radiographs demonstrating air–fluid levels in the intestine and no gas in the rectum. This is suggestive for Hirschsprung's disease. (*Courtesy of* Loren G. Yamamoto, MD, Honolulu, Hawaii.)

classic finding of a normal-caliber rectum or narrow distal segment, a funnel-shaped dilatation at the level of the transition zone, and a marked dilation of the proximal colon [69]. In addition, the prolonged retention of contrast in the colon for greater than 24 hours following an enema may suggest Hirschsprung's disease [63,70]. The preferred method of diagnosis is a suction biopsy from the rectum [71,72]. Microscopic proof can diagnose Hirschsprung's disease by showing an absence of ganglion cells, hypertrophy and hyperplasia of nerve fibers, and an increase in acetylcholinesterase-positive nerve fibers in the lamina propria and muscularis mucosa [72].

Ill-appearing neonates and infants should be considered septic, and a sepsis evaluation may be warranted. The physician should consider coagulopathy studies to rule out disseminated intravascular coagulopathy (DIC) and a blood gas with a lactate level to evaluate acid–base status.

Management

Neonates presenting in extremis require aggressive fluid resuscitation, broad-spectrum antibiotics, and supportive care. Placement of an NG tube to decompress the stomach and a rectal tube to decompress the rectum is warranted. Abdominal radiographs are also important in the initial evaluation. An early pediatric surgical consultation is warranted for potential complications of enterocolitis, such as perforation of a bowel wall, or for possible surgical exploration.

Infants

Hypertrophic pyloric stenosis

Pathophysiology

Hypertrophic pyloric stenosis (HPS) first was described in 1888 by Hirschsprung's [73]. Intraoperatively, an abnormally enlarged pyloric muscle usually measures 2 cm to 2.5 cm in length and 1 cm to 1.5 cm in diameter [74,75]. The hypertrophic changes result in partial or complete obstruction of the pyloric channel. The etiology of the abnormal pyloric muscle remains unclear. Exposure to macrolides has been linked and is considered a possible risk factor in the development of HPS [76]. Other researchers have suggested that growth factors, such as hormones and peptides [77,78], or gastric acid hypersecretion may play a role [79].

Epidemiology

HPS is the leading etiology for nonbilious emesis requiring a pediatric surgical intervention [75]. Its prevalence is estimated to be between 1.5 to 4 per 1000 live births [75]. It is two to five times more common in males [80] and more prevalent in white infants [81]. It is believed that firstborn males have a 30% risk for developing HPS [75], although this assertion is controversial. A child of an affected parent has an increased risk of HPS, with the risk being still higher if the mother is affected [82]. The peak age of presentation in an infant is between 3 to 6 weeks of age [83]. Reports also have described early and late presentations of 2 to 8 weeks of age, respectively [75]. HPS can occur at birth. Premature infants also have been described, but they typically present with projectile vomiting 2 weeks later than term infants.

Clinical presentations

Projectile, nonbilious vomiting is the classic description of an infant with HPS. Early in the course of the disease, vomiting is nonprojectile and often is mistaken for GER [84]. As time continues, the pylorus channel narrows, and the vomiting increases in frequency and intensity. Coffee ground emesis may occur secondary to gastritis or esophagitis [85]. Some infants will have diarrhea known as starvation stools, and may be mistaken as gastroenteritis [75]. Significant delays in diagnosis will lead to severe dehydration. Hyperbilirubinemia is described in 2% to 5% of infants and is attributed to a glucuronyl transferase deficiency [75,86]. Indirect bilirubin levels can be as high as 15 to 20 mg/dL [87].

Physical examination and palpation of the abdomen are performed best while the infant is sucking on a pacifier, a sugar plum, or dextrose water. The infant should be warm and relaxed. Observation of the infant's abdomen may reveal peristaltic waves in the left upper quadrant moving left to right. Palpation of the hypertrophic pyloric muscle, also known as the olive, can be difficult even for the most experienced clinician. Decompression of the stomach may be necessary prior to examination. The physician should palpate near the right upper quadrant, feeling along the edge of the liver and moving caudally in the midline a third of the distance between the xiphoid and the umbilicus. This examination should reveal a palpable olive [75,88].

Differential diagnosis

The most common nonsurgical cause for nonbilious vomiting is GER. Other causes for nonbilious vomiting are food allergies, intracranial diseases, appendicitis, inborn errors of metabolism, pyloric duplication, pyelonephritis, and duodenal antral web [89,90].

Laboratory and imaging diagnostics

Electrolytes with a renal panel are essential. The classic, but often late finding of HPS is hypokalemic, hypochloremic alkalosis [91]. These laboratory tests also will confer the severity of dehydration (BUN/Cr ratio). If the infant appears jaundiced, then liver function studies are prudent.

Ultrasound is the preferred modality to diagnose HPS [92]. Ultrasound will document an enlarged pyloric muscle with a thickness of 3.5 mm to 4 mm and a pyloric channel length of 16 mm or greater [74,92,93]. The mnemonic for π (3.14) is useful to remember the ultrasound criteria for

HPS: greater then 3 mm for thickness and longer than 14 mm [74]. With experienced ultrasonographers, the sensitivity approaches 100%, with a 99.5% sensitivity and a 100% specificity [92]. If the ultrasound is inconclusive, an UGI is warranted, which will show the classic string sign [94].

Management

Most infants will require a fluid bolus of normal saline at 20 mL/kg to correct initial fluid deficits, followed by a slow correction for the metabolic alkalosis and any remaining deficiency using 1.5 times maintenance of D5 0.45 normal saline. The addition of potassium chloride, 10 to 20 mEq/L, should be initiated after the infant demonstrates urine output. Infants who have HPS do not require an NG tube, because this will exacerbate the metabolic alkalosis [75]. Serum bicarbonate of less than 28 mEq/L and serum chloride over 100 mEq/L generally are required for safe anesthesia [75]. Once the patient is stable, a pediatric surgery consultation is required.

Incarcerated inguinal hernias

Pathophysiology

It is estimated that 80% to 100% of newborn infants have a patent vaginalis that should close within the first 6 months of life [95]. A failure to close results in an indirect hernia. Interesting, the left side appears to close earlier that the right [96], and not surprising, most hernias occur on the right side [97]. The following medical and postsurgical conditions have been associated with the development of congenital inguinal hernias: undescended testis, birth prematurity, ascites, and a ventriculoperitoneal shunt, to name a few [96]. Genetic connective tissue conditions such as Ehlers-Danlos syndrome, Hunter-Hurler syndrome, Marfan's syndrome, and mucopolysaccharidosis are described as placing a child at risk for inguinal hernias [96]. Any infant who has an inguinal hernia risks having their bowels becoming incarcerated, and in severe cases, enstrangulated.

Epidemiology

Inguinal hernia surgery is the most common operation performed by pediatric surgeons [98]. The prevalence ranges from 0.8% to 4.4% [99]. The first year of life is the typical age of presentation for asymptomatic inguinal hernias [96,99]. Males are more likely to develop an asymptomatic hernia, and there is a 3:1 male to female ratio [99]. Most hernias are right-sided, and about 11% of families have a history of hernias [96,99].

The overall incidence of an incarcerated hernia occurs in about 31% of the general population and between 6% to 18% in the pediatric population [100]. Incarcerations are most likely to occur in the first year of life, with a rate of 10% to 31% [101–104]. In fact, most incarcerations will present within the first 2 months of life [97,100].

Clinical presentations

Most inguinal hernias are asymptomatic. Once the bowel and other viscera become incarcerated, however, typically at the level of the internal ring, infants will present with a myriad of signs and symptoms. Early in the course, the infant will become fussy or may be described as being irritable. As the disease progresses to strangulation, abdominal distention, vomiting and obstipation will occur [105]. Physical examination will reveal a mass in the inguinal area with or without a scrotal mass.

If the incarcerated inguinal hernia is left unreduced, these infants progress rapidly to strangulation [106]. Ischemia to the testes and ovaries also is described [107]. Patients who have strangulated bowel present extremely irritable. The abdominal distention and vomiting can be pronounced. On examination, a tender, tense, nonfluctuant mass is found in the inguinal area. Late signs of strangulation are shock, blood per rectum, and peritonitis [108]. An abdominal radiograph will show a partial or complete bowel obstruction (Fig. 7). If the bowel extends into the scrotum, air–fluid levels may be seen in the scrotum.

Differential diagnosis

The diagnosis is difficult to confuse given the physical findings. Surgical conditions that may present with abdominal distension and vomiting include: necrotizing enterocolitis, abuse, Hirschsprung's disease, appendicitis, and malrotation with volvulus. Medical conditions presenting as a tender mass include an abscess or tumor.

Laboratory and imaging studies

As mentioned previously, air–fluid levels may be found on abdominal radiographs (see Fig. 7), indicating a partial or complete bowel obstruction.

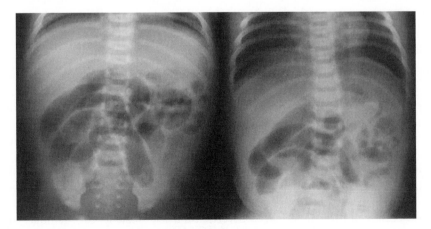

Fig. 7. A neonate with an inguinal mass and bilious vomiting. Abdominal radiograph showing small bowel obstruction. (*Courtesy of* Loren G. Yamamoto, MD, Honolulu, Hawaii.)

Ultrasound has become the modality of choice in determining inguinal hernias by differentiating among other causes for inguinal masses such as abscess, tumors, and a hydrocele. The accuracy rate approaches 97% and becomes higher with an associated history [109].

Management

Most patients who present with an incarcerated hernia can be managed nonoperatively. Manuel reduction with manipulation can occur without sedation, but the author advocates analgesics with sedation. Several effective techniques have been described. A well-known, time-honored, method is to have the infant in Trendelenburg position after sedation [108]. This method allows the mesentery, by gravity, to pull the bowel out of the hernia [108], although it may take time. Another technique is manual reduction. This requires the retraction of the hernia mass with one hand, while the free hand guides the tissue through the inguinal defect [96]. With proper analgesics and sedation, gentle compression has been shown to be effective. Other techniques have been described. Bedside ultrasound also has been described to increase the reduction rate by assisting the physician in the direction and location of the hernia defect [109]. Approximately 85% of all incarcerated hernias will be reduced [110,111]. Once the hernia is reduced, surgical follow-up is advised, usually within 2 days [96,112]. About 15% to 21% will recur; thus prompt operative herniorrhaphy is recommended [110,112,113]. Of note, early surgical repair will reduce recurrence rates by 25% [112].

If the incarcerated hernia cannot be reduced, or if the infant is suspected of having a strangulated inguinal hernia, a pediatric surgical consultation is required. Infants who have gangrenous bowel often are toxic, febrile, and present with an inguinal mass and abdominal distention. ED management should focus on aggressive fluid resuscitation, initiation of broad-spectrum antibiotics, and attention to airway, breathing, and circulation.

Meckel's diverticulum

Pathophysiology

A diverticulum is defined as an outpouching of a hollow or fluid-filled structure [114]. During the fifth week of fetal development, the vitelline duct normally is reabsorbed. When it fails to reabsorb, a diverticulum is formed. About 50% of intestinal diverticula will contain ectopic tissue such as gastric, colonic, or pancreatic mucosa [115]. Most ectopic tissue is comprised of gastric mucosa [116]. Diverticula containing gastric mucosa may ulcerate its own tissue layers and blood vessels, producing rectal bleeding. If the ulceration is severe, perforation will occur [117]. Two less common complications of Meckel's diverticulum are obstruction secondary to fixation of the omphalomesenteric duct remnants to the abdominal wall and inflammation [117].

Epidemiology

Meckel's diverticulum occurs in about 2% of the population, making it the most common congenital GI abnormality [118]. It is more symptomatically found in males, but is equally distributed among females and males [119]. It is generally located about 60 cm from the ileocecal valve. In pediatrics, it is a common cause of painless rectal bleeding and often presents in infants [120], although Shalaby noted a mean age of 5 years of age [121]. The rule of two is a common mnemonic to recall the basic information of Meckel's diverticulum. The diverticulum is within 2 in of the end of the small intestine, is 2 in in length, occurs in 2% of the population, is twice as common in males than females, and contains two types of ectopic mucosa, gastric and pancreatic [119]. The usual age of symptomatic presentation is within the first 2 years of life, but a percentage of patients will present in the first 2 decades of life [114].

Clinical presentations

An infant who has a diverticula containing gastric mucosa often will present with relatively painless rectal bleeding [120]. This is the most common presentation of Meckel's diverticulum and accounts for about 20% to 30% of all complications [122]. The bleeding is usually trivial; however, reports of massive bleeding are described [122–124]. Intestinal wall perforation also is described, and patients often present with an acute abdomen [125].

Intestinal obstruction occurs in about 10% to 20% of patients from either the Meckel's diverticulum-inducing intussusception as a pathological lead point, which is the most common, or secondary to an anatomic obstruction from bands attaching the diverticula to the abdominal wall [106,107,126]. These patients often will present with intermittent abdominal pain and vomiting [127].

Differential diagnosis

As a presenting sign of rectal bleeding, the differential diagnosis includes the following: polyp, peptic ulcer disease, underlying coagulopathy, nodular lymphoid hyperplasia, arteriovenous malformations, Hirschsprung's disease, and intussusception [120,127]. The differential diagnosis for abdominal pain and bilious vomiting includes the following surgical conditions: necrotizing enterocolitis, midgut volvulus, appendicitis, abuse, and intussusception. Medical conditions such as pyelonephritis and severe GER also should be considered.

Laboratory and imaging diagnostics

There are no specific laboratory studies to diagnose Meckel's diverticulum. In the overall evaluation of an infant with rectal bleeding, however, a CBC, coagulopathy panel, and LFTs, are recommended. If severe bleeding is noted, type and cross are mandatory. In infants or neonates presenting with vomiting and abdominal pain, a catheterized urine analysis is also warranted to rule out infection. The most commonly used study to diagnose Meckel's diverticulum is a Technetium-99 m pertechnetate scintigraphy, more commonly known as a Meckel's scan [128]. The radionucleotide, technetium-99, is absorbed by the gastric mucosa and results in an abnormal uptake (Fig. 8). Administering cimetidine, gastrin, or glucagons can enhance the absorption [129]. In the pediatric population, the positive predictive value (PPV) is 0.93, and the negative predictive value (NPV) is 0.93 [128]. Of interest, the same authors and others have found that the NPV falls sharply with children who have anemia, described as hemoglobin lower than 11 mg/dL [129]. This subset of patients subsequently was diagnosed with endoscopy or laparoscopic surgery. Ultrasound has been found effective in the diagnosis of Meckel's diverticulum associated with intussusception.

Abdominal radiographs are rarely useful with Meckel's diverticulum and rectal bleeding. In infants who present with bilious vomiting, however, a radiograph may show a small bowel obstruction or intussusception. Free air also may be noted if perforation of the diverticulum has occurred.

Management

Stable patients will require laboratory studies as noted. An intravenous catheter is prudent to begin fluid rehydration. For patients presenting with signs and symptoms of hemorrhagic or hypovolemic shock, aggressive fluid resuscitation is required. Blood products also may be required. Early pediatric surgical consultation is suggested. For symptomatic bleeding

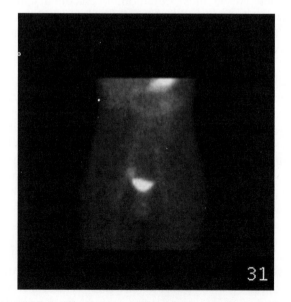

Fig. 8. An abnormal Meckel's scan. Note the increase area of uptake at the right iliac vessel indicating a Meckel's appendage. (*Courtesy of* David Cox, MD, St. Paul, Minnesota.)

with an inconclusive Meckel's scan, laparoscopic surgery has been proven to be safe and cost-effective for definitive diagnosis and care for rectal bleeding [121,130]. Infants presenting with abdominal pain and vomiting and subsequently found to have an obstruction will require an extensive work-up and eventual surgery. Patients with intussusception will require air-contrast enema for reduction.

Intussusception

Pathophysiology
Intussusception is the involution of one part of intestine into another. The word, intussusception is derived from the Latin words intus, meaning within, and suscipere, meaning to receive [131]. Thus, intussusception is the intestine's ability, by means of peristalsis, to invaginate over itself. In doing so, the intestine also carries the mesentery blood vessels into the intussusception. Shortly after, the blood vessels become congested. The clinical sign of current jelly stool is thought to be secondary to venous congestion and intestinal production of mucus [132]. As edema and swelling increase, arterial blood flow will be forfeited, leading to ischemia and bowel necrosis.

Epidemiology
Intussusception is the most common etiology for bowel obstruction in children younger than 2 years of age [133]. It is estimated to occur in about 1 in 2000 infants and children [133]. The typical age distribution is between 3 months to 6 years of age, and the peak incidence is 5 months to 12 months of age [22,134]. There is a 3:2 male to female distribution [135,136].

About 90% of intussusceptions are ileocolic and do not have a pathologic lead point [132]. A pathologic lead point is a lesion that is thought to cause the intussusception. Common lead points include: appendix, lipoma, intestinal polyp, a Meckel's diverticulum, enlarged Peyer's patch, and Henoch-Schonlein purpura (HSP)-associated submucosal hematomas [1,132,136]. The second common type, representing 4% of intussusceptions, is ileoileocolic [137]. Approximately 40% of ileoileocolic intussusceptions will have a pathologic lead point. Because of the anatomical location, these are more difficult to reduce and often present with an abdominal radiograph consistent of a small bowel obstruction [132,138]. Appendicocolic, cecocolic, colocolic, jejunojejunal and ileoileal also are described [132] and typically involve older patients. Pathologic lead points commonly are found with these anatomic variations of intussusceptions [132,139,140].

Clinical presentation
The most common signs and symptoms of intussusception are well documented: abdominal mass, rectal bleeding, vomiting, and colicky abdominal pain that bring the child's knees to the chest [137,139]. It is estimated that only 30% of children will have all four classic symptoms

[141]. Thus, relying on all four symptoms will delay the diagnosis [137]. Vomiting and colicky abdominal pain lasting for minutes are the most common and well-described clinical symptoms [141]. Another symptom is lethargy following abdominal pain (and vomiting), which Justice noted to be present in 75% of infants [142]. Finally, there is a subset of infants, estimated to be 15%, who do not have any history of abdominal pain [143]. These patients will have vomiting and will present listless, pale, and ill [143–145].

Rectal bleeding, although thought to be a late sign, is found more frequently than an abdominal mass [1,137]. Losek noted that 75% of cases with intussusception had stool that was guaiac-positive [146]. An abdominal mass typically is found in 22% of cases [147] and is palpated in the right upper quadrant. The mass is believed to be a displaced malpositioned colon occurring during intussusception. When this happens, a vacant space may be seen in the right lower quadrant. Concavity of the right lower quadrant and palpation of a right upper quadrant mass are known as the signe de Dance of intussusception [15,148].

Clearly, intussusception can be a difficult diagnosis. The most sensitive signs and symptoms are vomiting and abdominal pain, which are indistinguishable from gastroenteritis. Kupperman and colleagues developed a predictive model and found that rectal blood, male sex, and a highly suggestive radiographic finding were associated with sensitivities of 88%, 69%, and 86%, respectively. The negative predictive values were 76%, 49% and 79%, respectively. They argue that the presence of these variables should prompt the clinician to order an air contrast enema [133].

Differential diagnosis

The following life-threatening etiologies and common medical conditions should be considered in the differential diagnosis for abdominal pain and vomiting: incarcerated inguinal hernia, malrotation with volvulus, Hirschsprung's disease, abuse, gastroenteritis, constipation, appendicitis, and urinary tract infections.

Laboratory and diagnostic studies

The standard of care suggests obtaining a two-view abdominal film in the initial work-up for abdominal pain [132]. For intussusception, however, the use of plain radiographs remains controversial [149,150], because the diagnostic accuracy is about 25% to 50% [147,151,152]. Nevertheless, the following radiographic findings have become almost pathognomonic for intussusception:

- A soft tissue mass in the right upper quadrant effacing the liver edge
- The meniscus sign, which is a crescent of gas within the colonic lumen that outlines the apex of the intussusception

- The target sign, which is a soft-tissue mass outlined by a lucency of peritoneal fat (Fig. 9) [153]

These findings, unfortunately, are not common [154], and, more importantly, an infant with intussusception may have a normal radiograph.

Sonography is becoming the modality of choice in diagnosing intussusception. It offers the absence of radiation. It is noninvasive and has a 100% accuracy rate [155,156]. The ultrasound finding is distinct; on cross section, a 3 cm to 5 cm diameter mass is seen in the shape of a target or donut [157]. Sonography also has been shown to be effective in diagnosing pathologic lead points and determining other true causes of abdominal pain in children such as ovarian torsion and small bowel volvulus [157,158].

Management

Once the diagnosis is apparent or suspected, an air contrast enema is required to reduce the intussusception. Sedation is not required. Unsuccessful reduction or bowel wall perforation is uncommon. At the author's institution, a pediatric surgery consultation is not required prior to the air contrast enema. A surgery consultation is obtained if the pediatric radiologist is unable to reduce the intussusception or if perforation occurs.

Air contrast enema has replaced barium enema for several reasons: because perforation with contrast carries serious consequences, and the recurrence rate is higher with contrast [159]. Ultrasonography also has been shown to increase the success rate during difficult reductions [160].

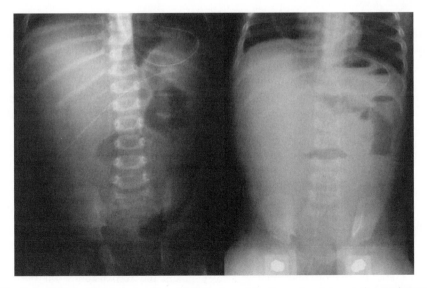

Fig. 9. An infant with intussusception. Note the loss of the liver edge. A target also can be seen in the right upper quadrant. (*Courtesy of* Loren G. Yamamoto, MD, Honolulu, Hawaii.)

Appendicitis

Pathophysiology

In neonates and infants, fecaliths are not causative agents in the development of appendicitis [161]. Pathologic obstruction of the appendiceal lumen from Hirschsprung's disease, an inguinal hernia, or emboli from congenital heart disease has been implicated [162,163]. A lack of physiologic and immunologic reserve, a small abdominal cavity allowing an intra-abdominal infection to easily spread, a relatively small omentum that cannot wall off an infection, and a thin-walled appendix have been cited to increase morbidity and mortality for appendicitis for this young age group [164].

Epidemiology

Appendicitis in infancy is rare, and, as a surgical procedure, represents less than 2% of all pediatric appendectomies [165]. The incidence is about 0.4% for children younger than 12 months of age [165,166]. By the time of diagnosis, appendiceal perforation typically has occurred, with notable rates from 37% to 94% [167,168]. In fact, perforation rates exceed 95% within only 48 hours of symptoms [168]. In a recent study by Lin, perforation rates were 100%, and one infant died out of a total of seven infants during a 10-year period [169]. Without aggressive management with surgery and antibiotics, mortality rates for infants and neonates were 29% and 81%, respectively [162,165].

Clinical presentation

The high perforation rate implies nonspecific clinical findings or a lack of attention by providers or caregivers. Early diagnosis is challenging, and the most common sign and symptom are nonspecific and ubiquitous: fever, vomiting, anorexia, and diarrhea [169,170]. As a result, the average time to correctly diagnosis appendicitis is 4 days [171]. As the appendiceal inflammation continues, irritability and lethargy may be noted in the infant or neonate [1,172]. Grunting respirations and parental concerns for their infant's right hip may be noted [6,173]. Eighty-four percent of infants will have fevers [165,168,173]. Once perforation occurs, abdominal pain and distention will be noted [169]. A right lower quadrant mass will develop as inflammation and infection worsens [174]. In severe peritonitis, abdominal wall cellulitis may be visible [169].

A high clinical suspicion is needed to diagnose a neonate or infant with appendicitis. In 1947, Howard Williams noted:

> "[a] history from the mother of a continued bellyache or discomfort and repeated vomiting should be presumptive evidence of appendicitis. I am in opinion that such a history places the responsibility on the medical attendant of suspecting appendicitis and of acting accordingly" [175].

Differential diagnoses

Medical and surgical conditions mimicking appendicitis include AGE, GER, malrotation with volvulus, Hirschsprung's disease, Meckel's diverticulum with a Ladd's band, and NEC. Nonintentional trauma always should be considered with abdominal distention and vomiting.

Laboratory and diagnostic imaging

No laboratory studies will diagnose appendicitis. White cell blood counts have been noted to be normal among infants with perforated appendicitis [169]. For ill-appearing patients, a sepsis work-up should be considered. The evaluation of appendicitis with ultrasound and CT has not been studied in neonates or infants. CT scans have a high sensitivity and specificity in older children and adults [176]. Neonates and infants, however, have relatively little body fat and a small appendix; thus diagnosing a nonperforated appendix may be difficult [177]. In addition, exposing infants to radiation should not be taken lightly. Researchers strongly urge more restrictive use of CT scanning of children [178,179]. This is based on the following factors:

Children are more inherently sensitive to radiation, because they have more cells in mitosis.

- The overall radiation dose is much greater than adults.
- Children are more likely to have additional CT scans over their life time, and the carcinogenetic effects from radiation are cumulative.
- Children have long lives and have more time to express cancer [180,181].

Hall estimated that the lifelong risk of developing cancer after a single abdominal CT was 1/1000 [181]. To put this into perspective, an estimate 2.7 million CT scans are performed in children each year [182]. The public health implications are staggering. With this being noted, the author advocates the use of abdominal CT when indicated, but also reminds physicians to use it judiciously.

Ultrasound has proven to be a valuable modality in diagnosing appendicitis, especially in the hands of a well-trained ultrasonographer [183]. It has the added value of being noninvasive (no intravenous catheter or the need for oral contrast), not exposing the child to radiation, and not requiring sedation. The sensitivities and specificities are good and have been reported to range from 44% to 95% and 47% to 95%, respectively [184]. The inability to visualize the appendix is the most common cause for the false-negative rate [185].

As mentioned before, neonatal and infant perforation rates are high and have not changed in recent years. Similarly, perforation rates for older children and adolescents have not changed [186]. So how does one proceed? Kosloske and colleagues proposed a clinical pathway that was effective at reducing radiation exposure from CT scans without compromising accuracy. In their study, they reported an accuracy of 97%, which was higher than using a CT scan or ultrasound alone [187], when a pediatric surgeon performed an abdominal examination on each patient. Other researchers have proposed using an ultrasound to screen suspected cases [188]. Morrow and other researchers suggest that if the combination of history, physical examination, laboratory studies, and ultrasound are inconclusive, then the patient could undergo a CT scan or be admitted for serial abdominal examinations [170,189].

Management

If appendicitis is suspected, early pediatric consultation is warranted. Intravenous access for aggressive fluid resuscitation is critical, given that most infants will have perforated once the diagnosis is made. Broad-spectrum antibiotics should be initiated early in the evaluation if the neonate or infant appears ill. One should consider performing a full sepsis work-up and also obtaining coagulopathy, type and screen, and VBG laboratory tests. Supporting the airway, breathing, and circulation is the dictum until definitive surgical repair or transfer to the critical care unit.

Summary

Neonatal and infant abdominal emergencies can present with a myriad of signs and symptoms. There are, however, common themes with each disease. For example, bilious vomiting always should be considered a life-threatening emergency, and it can be seen in all of the conditions discussed including, malrotation with volvulus, necrotizing enterocolitis, Hirschsprung's disease, incarcerated inguinal hernia, omphalitis, and appendicitis except hypertrophic pyloric stenosis. Abdominal distention also can be seen in all but HPS. A thorough physical examination will diagnose omphalitis and incarcerated inguinal hernia. To some extent, abdominal radiographs can be very helpful, especially if vomiting and abdominal distention are present. Rectal bleeding or guaiac positive stool can be seen with Meckel's diverticulum, Hirschsprung's disease, necrotizing enterocolitis, and intussusception. Table 2 is a quick reference guide for the clinician when presented with neonates and infants who may have an abdominal emergency.

Ill-appearing patients with vomiting, fever, and abdominal distention are late presentations of malrotation with volvulus, necrotizing enterocolitis, omphalitis, Hirschsprung's disease, incarcerated inguinal hernia, intussusception, and appendicitis. These patients require aggressive fluid resuscitation, broad-spectrum antibiotics, attention to the ABCs, and a pediatric surgery consultation.

The use of technology has changed patient care. Ultrasound and CT have saved countless lives and decreased morbidity, especially for appendicitis. Adversely, it now seems that radiation exposure from CT scans may have consequences to all children. Obviously, the benefit of the CT scan outweighs the risk for most situations. Physicians must strive to protect patients as best possible.

Table 2
A brief guide to determining the diagnosis of neonatal and infant abdominal emergencies

Age	Disease	Clinical presentation	Determining the diagnosis	Adjunct studies
Neonate	Malrotation with volvulus	Bilious vomiting	H, PE, UGI	
	Necrotizing enterocolitis	Vomiting, abdominal distention	H, PE, AXR	
	Omphalitis	Erythema of umbilicus	H, PE	US or CT
	Hirschsprung's disease	Abdominal distention, diarrhea	H, PE, AXR, RB	CE
Infant	Hypertrophic pyloric stenosis	Projectile, nonbilious vomiting	H, PE, US	UGI
	Incarcerated inguinal hernia	Inguinal mass, vomiting	H, PE	
	Meckel's diverticulum	Rectal bleeding or bilious vomiting	H, PE	MS or UGI
	Intussusception	Vomiting, colicky abdominal pain, listless	H, PE, A-CE	
	Appendicitis	Vomiting, anorexia, fussy	H, PE, US	CT or EL

Abbreviations: H, history; PE, physical exam; UGI, upper gastrointestinal; AXR, abdominal radiograph; US, ultrasound; RB, rectal biopsy; A–CE, air–contrast enema; MS, Meckel's scan; EL, exploratory laparotomy.

Acknowledgements

The author is indebted to Suzanne Remington, JD, and Sheryl Louie, MD, for their help in the preparation and editing of this manuscript. The author is also thankful for Loren G. Yamamoto, MD, and Dave Cox, MD, for allowing access to their radiographic libraries. The reader is invited to view more of Dr. Yamamoto's teaching files at: www.hawaii.edu/medicine/pediatrics. The author also appreciates Joe Arms, MD, and Amy Schirmer for their assistance.

References

[1] Pollack ES. Pediatric abdominal surgical emergencies. Pediatr Ann 1996;25:448–57.
[2] Samuel Bard. A discourse on the duties of a physician: address to the first graduating class at the medical school established in affiliation with what was then known as King's College, New York. New York: A&J Robertson; 1769 [As cited in Tabott JH, A biographical history of medicine, p. 356 (q.v.)]. LEARNING 1328.
[3] De Bruin WJ, Greenwald BM, Notterman DA. Fluid resuscitation in pediatrics. Crit Care Med 1992;8:423–38.
[4] Carcillo JA, Tasker RC. Fluid resuscitation of hypovolemic shock: acute medicine's great triumph for children. Intensive Care Med 2006;32:958–61.
[5] Rosival V. Hyperventilation in severe diabetic ketoacidosis. Pediatr Crit Care Med 2005;6:405–11.

[6] Singer JI, Losek JD. Grunting respirations: chest or abdominal pathology? Pediatr Emerg Care 1992;8:354–8.

[7] Hanna GL, Fischer DJ, Fluent TE. Separation anxiety disorder and school refusal in children and adolescents. Pediatr Rev 2006;27:56–62.

[8] Filston HC, Kirks DR. Malrotation—the ubiquitous anomaly. J Pediatr Surg 1981;16:614–20.

[9] Cywes S, Millar AJW. Embryology and anomalies of the intestine. In: Haubrich WS, Schaffner F, Berke JE, editors. Bockus gastroenterology. 5th edition. Philadelphia: WB Saunders; 1995. p. 899–929.

[10] Dott NM. Anomalies of intestinal rotation: their embryology and surgical aspects with five cases. Br J Surg 1923;11:251–86.

[11] Louw JH, Barnard CN. Congenital intestinal atresia: observations on its origins. Lancet 1955;2:1065–7.

[12] Millar AJW, Rode H, Cywes S. Malrotation and volvulus in infancy and childhood. Semin Pediatr Surg 2003;12:229–36.

[13] Ladd WE. Surgical disease of the alimentary tract in infants. N Engl J Med 1936;215:705–8.

[14] Skandalakis JE, Gray SW, Ricketts R, et al. The small intestines. In: Skandalakis JE, Gray SW, editors. Embryology for surgeons. 2nd edition. Baltimore (MD): Williams & Wilkins; 1994. p. 184–241.

[15] Irish MS, Pearl RH, Caty MG, et al. The approach to common abdominal diagnoses in infants and children. Pediatr Clin North Am 1998;45:729–72.

[16] Spingand N, Brandt ML, Yazbeck S. Malrotation presenting beyond the neonatal period. J Pediatr Surg 1990;25:1139–42.

[17] Garg P, Singh M, Marya SK. Intestinal malrotation in adults. Indian J Gastroenterol 1991; 10:103–4.

[18] Seashore JH, Touloukian RJ. Midgut volvulus: an ever-present threat. Arch Pediatr Adolesc Med 1994;148:43–6.

[19] Bonadio WA, Clarkson T, Naus J. The clinical features of children with malrotation of the intestine. Pediatr Emerg Care 1991;7:348–9.

[20] Maxson RT, Franklin PA, Wagner CW. Malrotation in the older child: surgical management, treatment, and outcome. Am Surg 1995;61:135–8.

[21] Millar AJW, Rode H, Brown RA, et al. The deadly vomit: malrotation and midgut volvulus. Pediatr Surg Int 1987;2:448–53.

[22] Felter RA. Nontraumatic surgical emergencies in children. Emerg Med Clin North Am 1991;9:589–610.

[23] Godbole P, Stringer MD. Bilious vomiting in the newborn: how often is it pathologic? J Pediatr Surg 2002;6:909–11.

[24] Lilien LD, Srinivasan G, Pyati SP, et al. Green vomiting in the first 72 hours in normal infants. Am J Dis Child 1986;140:662–4.

[25] Swischuk LE, Volvulus. In: Jones KL, Smith DW, editors. Emergency radiology of the acutely ill or injured child. 5th edition. Baltimore (MD): Williams & Wilkins; 1994. p. 289–98.

[26] Dufour D, Delaet MH, Dassonville M, et al. Midgut malrotation: the reliability of sonographic diagnosis. Pediatr Radiol 1992;22:21–3.

[27] Orzech N, Navarro OM, Langer JC. Is ultrasonography a good screening test for intestinal malrotation? J Pediatr Surg 2006;41:1005–9.

[28] Kim SS, Albanese CT, et al. Necrotizing enterocolitis. In: Grosfeld JL, O'Neill JA, Coran AG, editors. Pediatric surgery. 6th edition. St. Louis (MO): Mosby; 2006. p. 1427–52.

[29] Rodin AE, Nichols MM, Hsu FL. Necrotizing enterocolitis occurring in full-term neonates at birth. Arch Pathol 1973;96:335–8.

[30] Maayan-Metzger A, Itzchak A, Mazkereth R, et al. Necrotizing enterocolitis in full-term infants: case control study and review of the literature. J Perinatol 2004;24:494–9.

[31] Ostie DJ, Spilde TL, St. Peter SD, et al. Necrotizing enterocolitis in full-term infants. J Pediatr Surg 2003;7:1039–42.

[32] Tannuri U, Gomes VA, Troster EJ. Concomitant involvement of the small intestine and the distal esophagus in an infant with massive necrotizing enterocolitis. Rev Hosp Clin Fac Med Sao Paulo 2004;59:131–4.

[33] Hostetler MA, Schulman M. Necrotizing enterocolitis presenting to the emergency department: case report and review of the differential considerations for vomiting in the neonate. J Emerg Med 2001;21:165–70.

[34] Kosloske AM, Musemeche CA, Ball WS, et al. Necrotizing enterocolitis: value of radiographic findings to predict outcome. Am J Roentgenol 1988;151:771–4.

[35] Silva CT, Daneman A, Navarro OM, et al. Correlation of sonographic findings and outcome in necrotizing enterocolitis. Padiatr Radiol 2007;37:274–83.

[36] Faingold R, Daneman A, Tomlinson G, et al. Necrotizing enterocolitis: absent of bowel viability with color Doppler US. Radiology 2005;235:587–94.

[37] Rowe MI, O'Neill JA, Grosfeld JL, et al. Disorders of the umbilicus. In: Rowe MI, O'Neill AJ, Grosfeld JL, et al, editors. Essentials of pediatric surgery. St. Louis (MO): Mosby; 1995. p. 245–55.

[38] Weber DM, Freeman NV, Elhag KM, et al. Periumbilical necrotizing fasciitis in the newborn. Eur J Pediatr Surg 2001;11:86–91.

[39] Kosloske AM, Cushing AH, Borden TA, et al. Cellulitis and necrotizing fasciitis of the abdominal wall in pediatric patients. J Pediatr Surg 1981;16:246–51.

[40] McKenna H, Johnson D. Bacteria in neonatal omphalitis. Pathology 1977;9:111–3.

[41] Hsieh W, Yang P, Chao H, et al. Neonatal necrotizing fasciitis: a report of three cases and review of the literature. Pediatrics 1999;103:e53.

[42] Samuel M, Freeman N, Vaishnav A, et al. Necrotizing fasciitis: a serious complication of the omphalitis in neonates. J Pediatr Surg 1994;29:1414–6.

[43] Sawardekar KP. Changing spectrum of neonatal omphalitis. Pediatr Infect Dis 2004;23: 22–6.

[44] Janssen PA, Selwood BL, Dobson SR, et al. To dye or not to dye: a randomized, clinical trial of a triple-dye/alcohol regime versus dry cord care. Pediatrics 2003;111:15–20.

[45] Dore S, Buchan D, Coulas S, et al. Alcohol versus natural drying for newborn cord care. J Obstet Gynecol Neonatal Nurs 1998;27:621–7.

[46] Weathers L, Takagishi J, Rodriguez L, et al. Umbilical cord care. Pediatrics 2004;113:625–6.

[47] Mullany LC, Darmstadt GL, Khatry SK, et al. Impact of umbilical cord cleansing with 4.0% chlorhexidine on time to cord separation among newborns in southern Nepal: a cluster-randomized, community-based trial. Pediatrics 2006;118:1464–71.

[48] Cushing AH. Omphalitis: a review. Pediatr Infect Dis J 1985;4:282–5.

[49] Simon NP, Simon MW. Changes in newborn bathing practices may increase the risk for omphalitis. Clin Pediatr (Phila) 2004;43:763–7.

[50] Bauer TR, Gu YC, Creevy KE, et al. Leukocyte adhesion deficiency in children and Irish setter dogs. Pediatr Res 2004;55:363–7.

[51] Etzioni A, Tonetti M. Leukocyte adhesion deficiency II—from A to almost Z. Immunol Rev 2000;178:138–47.

[52] Donolon CR, Furdon SA. Assessment of the umbilical cord outside of the delivery room. Part 2. Adv Neonatal Care 2002;2:187–97.

[53] Khati NJ, Enquist EG, Javitt MC. Imaging of the umbilicus and periumbilical region. Radiographics 1998;18:413–31.

[54] Holschneider AM, Ure BM. Hirschsprung's disease. In: Ashcraft KW, Holcom GW, Murphy JP, editors. Pediatric surgery. 4th edition. Philadelphia: WB Saunders; 2005. p. 477–95.

[55] Whitehouse F, Kernohan J. Myenteric plexuses in congenital megacolon; study of 11 cases. Arch Intern Med 1948;82:75–7.

[56] Bodian M, Carter C. A family study of Hirschsprung's disease. Ann Hum Genet 1963;26: 261–77.

[57] Badner JA, Sieber WK, Garver KL, et al. A genetic study of Hirschsprung's disease. Am J Hum Genet 1990;46:568–80.

[58] Amiel J, Lyonnet S. Hirschsprung's disease, associated syndromes, and genetics: a review. J Med Genet 2001;38:729–39.

[59] Jones KL. Hirschsprung aganglionosis. In: Jones KL, Smith DW, editors. Smith's recognizable patterns of human malformation. 5th edition. Philadelphia: WB Saunders; 1997. p. 832–3.

[60] Swenson O, Sherman JO, Fisher JH. Diagnosis of congenital megacolon: an analysis of 501 patients. J Pediatr Surg 1973;8:587–94.

[61] Khan AR, Vujanic GM, Huddart S. The constipated child: how likely is Hirschsprung's disease. Pediatr Surg Int 2003;19:439–42.

[62] Lewis NA, Levitt MA, Zallen GS, et al. Diagnosing Hirschsprung's disease: increasing the odds of a positive rectal biopsy. J Pediatr Surg 2003;38:412–6.

[63] Puri P, Wester T. Enterocolitis complicating Hirschsprung's disease. In: Holschneier AM, Puri P, editors. Hirschsprung's disease and allied disorders. 2nd edition. London: Harwood Academic Publishers; 2000. p. 165–75.

[64] Elhalaby EA, Coran AG, Blane CE, et al. Enterocolitis associated with Hirschsprung's disease. A clinical–radiological characterization of 168 patients. J Pediatr Surg 1995;30:76–83.

[65] Imamura A, Puri P, O'Briain DS, et al. Mucosal immune defense mechanisms in enterocolitis complicating Hirschsprung's disease. Gut 1992;33:801–6.

[66] Sherman JO, Snyder ME, Weitzman JJ, et al. A 40-year multinational retrospective study of 880 Swenson procedures. J Pediatr Surg 1989;24:833–8.

[67] Carcassone M, Guys JM, Morrisson-Lacombe G, et al. Management of Hirschsprung's disease: curative surgery before 3 months of age. J Pediatr Surg 1989;24:1032–4.

[68] Blane CE, Elhalaby E, Coran AG. Enterocolitis following endorectal pull-through procedure in children with Hirschsprung's disease. Pediatr Radiol 1994;24:164–6.

[69] Swenson O, Neuhauser EBD, Pickett LK. New concepts of the etiology, diagnosis, and treatment of congenital megacolon (Hirschsprung's disease). Pediatrics 1949;4:201–9.

[70] Swenson O. Hirschsprung's disease: a review. Pediatrics 2002;109:914–8.

[71] Swenson O, Fisher JH, MacMahon HE. Rectal biopsy as an aid in the diagnosis of Hirschsprung's disease. N Engl J Med 1955;253:632–5.

[72] Lake BD, Puri P, Nixon HH, et al. Hirschsprung's disease: an appraisal of histochemically demonstrating acetylcholinesterase activity in suction biopsy specimens as an aid to diagnosis. Arch Pathol Lab Med 1978;102:244–7.

[73] Hirschsprung H. Falle von angeborener pyloric stenose. J Kinderheilk 1888;27:61–8.

[74] Keller H, Waldmann D, Greiner P. Comparison of preoperative sonography with intraoperative findings in congenital hypertrophic pyloric stenosis. J Pediatr Surg 1987;22:950–2.

[75] Schwartz M, et al. Hypertrophic pyloric stenosis. In: Grosfeld JL, O'Neill JA, Coran AG, editors. Pediatric surgery. 6th edition. St. Louis (MO): Mosby; 2006. p. 1215–24.

[76] Honein MA, Paulozzi LJ, Himelright IM, et al. Infantile hypertrophic pyloric stenosis after pertussis prophylaxis with erythromycin: a case review and cohort study. Lancet 1999;35: 2101–5.

[77] Christofides ND, Mallet E, Ghatei MA, et al. Plasma enteroglucagon and neurotensin in infantile pyloric stenosis. Arch Dis Child 1983;58:52–5.

[78] Dick AC, Ardill J, Potts SR, et al. Gastrin, somatostatin, and infantile hypertrophic pyloric stenosis. Acta Paediatr 2001;90:879–82.

[79] Rogers IM. The true cause of pyloric stenosis is hyperacidity. Acta Paediatr 2006;95:132–6.

[80] Schecter R, Torfs CP, Bateson TF. The epidemiology of infantile hypertrophic pyloric stenosis. Paediatr Perinat Epidemiol 1997;11:407–11.

[81] Mitchell LE, Risch N. The genetics of infantile hypertrophic stenosis. Am J Dis Child 1993; 147:1203–11.

[82] Carter CO, Evans KA. Inheritance of congenital pyloric stenosis. J Med Genet 1969;6:233–54.

[83] Naik-Mathuria B, Olutoye OO. Foregut abnormalities. Surg Clin North Am 2006;86: 261–84.

[84] Spitz L, McLeod E. Gastroesophageal reflux. Semin Pediatr Surg 2003;12:237–40.

[85] Benson CD, Lloyd JR. Infantile pyloric stenosis. Am J Surg 1964;107:429–33.

[86] Lippert MM. Jaundice with hypertrophic pyloric stenosis. J Pediatr 1990;117:168–9.

[87] Roth B, Statz A, Heinisch HM, et al. Elimination of indocyanine green by the liver of infants with hypertrophic pyloric stenosis and the icteropyloric syndrome. J Pediatr 1981; 99:240–3.

[88] Aktug T, Akgur FM, Olguner M. Analyzing the diagnostic efficiency of olive palpation for hypertrophic pyloric stenosis. J Pediatr Surg 1999;34:1585–6.

[89] Bell MJ, Ternberg JL, McAlister W, et al. Antral diaphragm—a cause of gastric outlet obstruction in infants and children. J Pediatr 1977;90:196–200.

[90] Murray KF, Christie DL. Vomiting. Pediatr Rev 1998;19:337–41.

[91] Chesney RW, Zelikovic I. Pre- and postoperative fluid management in infancy. Pediatr Rev 1989;11:153–8.

[92] Hernanz-Schulman M, Sells LL, Ambrosino MM, et al. Hypertrophic pyloric stenosis in the infant without a palpable olive: accuracy of sonographic diagnosis. Radiology 1994; 193:771–6.

[93] Blumhagen JD, Noble HG. Muscle thickness in hypertrophic pyloric stenosis: sonographic determination. Am J Roentgenol 1983;140:221–3.

[94] Garcia VF, Randolph JG. Pyloric stenosis: diagnosis and management. Pediatr Rev 1990; 11:292–6.

[95] Synder W Jr, Greaney E Jr, et al. Inguinal hernia. In: Benson C, Mustard W, Ravitch M, editors. Pediatric surgery. Chicago: Year Book Medical Publishers; 1962. p. 573–87.

[96] Glick PL, Boulanger SC, et al. Inguinal hernias and hydroceles. In: Grosfeld JL, O'Neill JA, Coran AG, editors. Pediatric surgery. 6th edition. St. Louis (MO): Mosby; 2006. p. 1172–92.

[97] Rowe MI, Clatworthy HW. Incarcerated and strangulated hernias in children: a statistical study of high risk factors. Arch Surg 1970;101:136–9.

[98] Snyder CL. Preface. Semin Pediatr Surg 2007;16:1–2.

[99] Bronsther B, Abrams MW, Elboim C. Inguinal hernias in children—a study of 1000 cases and a review of the literature. J Am Med Womens Assoc 1972;27:522–5.

[100] Rescorla FJ, Grosfeld JL. Inguinal hernia repair in the perinatal period and early infancy: clinical considerations. J Pediatr Surg 1984;19:832–7.

[101] Niedzielski J, Krol R, Gawlowska A. Could incarnation on inguinal hernia in children be prevented? Med Sci Monit 2003;9:C R16–8.

[102] Stephens BJ, Riice WT, Koucky CJ, et al. Optimal timing of elective indirect inguinal hernia repair in healthy children: clinical considerations for improved outcome. World J Surg 1992;16:952–6.

[103] Grosfeld JL. Current concepts in inguinal hernia in infants and children. World J Surg 1989;13:506–15.

[104] Thorndike AJ, Ferguson C. Incarcerated inguinal hernia in infancy and childhood. Am J Surg 1938;39:429.

[105] Mastagas MI, Fatouros M, Koulouras B, et al. Incidence, complications, and management of Meckel's diverticulum. Arch Surg 1995;130:143–6.

[106] Meguid M, Canty T, Eraklis AJ. Complications of Meckel's diverticulum in infants. Surg Gynecol Obstet 1974;139:541–4.

[107] Harkins H. Intussusception due to invaginated Meckel's diverticulum. Am J Surg 1933;98: 1070–95.

[108] Gilchrist BF, Scriven RJ, Lessin MS, et al. Frequently encountered problems in pediatric surgery I: neonatal problems. HP general surgery board review manual Hosp Physician 1998;4:1–12. www.turner-white.com.

[109] Chen SC, Lee CC, Liu YP, et al. Ultrasound may decrease the emergency surgery rate of incarcerated inguinal hernia. Scand J Gastroenterol 2005;40:721–4.

[110] Stylianos S, Jacir NN, Harris BH. Incarceration of inguinal hernias in infants prior to elective repair. J Pediatr Surg 1993;28:582–3.

[111] Goldman RD, Balasubramanian S, Wales O, et al. Pediatric surgeons and pediatric emergency medicine physicians' attitudes towards analgesia and sedation for incarcerated inguinal hernia reduction. J Pain 2005;6:650–5.

[112] Lau S, Yi-Horng L, Caty MG. Current management of inguinal hernias and hydroceles. Semin Pediatr Surg 2007;16:50–7.

[113] Schmidt M, Peiffert B, de Miscault G, et al. Compilations of inguinal hernia in children. Cir Pediatr 1987;28:193–6.

[114] Snyder CL, et al. Meckel's diverticulum. In: Grosfeld JL, O'Neill JA, Coran AG, editors. Pediatric surgery. 6th edition. St. Louis (MO): Mosby; 2006. p. 1304–12.

[115] Turgeon DK, Barnett JL. Meckel's diverticulum. Am J Gastroenterol 1990;85:777–81.

[116] St-Vil D, Brandt ML, Panic S, et al. Meckel's diverticulum in children: a 20-year review. J Pediatr Surg 1991;26:1289–92.

[117] Sai Prassad TR, Chui CH, Singaporewalla FR, et al. Meckel's diverticulum complications in children: is laparoscopy the order of the day? Pediatr Surg Int 2007;23:141–7.

[118] Brown KL, Glover DM. Persistent omphalomesenteric duct; incidence relative to Meckel's diverticulum. Am J Surg 1952;83:680–5.

[119] Brown RL, Azizkhan RG. Gastrointestinal bleeding in infants and children: Meckel's diverticulum and intestinal duplication. Semin Pediatr Surg 1999;8:202–9.

[120] Teach SJ, Fleisher GR. Rectal bleeding in the emergency department. Ann Emerg Med 1994;23:1252–8.

[121] Shalaby RY, Soloman SM, Fawy M, et al. Laparoscopic management of Meckel's diverticulum in children. J Pediatr Surg 2005;40:52–7.

[122] Rutherford RB, Akers DR. Meckel's diverticulum: a report of 148 pediatric patients, with special reference to the pattern of bleeding and to mesodiverticular vascular bands. Surgery 1966;59:618–26.

[123] Vane DW, West KW, Grosfeld JL. Vitelline duct anomalies. Experience with 217 childhood cases. Arch Surg 1987;122:542–7.

[124] Jan IA, Mirza FM, Ali M, et al. Meckel's diverticulum causing exsanguinating haemorrhage. J Coll Physicians Surg Pak 2004;14:300–1.

[125] Gandy J, Byrne P, Lees G. Neonatal Meckel's diverticular inflammation with perforation. J Pediatr Surg 1997;32:750–1.

[126] Aitken J. Remnants of the vitello–intestinal duct; a clinical analysis of 88 cases. Arch Dis Child 1953;28:11–7.

[127] Rayorn N, Thrall C, Silber G. A review of the causes of lower gastrointestinal tract bleeding in children. Gastroenterol Nurs 2001;24:77–82.

[128] Swaniker F, Soldes O, Hirschl RB. The utility of technetium 99m pertechnetate scintigraphy in the evaluation of patients with Meckel's diverticulum. J Pediatr Surg 1999;34:760–5.

[129] Sfakianakis GN, Conway JJ. Detection of ectopic gastric mucosa in Meckel's diverticulum and in other aberrations by scintigraphy. II. Indications and methods—a 10-year experience. J Nucl Med 1981;22:732–8.

[130] Lee KH, Yeung CK, Tam YH, et al. Laparoscopy for definitive diagnosis and treatment of gastrointestinal bleeding of obscure origin in children. J Pediatr Surg 2000;35:1291–3.

[131] Hamby LS, Fowler CL, Pokorny WJ. Intussusception. In: Donnellan WL, editor. Abdominal surgery of infancy and childhood. Australia: Harwood; 1996. p. 1. 1407–8.

[132] Ein SH, Daneman A, et al. Intussusception. In: Grosfeld JL, O'Neill JA, Coran AG, editors. Pediatric surgery. 6th edition. St. Louis (MO): Mosby; 2006. p. 1313–41.

[133] Kupperman N, O'Dea T, Pinckney L, et al. Predictors of intussusception in young children. Arch Pediatr Adolesc Med 2000;154:250–5.

[134] Buchart GS. Abdominal pain in children: an emergency practitioner's guide. Emerg Med Clin North Am 1989;7:497–517.

[135] Stevenson RJ. Intussusception. In: Rudolph CD, Rudolph AM, Hostetter MK, et al, editors. Rudolph's pediatrics. 21st edition. Ohio (OH): McGraw-Hill; 2002. p. 1407–9.

[136] Nelson KA, Hostetler MA. A listless infant with vomiting. Hosp Physician 2002;38:40–6, www.turner-white.com.

[137] Ein SH, Stephens CA. Intussusception: 354 cases in 10 years. J Pediatr Surg 1971;6:16–27.

[138] Ein SH, Mercer S, Humphry A, et al. Colon perforation during attempted barium enema reduction of intussusception. J Pediatr Surg 1981;16:313–5.

[139] Stringer M, Pablot S, Brereton R. Paediatric intussusception. Br J Surg 1992;79: 867–76.

[140] Valman HB. ABC of 1 to 7: acute abdominal pain. Br Med J (Clin Res Ed) 1981;282: 1858–60.

[141] Sparnon AL, Little KE, Morris LL. Intussusception in childhood: a review of 139 cases. Aust NZ J Surg 1984;54:353–6.

[142] Justice FA, Auldist AW, Bines JE. Intussusception in the clinical presentation and management. J Gastroenterol Hepatol 2006;21:842–6.

[143] Ein SH, Stephens CA, Minor A. The painless intussusception. J Pediatr Surg 1976;11: 563–4.

[144] West KW, Stephens B, Vane DW, et al. Intussusception: current management in infants and children. Surgery 1987;102:704–10.

[145] Ravitch MM, et al. Intussusception. In: Welsh KJ, Randolph JG, Ravitch MM, editors. Pediatric surgery. 4th edition. Chicago: Year Book; 1986. p. 868–82.

[146] Losek JD, Fiete RL. Intussusception and the diagnostic value of testing stool for occult blood. Am J Emerg Med 1991;9:1–3.

[147] Losek DJ. Intussusception: don't miss the diagnosis!. Pediatr Emerg Care 1993;9:46–51.

[148] Gross RE. Intussusception. In: Gross RE, editor. The surgery of infancy and childhood. 1st edition. Philadelphia: WB Saunders; 1953. p. 281–98.

[149] Daneman A, Alton DJ. Intussusception: issues & controversies related to diagnosis and reduction. Radiol Clin North Am 1996;34:743–56.

[150] Littlewood TR, Vogel SA. Intussusception: the paediatric radiologist's perspective. Pediatr Surg Int 1998;14:158–68.

[151] Smith SS, Bonadio WA, Losek JD. The role of abdominal x-rays in the diagnosis and management of intussusception. Pediatr Emerg Care 1992;8:324–7.

[152] Bolin H. Conventional roentgenography in diagnosis of intussusception. Acta Radiol Diagn (Stockh) 1964;2:32–40.

[153] del-Pozo G, Albillos JC, Tejedor D, et al. Intussusception in children: current concepts in diagnosis and enema reduction. Radiographics 1999;19:299–319.

[154] Ratcliffe JF, Fong S, Cheong I, et al. Plain film diagnosis of intussusception. Am J Radiol 1992;158:619–21.

[155] Harrington L, Connolly B, Hu X, et al. Ultrasonography and clinical predictors of intussusception. J Pediatr 1998;132:836–9.

[156] Verschelden P, Filiatrault D, Garel L, et al. Intussusception in children: reliability of US in diagnosis—a prospective study. Radiology 1992;184:741–4.

[157] Daneman A, Navarro O. Intussusception. Part 1: a review of diagnostic approaches. Pediatr Radiol 2003;33:79–85.

[158] Navarro O, Dugougeat F, Kornecki A, et al. The impact of imaging in the management of intussusception owing to pathologic lead points in children. A review of 43 cases. Pediatr Radiol 2000;30:594–603.

[159] Daneman A, Alton DJ, Lobo E. Patterns of recurrence of intussusception in children: a 17-year review. Pediatr Radiol 1998;28:913–9.

[160] Yoon CH, Kim HJ, Goo HW, et al. US-guided pneumatic reduction—initial experience. Radiology 218(1):85–8.

[161] Bryant LR, Trinkle JK, Noonan JA, et al. Appendicitis and appendiceal perforation in neonates. Am Surg 1970;36:523–5.

[162] Parsons JM, Miscall BG, McSherry CK. Appendicitis in the newborn infant. Surgery 1970; 67:841–3.

[163] Schorlemner GH, Herbst CA. Perforated neonatal appendicitis. South Med J 1983;76: 536–7.

[164] Bax NM, Pearse RG, Dommering N, et al. Perforation of the appendix in the neonatal period. J Pediatr Surg 1980;15:200–2.

[165] Bartlett RH, Eraklis AJ, Wilkerson RH. Appendicitis in infancy. Surg Gynecol Obstet 1970;130:99–104.

[166] Gryboski J, Walker WA. The colon, rectum and anus. In: Gryboski J, Walker WA, editors. Gastrointestinal problems in the infant. Philadelphia: WB Saunders; 1983. p. 511–3.

[167] Rappaport WD, Petersen M, Stanton C. Factors responsible for the high perforation rate seen in early childhood appendicitis. Am Surg 1989;55:602–5.

[168] Grossfeld JL, Weinburger M, Clatworthy HW. Acute appendicitis in the first two years of life. J Pediatr Surg 1973;8:285–93.

[169] Lin YL, Lee CH. Appendicitis in infancy. Pediatr Surg Int 2002;19:1–3.

[170] Morrow SE, Newman KD. Current management of appendicitis. Semin Pediatr Surg 2007; 16:34–40.

[171] Horwitz JR, Gursoy M, Jaksic T, et al. Importance of diarrhea as a presenting symptom of appendicitis in very young children. Am J Surg 1997;173:80–2.

[172] Buntain WL, Krempe RE, Kraft JW. Neonatal appendicitis. Ala J Med Sci 1984;21:295–8.

[173] Puri P, O'Donnell B. Appendicitis in infancy. J Pediatr Surg 1978;13:173–4.

[174] Barker AP, Davey RB. Appendicitis in the first three years of life. Aust N Z J Surg 1988;58: 491–4.

[175] Williams H. Appendicitis in infancy. BMJ 1947;2:730.

[176] Jabra AA, Shalaby-Rana EI, Fishman EK. CT of appendicitis in children. J Comput Assist Tomogr 1997;21:661–6.

[177] Friedland JA, Siegel MJ. CT appearance of acute appendicitis in children. AJR Am J Roentgenol 1997;168:439–42.

[178] Donnelly LF, Emery KH, Brody AS, et al. Minimizing radiation dose for pediatric body application of single-detector helical CT: strategies at a large children's hospital. AJR Am J Roentgenol 2001;176:303–6.

[179] The ALARA (as low as reasonably achievable) concept in pediatric CT intelligent dose reduction. Multidisciplinary conference organized by the Society of Pediatric Radiology. Pediatr Radiol 2002;32:217–313.

[180] Brenner DJ. Estimating cancer risks from pediatric CT: going from the qualitative to the quantitative. Pediatr Radiol 2002;32:228–31.

[181] Hall EJ. Lessons we have learned from our children: cancer risks from diagnostic radiology. Pediatr Radiol 2002;32:700–6.

[182] Mettler FA, Wiest PW, Locken JA, et al. CT scanning: patterns of use and dose. J Radiol Prot 2000;20:353–9.

[183] Schulte B, Beyer D, Kaiser C, et al. Ultrasonography in suspected acute appendicitis in childhood—report of 1285 cases. Eur J Ultrasound 1998;8:177–82.

[184] Sivit CJ, Siegel MJ, Applegate KE, et al. When appendicitis is suspected in children. Radiographics 2001;21:247–62.

[185] Hahn HB, Hoepner FU, Kalle T, et al. Sonography of acute appendicitis in children: 7 years experience. Pediatr Radiol 1998;28:147–51.

[186] Partrick DA, Janik JE, Janik JS, et al. Increased CT scan utilization does not improve the diagnostic accuracy of appendicitis in children. J Pediatr Surg 2003;39:659–62.

[187] Kosloske AM, Love CL, Rohrer JE, et al. The diagnosis of appendicitis in children: outcome of a strategy based on pediatric surgical evaluation. Pediatrics 2004;113:29–34.

[188] Rice HE, Arbesman M, Martin DJ, et al. Does early ultrasonography affect management of pediatric appendicitis? A prospective analysis. J Pediatr Surg 1999;34:754–9.

[189] Peña BM, Taylor GA, Fishman SJ, et al. Costs and effectiveness of ultrasonography and limited computed tomography for diagnosing appendicitis in children. Pediatrics 2000; 106:672–6.

ELSEVIER
SAUNDERS

Emerg Med Clin N Am
25 (2007) 1041–1060

EMERGENCY
MEDICINE
CLINICS OF
NORTH AMERICA

Metabolic Emergencies

Kenneth T. Kwon, MD, RDMS, FACEP, FAAP[a,b,*],
Virginia W. Tsai, MD[a]

[a]Department of Emergency Medicine, University of California, Irvine School of Medicine,
Route 128, 101 The City Drive South, Orange, CA 92868, USA
[b]Pediatric Emergency Services, Mission Regional Medical Center/Children's Hospital
of Orange County at Mission, 27700 Medical Center Road, Mission Viejo, CA 92691, USA

Children with metabolic disturbances frequently present with symptoms similar to those with other emergencies, particularly in the newborn period and early infancy. Initial consideration of a metabolic disease in the differential diagnosis is important, especially in previously healthy neonates with acute deterioration. Metabolic disorders, either acquired or congenital, comprise a variety of entities which cause derangement in normal physiology and metabolism. These disorders may include diseases related to electrolyte imbalances, endocrine dysfunction, or inborn errors of metabolism. Although some use the term metabolic disorder only in relation to inherited inborn errors as first described by Garrod in 1902, this article focuses on pediatric metabolic disorders in the general sense.

Metabolic diseases can vary as much in clinical presentation as they can in classification. Because the symptomatology of these disorders is also associated with a variety of non-metabolic diseases, many metabolic conditions are missed in the emergency department. A definitive diagnosis is frequently not possible or necessary during the emergency department course, but proper initial management based on the probable diagnosis can be life-saving or reduce neurologic sequelae. Disorders which are responsive to emergency department treatment are highlighted herein.

Infants with metabolic disorders frequently present with nonspecific symptoms similarly seen in other infectious, neurologic, and toxicologic emergencies. Differences in presentation can be subtle, especially in the neonatal period. Vomiting, alterations in neurologic status, and feeding difficulties are perhaps the most prominent features of metabolic diseases.

* Corresponding author. Department of Emergency Medicine, University of California, Irvine School of Medicine, Route 128, 101 The City Drive South, Orange, CA 92868.
E-mail address: kwonk@uci.edu (K.T. Kwon).

0733-8627/07/$ - see front matter © 2007 Elsevier Inc. All rights reserved.
doi:10.1016/j.emc.2007.07.009   *emed.theclinics.com*

Characteristic clinical manifestations of specific disorders are discussed in the following sections.

Hypoglycemia

Hypoglycemia is one of the most commonly encountered metabolic problems, especially in the neonatal period. The definition of hypoglycemia is somewhat controversial and age dependent. In children, infants, and term neonates older than 1 to 2 days of life, hypoglycemia is usually defined as a serum glucose concentration less than 40 to 45 mg/dL [1,2]. In term and premature neonates within 1 day of life, levels as low as 30 mg/dL are considered by some to be normal. The laboratory value should be interpreted in the context of the clinical presentation, because symptoms may occur within a continuum of low glucose levels. Glucose levels of 50 to 60 mg/dL with symptoms of hypoglycemia may warrant treatment.

Glucose is the main energy substrate for the brain, and its levels represent a balance between exogenous supply and endogenous gluconeogenesis and glycogenolysis. Mobilization and use of glucose is mediated by hormones, primarily insulin. Insulin stimulates glucose uptake in cells and glycogen synthesis, and its actions are opposed by epinephrine, glucagon, cortisol, and growth hormone. Hypoglycemia can occur when imbalances exist between exogenous and endogenous substrate supply which may involve these hormonal abnormalities. Causes of hypoglycemia in the pediatric population are listed in Box 1. Important etiologies in the emergency department include infection, adrenal insufficiency, inborn errors, and medication-induced causes. Hyperinsulinemia, particularly persistent hyperinsulinemic hypoglycemia of infancy, should be considered as a potential cause of intractable hypoglycemia from the newborn period to 6 months of age.

Symptoms of hypoglycemia generally fall into two categories: (1) those associated with activation of the autonomic nervous system (adrenergic), and (2) those associated with decreased cerebral glucose use (neuroglycopenic). Adrenergic symptoms are usually seen early with a rapid decline in blood glucose and include tachycardia, tachypnea, vomiting, and diaphoresis. Because most of these patients are hypoglycemic before arrival to the emergency department, these symptoms are frequently absent. More familiar are the neuroglycopenic symptoms, which are usually associated with slower or prolonged hypoglycemia. These symptoms include poor feeding, altered mental status, lethargy, and seizures. These classic symptoms are usually evident in older children and adults; in infants, the presentation may be subtle and include only hypotonia, hypothermia, jitteriness, exaggerated primitive reflexes, or feeding difficulties.

Early detection of hypoglycemia is critical because permanent brain damage may begin shortly after symptoms develop, particularly in newborns and infants. Bedside glucose testing should be performed on all

---

Box 1. Causes of hypoglycemia

Decreased production/availability of glucose
Low glycogen stores
    Small for gestational age, prematurity
Malnutrition/fasting
Malabsorption/diarrhea

Increased use of glucose
Hyperinsulinemic states
    Infant of diabetic mother
    Persistent hyperinsulinemic hypoglycemia of infancy
        Nesidioblastosis
        Islet cell adenoma/hyperplasia
    Beckwith-Wiedemann syndrome
Stress
    Infection/sepsis

Combined or other mechanism
Inborn errors of metabolism
Hormone deficiency
    Adrenal (glucocorticoid) insufficiency
    Growth hormone deficiency
    Glucagon deficiency
Iatrogenic
    Insulin/oral hypoglycemic therapy
    Poisoning (ethanol, propanolol, salicylates)
    Reye's syndrome

---

pediatric patients who appear seriously ill or altered. Hypoglycemia occurring in children requiring resuscitation care is associated with increased mortality [3].

Acute treatment for hypoglycemia begins with intravenous glucose bolus replacement. The recommended dose ranges from 0.2 to 1 g/kg; a midlevel range of 0.4 to 0.5 g/kg glucose translates to approximately 4 mL/kg of 10% dextrose or 2 mL/kg of 25% dextrose. Some advocate a smaller bolus of 0.2 g/kg (2 mL/kg of 10% dextrose) to minimize hyperglycemia and resultant insulin secretion and possible prolonged hypoglycemia [4]. Generally, a 10% solution is used in neonates and infants, whereas a 25% solution is used in toddlers and children. More dilute solutions are used in younger patients to minimize vascular injury caused by more concentrated fluids. Continuous glucose infusion should follow bolus administration to maintain normal glucose homeostasis, especially in neonates. The normal glucose requirement in a neonate is 6 to 10 mg/kg/min, which is roughly equivalent to an infusion of 10% dextrose-containing solution at 1.5 times the maintenance rate. Glucose levels should be rechecked frequently (every 1–2 hours) and the infusion rate adjusted accordingly.

If hypoglycemia persists despite boluses and infusions, a hyperinsulinemic state should be considered. Glucagon, 0.1 to 0.2 mg/kg (up to 1 mg) parenterally, can be given to infants for refractory hypoglycemia. Because it can be given intramuscularly, glucagon can be particularly helpful when intravenous access is difficult or delayed. Glucagon will not be effective in patients lacking adequate glycogen stores, such as those with inherited storage diseases [5]. Hydrocortisone, 2 to 3 mg/kg or 25 to 50 mg/m^2, can also be considered for refractory hypoglycemia [6].

Hyperglycemia and diabetic ketoacidosis

Hyperglycemia is typically defined as a glucose concentration of greater than 125 to 150 mg/dL. It is often seen in critically ill, non-diabetic patients of all ages and can signify increased mortality. Hyperglycemia is frequently seen in the first week of life and is inversely correlated to gestational age, with up to 18 times greater occurrence in neonates with birth weights less than 1000 g [7,8]. It is also seen in infants who are acutely stressed or septic, receiving high rates of glucose infusion, or being treated with corticosteroids or other drugs. In non-iatrogenic conditions, hyperglycemia is a consequence of physiologic stress and increased levels of counterregulatory hormones including glucagon, catecholamines, cortisol, and growth hormones. Mechanisms of hyperglycemia include immaturity in the neonatal period, absolute or relative insulin insufficiency, and hepatic and peripheral insulin resistance. Owing to their small mass of insulin-dependent tissue, namely, muscle and fat, infants have limited glucose use when compared with larger children and adults [7,8]. The greatest risk of hyperglycemia is dehydration secondary to the resulting urinary loss of glucose and osmotic diuresis. The hyperosmolarity and osmotic shifts that occur can increase the risk of cerebral bleeding due to brain cell dehydration, dilation of capillaries, and an inability to autoregulate cerebral blood pressure. It is unknown whether infants with stress-induced hyperglycemia are at risk for later development of diabetes mellitus [9,10].

Insulin-dependent diabetes mellitus (IDDM) diagnosed in the newborn or during the first 6 months of life is extremely rare, affecting approximately 1 in 500,000 births [7,8]. More common is a temporary form called transient neonatal diabetes mellitus. It resembles permanent diabetes mellitus but resolves within several weeks or months. Patients affected with the transient form during infancy may have diabetes mellitus recur later in life [8]. The ultimate cause of neonatal diabetes remains unclear; however, many theories have related to immature metabolic pathways. Most children studied do have a low birth weight for gestational age, with some full-term infants weighing less than 1500 g. Other possible associations include short-term maternal enterovirus infection, autoimmune enterocolitis, congenital absence of the islet of Langerhans, rare genetic disorders, and pancreatic agenesis [7–9]. Patients in whom IDDM develops after the first 180 days of life have genetic profiles and a clinical course similar to patients in whom IDDM develops later in life [8].

Diagnosing IDDM in the young infant can be difficult for obvious reasons. Polydipsia cannot be communicated by the nonverbal infant, new absorbent diapers may mask polyuria, and oral rehydration may conceal acute weight loss. Recurrent cutaneous candidiasis, although common in infants, can be considered an indication for the clinician to check blood glucose levels [9–11]. Infants are often misdiagnosed with pneumonia, asthma, or bronchiolitis and undergo treatment with corticosteroids that will only aggravate the metabolic derangements of IDDM. These difficulties help explain why the younger the patient presents with IDDM, the more likely they will present with severe decompensation, including acidosis, obtundation, and possibly cerebral edema [9].

Diabetic ketoacidosis (DKA) is defined as a glucose level greater than 200 mg/dL with either a bicarbonate level less than 15 mEq/L or a venous pH less than 7.3. It is more difficult to recognize and treat in younger patients for several reasons. The higher basal metabolic rate and larger surface area to body mass ratio in infants require stricter amounts of fluid and electrolyte repletion. The smaller patient is also at greater risk for cerebral edema owing to the immaturity of autoregulatory mechanisms. Cerebral edema is thought to occur in about 0.5% to 1% of all children with DKA and is the most likely cause of morbidity, with death in 20% to 25% of these patients and pituitary insufficiency in 10% to 25% of survivors [9,11–13]. Other causes of mortality in infants with DKA include concomitant pneumonia, sepsis, pulmonary edema, and cardiac arrhythmias associated with electrolyte imbalances.

The pathophysiology of DKA can be condensed to a blend of insulin deficiency and antagonism during physiologic stress with the actions of counterregulatory hormones. Increased glucose production from glycogenolysis and gluconeogenesis coupled with the incapacity to use glucose lead to hyperglycemia, osmotic diuresis, loss of electrolytes, hyperosmolarity, and dehydration. This vicious cycle occurs concurrently with lipolysis as the body senses a starvation mode and enters oxidative metabolism with resultant ketone (beta-hydroxybutyrate) formation and metabolic acidosis. Lactic acid also contributes to the acidosis as tissues undergo anaerobic metabolism with inadequate perfusion. Clinically, the infant will most likely present with vomiting, lethargy or frank coma, polyuria, deep Kussmaul's respirations, and severe dehydration. DKA can be categorized as mild with a venous pH of 7.2 to 7.3, moderate with a venous pH of 7.1 to 7.2, and severe with a venous pH less than 7.1.

Assessment starts with the suspicion of DKA if the young infant did not previously carry the diagnosis of diabetes. Clinical examination should focus on volume status as well as a search for a source of infection, although this may not be the precipitating cause in first time presentations. The patient should be carefully weighed and measured for accurate fluid therapy calculations. Previously known weights should not be used because the patient may have sustained an unnoticed amount of weight loss. Airway protection with intubation may be necessary in the unresponsive infant or with impending respiratory failure. Care must be taken to set the respiratory rate on the ventilator to match the infant's previous natural rate to compensate for the metabolic acidosis; however, aggressive hyperventilation (to P_{CO2} <22) is associated with poorer neurologic outcomes and is not recommended [9,11,12]. Initial diagnostic tests should include blood draws for serum electrolyte levels, glucose, osmolality, pH, complete blood count, beta-hydroxybutyrate and acetone levels, and blood cultures. Blood gases from venous or capillary origin are generally regarded as acceptable in non-intubated and well-perfused infants [14,15]. Catheterized urinalysis and culture should also be performed. An electrocardiogram can be obtained as a rapid way to assess the potassium level. Pseudohyponatremia is usually seen from the dilutional effect of hyperglycemia. Leukocytosis may be from a stress response rather than an underlying infection.

Initial management should focus on rapid expansion of the intravascular volume and improvement of acidosis, the two life-threatening circumstances; however, rapid fluid administration to improve glomerular filtration must be carefully monitored to avoid excessive hydration and augmenting the possibility of cerebral edema. Approximately, a 10% fluid deficit in infants with DKA can be assumed. Isotonic solutions of 0.9% saline or Ringer's lactate can be used with a volume of 10 to 20 mL/kg over 1 to 2 hours. If the infant remains severely dehydrated or hypotensive, this volume can be repeated. Once adequate intravascular volume is obtained, the remaining fluid deficit can be restored over the next 24 to 48 hours depending on the degree of initial hyperosmolality. The first 4 to 6 hours of replacing fluid deficit can be done with 0.9% normal saline or Ringer's lactate. Subsequent volumes should be replaced with a fluid of tonicity greater than 0.45% saline and added potassium or phosphate, provided that urine output is adequate [9].

Insulin therapy is key to resolving DKA and halting lipolysis and ketone generation. Insulin infusion should begin after the initial fluid bolus, about 1 to 2 hours after the start of resuscitation. Only intravenous routes should be considered, because subcutaneous and intramuscular absorption is irregular or inadequate in the dehydrated patient. Insulin bolus is not recommended in the pediatric population, because extensive evidence demonstrates this may exacerbate the risk of cerebral edema by dropping blood glucose levels too quickly. The dose of insulin should be 0.1 U/kg/h (or as low as 0.05 U/kg/h in some infants) with the rate of infusion adjusted to achieve a fall in blood glucose of about 50 to 90 mg/dL per hour. Once the blood glucose level falls to about 300 mg/dL, glucose should be added to the intravenous solution. As long as acidosis is present, insulin infusion should continue with the amount of added glucose adjusted to maintain levels between 150 and 200 mg/dL. Once acidosis has resolved and the patient can tolerate oral intake, subcutaneous insulin can be initiated, usually 1 to 2 hours before insulin infusion is discontinued. The dose for subcutaneous insulin is 0.25 U/kg [9,10].

DKA patients generally experience a potassium deficit of about 3 to 6 mEq/kg. Most of the potassium deficit is intracellular as the acidosis, lipolysis, hypertonicity, and glycogenolysis promote a general efflux of potassium out of cells. Extracorporeal losses through vomiting and urinary diuresis also contribute to total body potassium deficit. At presentation of DKA, the extracellular potassium level that is measured may be decreased, normal, or increased. Once insulin therapy is begun and acidosis is improved, potassium is forced back into cells, which may cause a precipitous drop in potassium levels and lead to cardiac arrhythmias. As a general guideline, potassium replacement is necessary early in treatment. If the potassium level is greater than 4 mEq/L, 40 mEq/L of potassium is added to the intravenous fluids after vascular competency and urine output are restored. If the initial potassium level is less than 4 mEq/L, replacement should be started after the fluid bolus and before insulin therapy. Should laboratory values be delayed, the electrocardiogram and cardiac monitor can serve as a way to estimate potassium levels. Potassium phosphate combined with potassium chloride or acetate can be used with the maximum infusion rate at 0.5 mEq/kg/h.

Phosphate depletion due to osmotic diuresis can also be expected in DKA patients, but the benefit of phosphate replacement is unclear. Although a few studies have not demonstrated a clinical benefit to phosphate repletion, severe hypophosphatemia exhibited by muscle weakness can be treated through supplementation. Calcium levels may decline, and phosphate infusion should be terminated if hypocalcemia occurs. Potassium phosphate has been shown to be safe for use with close observation of calcium levels [9].

Bicarbonate therapy in DKA and other acidotic states is discussed in the section on metabolic acidosis. Generally, bicarbonate is not recommended, because the acidosis should self-correct during fluid resuscitation and insulin therapy. Some advocate its use in DKA with a pH less than 6.9 or significant hyperkalemia or arrhythmias. The American Diabetic Association recommends consideration of bicarbonate in the pediatric patient if the pH remains less than 7.0 after the first hour of hydration [16]. If given for DKA, bicarbonate can be mixed as an isotonic solution (2 ampules of sodium bicarbonate in 0.45% normal saline) and given over 1 hour.

These treatment guidelines have been based on concerns of how to best avoid the development or worsening of cerebral edema. The pathophysiology of cerebral edema is not well described, but DKA and its treatment have both been implicated. Perhaps the most common theory involves fluid entry into the brain due to a rapid drop in serum osmolality concomitant with vigorous fluid resuscitation. One should not infuse more than 50 mL/kg over the first 4 hours of treatment because higher volumes have been associated with an increased risk of cerebral edema [13]. Recent studies also suggest a vasogenic, rather than cytotoxic, mechanism of cerebral edema [9,12,13]. Patients who are at greatest risk for cerebral edema tend to be those who present with extreme acidosis, have high levels of blood urea nitrogen, and hypocapnia. Cerebral edema can be present before the initiation of therapy or within 4 to 24 hours after treatment [9,11–13]. Radiographic imaging can be normal early on with later signs of focal or diffuse edema, hemorrhage, or infarction. Cerebral edema should be suspected in infants with persistent vomiting, bradycardia, hypertension, labile oxygen saturation, irritability, lethargy, or in the presence of neurologic findings. Treating cerebral edema has been attempted with mannitol (0.25–1.0 g/kg) or hypertonic saline (3%) given 5 to 10 mL/kg over a period of 30 minutes. Hyperventilation in intubated patients should not be beyond the patient's physiologic tendency.

Hyponatremia

Although not as common as hypoglycemia in the emergency department, hyponatremia is one of the most common electrolyte abnormalities in hospitalized children [17]. Hyponatremia can be caused by salt-losing states, such as vomiting or diarrhea, diuretic excess, and adrenal insufficiency, or by excess total body water states such as the infection-induced syndrome of inappropriate secretion of antidiuretic hormone (SIADH), nephrotic syndrome, and cirrhosis. Factitious, or pseudohyponatremia, can occur with hyperglycemia, hyperlipidemia, or hyperproteinemia. In infants, hyponatremia is commonly due to excess gastrointestinal loss from prolonged vomiting or diarrhea, or from inappropriately diluted formulas. Pyridoxine-dependent seizures are a rare cause of intractable seizures in neonates.

Hyponatremia is typically defined as a serum sodium level less than 125 to130 mEq/L, although clinical symptoms are not usually seen until serum sodium falls below 120 mEq/L. Manifestations include altered mental status, lethargy, vomiting, diarrhea, seizures, and circulatory collapse. Vomiting can be a cause and manifestation of hyponatremia. The presence of symptoms is dependent in part on the rate of change in serum sodium. A gradual or chronic progression of hyponatremia may not become clinically evident even at levels below 110 mEq/L. Conversely, less severe hyponatremia may be symptomatic if the decline in serum sodium is rapid.

Treatment should be geared toward the underlying cause. Aggressive treatment with 3% hypertonic saline (514 mL/kg) should only be initiated if significant symptoms are present, such as seizures or coma. A dose of

5 mL/kg over 10 to 15 minutes should raise the sodium level by approximately 5 mEq/L; smaller additional doses of 2 to 3 mL/kg can be considered if there is no clinical improvement. The exact sodium deficit can be calculated as follows: mEq Na^+ needed $= 0.6 \times$ weight (kg) $\times$ (Na^+ desired $- Na^+$ measured). Acute correction to a level of 125 mEq/L should alleviate symptoms in most cases. After acute correction for symptoms, the goal is to raise the sodium level slowly at a rate of 0.5 mEq/L per hour (maximum, 12 mEq/L per day) by using 0.9% normal saline infusion. If SIADH is suspected, one should consider fluid restriction to two-thirds maintenance and administration of furosemide, 1 to 2 mg/kg. Pyridoxine, 100 mg intravenously, should be considered for neonates with intractable seizures of unclear etiology [18].

Central pontine myelinolysis is a potential complication of hypertonic saline use, although it has been less well described in children than adults [17]. This observation may reflect the fact that hyponatremia in the pediatric population tends to occur acutely rather than chronically, and most cases of central pontine myelinolysis after a rapid rise of sodium are described in a setting of chronic hyponatremia. Infants can apparently tolerate rapid and large increases in sodium levels without sequelae.

Metabolic acidosis

Metabolic acidosis occurs via three major mechanisms: (1) loss of bicarbonate from the kidney or gastrointestinal tract, (2) excess acid from endogenous production or an exogenous source, or (3) underexcretion of acid by the kidneys. Neonates and infants are more susceptible than are older children to acidosis owing to their lower renal threshold for bicarbonate reabsorption and limited maximum net acid excretion. Young infants have a relatively limited compensatory mechanism for an excess acid load.

The presence of metabolic acidosis has important diagnostic considerations depending on the classification of acidosis as a normal anion gap or increased anion gap. The anion gap is calculated as the difference between serum sodium and the sum of serum chloride and bicarbonate [$Na^+ - (Cl^- + HCO_3^-)$]. A normal anion gap range is somewhat age dependent but in children is 12 ± 4, and an anion gap of greater than 16 is considered elevated. Causes of metabolic acidosis based on the anion gap are listed in Box 2. Lactic acidosis is the most common cause of an increased anion gap acidosis in critically ill neonates [19].

Clinical manifestations of metabolic acidosis are nonspecific and include altered mental status, vomiting, respiratory distress, and poor perfusion. An important sign, particularly in infants, that can alert the emergency department physician of metabolic acidosis is tachypnea, a compensatory mechanism creating a respiratory alkalotic response. This breathing can range from mild shallow tachypnea to deep Kussmaul respirations of severely acidotic patients.

Box 2. Causes of metabolic acidosis

Normal anion gap
Gastroenteritis/diarrhea
Renal tubular acidosis
Adrenal (mineralocorticoid) insufficiency

Increased anion gap
MUDPILES
    Methanol, uremia, DKA, paraldehyde, iron or isoniazid, lactic
      acidosis, ethylene glycol, salicylates
Inborn errors
    Carbohydrate, amino acid, or fatty acid metabolism
Starvation
Chronic renal insufficiency

Treatment is focused toward appropriate fluid resuscitation and specific therapy for the underlying cause of the acid-base disturbance. The use of sodium bicarbonate is controversial. Most clinicians would only recommend it if an inborn error is suspected or if the metabolic acidosis is causing significant arrhythmias or hemodynamic instability. Some advocate its use in DKA with a pH less than 6.9 or significant hyperkalemia or arrhythmias, or in non-DKA metabolic acidosis with a pH less than 7.1 refractory to other treatments. The dose of sodium bicarbonate is 1 to 2 mEq/kg given intravenously. Bicarbonate potentially improves cardiac output and blood pressure, but these benefits are thought to be only transient in neonates [20]. Bicarbonate therapy is potentially harmful because it shifts the oxygen-hemoglobin dissociation curve to the left and can worsen tissue hypoxia, particularly in hypovolemic patients. It can also cause hypernatremia, hypokalemia, and a paradoxical drop in central nervous system pH leading to decreased consciousness. A 5% albumin infusion in neonates has been shown to be less effective than bicarbonate in correcting metabolic acidosis [21].

Adrenal insufficiency

Adrenal insufficiency is due to primary adrenal disease or secondary to pituitary suppression and can be inherited or acquired. Congenital adrenal hyperplasia (CAH) is an important cause of primary adrenal insufficiency in the newborn period, whereas Addison's disease is a more common etiology in children and adolescents. Secondary adrenal insufficiency is more common in older children and almost always involves exogenous steroid use for a chronic disease with subsequent discontinuation. Acute adrenal insufficiency or crisis occurs when the adrenal glands fail to produce adequate glucocorticoid and mineralocorticoid in response to stress. The common emergency department presentation involves a newborn male with an uneventful birth history who presents within the first 2 weeks of life with apparent dehydration or sepsis and circulatory collapse unresponsive to fluid resuscitation.

The term *congenital adrenal hyperplasia* refers to a group of inherited autosomal recessive disorders with defects in adrenal biosynthesis of the glucocorticoid cortisol. The low cortisol production stimulates pituitary production of ACTH which causes the characteristic hyperplasia of the adrenal cortex. Depending on the affected enzyme, the synthesis of other steroids such as mineralocorticoids (aldosterone) and androgens may also be affected, and the clinical expression will vary depending on the accumulated biosynthetic precursors. Deficiency of 21-hydroxylase accounts for up to 95% of CAH cases, and the discussion herein is limited to this particular form of CAH. This disorder occurs in 1 in 10,000 to 15,000 live births worldwide [22]. Up to 75% of affected newborns have the classic salt-losing virilizing variant, which is associated with aldosterone deficiency and androgen overproduction (17-hydroxyprogesterone); up to 25% have the non–salt-losing simple virilizing type. The degree of virilization and other clinical signs are usually more pronounced and seen earlier in life in the salt-losing variant.

Many states now screen newborns for CAH; however, these results may not be available for several weeks, allowing for an acute adrenal crisis to occur during this time. Males are particularly prone to missed diagnosis because their genitalia may appear normal at birth. Females usually exhibit some degree of ambiguous genitalia, such as clitoral enlargement or fusion of the labial folds. Another physical examination sign is hyperpigmentation, which may be present in the axilla and scrotal/labial areas and is due to the accumulation of a corticotropin precursor that stimulates melanocytes. With the classic salt-losing type, symptoms may begin 1 to 2 weeks after birth and include weight loss, poor feeding, vomiting, polyuria, and dehydration. Progression can occur rapidly, particularly in the setting of infection or trauma, to altered mental status, hypotension, or death.

Acute adrenal insufficiency, whether acquired or from CAH, is associated with hyponatremia, hyperkalemia, and hypoglycemia. A normal anion gap metabolic acidosis is often seen due to aldosterone deficiency. Unexplained hypotension unresponsive to intravenous fluids is another sign of steroid deficiency. Treatment should be geared toward aggressive fluid resuscitation and rapid stress doses of corticosteroids. Before treatment, if possible, blood should be collected for non-emergent testing of specific endocrine hormones and metabolites.

Acute adrenal insufficiency is treated with stress doses of corticosteroids. Table 1 lists various options. Hydrocortisone is the steroid of choice because it has equal glucocorticoid and mineralocorticoid effects; cortisone is an

Table 1
Corticosteroids for adrenal insufficiency

Drug	Dose	Potency effect (per mg)	
		Glucocorticoid	Mineralocorticoid
Glucocorticoid			
Hydrocortisone	25–50 mg/m^2 IV/IM	1	1
	Infant: 25 mg		
	Child: 50 mg		
	Teen: 75 mg		
Cortisone	1 mg/kg IM	0.8	1
Dexamethasone	0.1–0.2 mg/kg IV/IM	40	None
Mineralocorticoid			
Fludrocortisone	0.1 mg PO daily	15	400

Abbreviations: IV/IM, intravenous/intramuscular; PO, by mouth.

alternative but cannot be given intravenously. The stress parenteral dose of hydrocortisone is 25 to 50 mg/m^2 (approximately 2–3 mg/kg), followed by 100 mg/m^2/d in divided doses. The typical dose in a neonate or young infant is 25 mg. Dexamethasone has no mineralocorticoid effect but is advocated by some over hydrocortisone in normotensive patients with an unconfirmed diagnosis owing to its noninterference with diagnostic ACTH stimulation testing. An oral mineralocorticoid such as fludrocortisone can be started after initial stabilization with intravenous fluids and glucocorticoids. Hyperkalemia should correct with fluids and steroid therapy and rarely needs individual correction, because neonates can tolerate elevated potassium levels better than children and adults.

Inborn errors of metabolism

This diverse group of hereditary disorders involves gene mutations, usually of a single enzyme or transport system, causing significant blocks in metabolic pathways and accumulation or deficiency of a particular metabolite. Due to the large number and complexity of inborn errors of metabolism (IEMs), the reported incidence of these disorders varies greatly, ranging from 1 in 1400 to 200,000 live births [23,24]. It is now possible to screen for many of these defects in the newborn as well as prenatal periods. Some IEMs manifest clinically in the newborn period or shortly thereafter, and failure of early diagnosis may lead to permanent neurologic sequelae and death if specific treatment is not initiated. Although collectively numerous, IEMs that are amenable to specific emergency medications are limited; however, the majority of them should respond to removal of the offending metabolite from the diet. The most common emergent clinical manifestations in the neonatal period include vomiting, neurologic abnormalities, metabolic acidosis, and hypoglycemia [25,26]. These nonspecific findings can mimic other disorders, such as sepsis or adrenal crisis, but an IEM should be considered in a previously normal neonate with acute clinical deterioration. Conversely, the presence of infection does not exclude the possibility of IEMs, because these patients frequently deteriorate and become septic quickly. Standard laboratory values, particularly blood ammonia, electrolytes, and urinalysis can be helpful in further classifying the IEM and tailoring treatment in the emergency department (Fig. 1).

IEMs can be divided into disorders of amino acid metabolism (phenylketonuria, nonketotic hyperglycinemia), fatty acid oxidation/metabolism (medium-chain acyl-CoA dehydrogenase deficiency, primary carnitine deficiency), energy metabolism (primary lactic acidemias), and carbohydrate metabolism (glycogen storage diseases, galactosemia). Organic acidemias and acidurias (methylmalonic, propionic, and isovaleric acidemias, maple syrup urine disease) refer to a specific group of disorders of amino and fatty acid metabolism in which high levels of non-amino organic acids accumulate in serum and urine.

Many patients with IEMs exhibit symptoms as newborns after feedings have been initiated, but a minority may go undetected into childhood with only psychomotor delay until a stressor causes acute deterioration. Recurrent vomiting, dehydration, and acute metabolic encephalopathy are common clinical manifestations. Neurologic symptoms can range from hypotonia to seizures to frank coma. Intractable seizures are characteristic of nonketotic hyperglycinemia and pyridoxine-dependent seizures. Hepatomegaly is a common finding on physical examination and can be

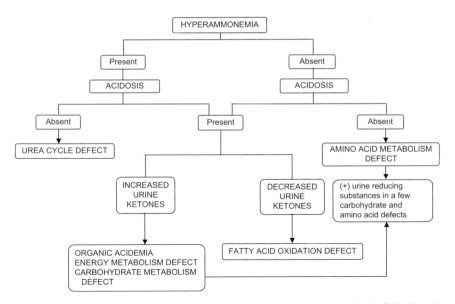

Fig. 1. Diagnostic pathway for inborn errors. (*Modified from* Brousseau T, Sharieff G. The critically ill newborn. Critical Decisions in Emergency Medicine 2003;18:5; with permission.)

pronounced in glycogen storage diseases and galactosemia, although it tends to be less evident in infancy. The risk of infection, particularly *Escherichia coli* sepsis, and liver failure are also increased in patients with galactosemia. A peculiar odor in body fluids can be associated with specific disorders and may offer an invaluable aid to diagnosis when present. Maple syrup urine disease is named for its characteristic sweet sugar odor, isovaleric acidemia is associated with a "sweaty feet" scent, and methylmalonic and propionic acidemias can exude a fruity ketotic odor similar to that of diabetic ketoacidosis. Metabolic acidosis with an increased anion gap is common in many IEMs and can aid in further classification. Hypoglycemia is also common and can be pronounced, particularly in glycogen storage diseases and defects of fatty acid oxidation [27]. Hyperammonemia is most commonly seen in organic acidemias and urea cycle defects.

Urea cycle defects are a specific classification of IEMs which lead to hyperammonemia due to the inability to detoxify ammonia to urea. Common disorders include ornithine transcarbamylase deficiency, arginase deficiency (argininemia), and argininosuccinic acid synthetase deficiency (citrullinemia). Clinical manifestations parallel those seen in other IEMs. Neonates frequently present after a few days of protein feeding of either breast milk or formula. Symptoms include vomiting, poor feeding, and post-prandial neurologic alterations. Older infants and children may present with recurrent vomiting, ataxia, or developmental delay. Tachypnea is common due to stimulation of the respiratory center by ammonia. The level of hyperammonemia tends to be higher than that seen in organic acidemias. Blood ammonia is usually above 200 µmol/L (normal, <35–50 µmol/L), with some complete enzyme defects reaching levels greater than 500 to 1000 µmol/L [28,29]. Although sicker infants tend to have higher ammonia levels, no strict correlation exists between ammonia levels and clinical findings. The degree of neurologic impairment is thought to be related more to the duration of hyperammonemia rather than the level itself. Blood urea nitrogen is usually low, but a normal level does not exclude a urea cycle defect. Metabolic acidosis does not occur with these disorders unless they are associated with a concurrent dehydrating illness. The lack of acidosis is helpful in differentiating urea cycle defects from many of the other IEMs.

Treatment for IEMs consists of general measures as well as specific medications if a probable type of IEM is suspected. Unless the infant has a known IEM and is already on a special formula, all dietary intake should be withheld and feedings reintroduced after consultation with a specialist. Intravenous fluid containing dextrose may be indicated, particularly if a urea cycle defect is suspected, because stimulating endogenous insulin will minimize protein catabolism and ammonia production. After appropriate fluid boluses of normal saline to correct shock, most IEMs can be managed with a standard intravenous fluid consisting of 10% dextrose in one-fourth normal saline at 1.5 times maintenance. Metabolic acidosis unresponsive to intravenous fluids should be treated with sodium bicarbonate boluses of

1 to 2 mEq/kg. Although controversial for other diseases, bicarbonate use for IEMs is indicated, but standard calculations of bicarbonate requirements will underestimate actual needs owing to ongoing production of acidic metabolites [28,30]. Correction of severe acidosis will often require large doses of bicarbonate, up to 20 mEq/kg in some organic acidemias [31]. Liberal use of bicarbonate should be performed in consultation with a metabolic specialist. The rapid removal of toxins may be life-saving in some cases, particularly with severe hyperammonemia. An ammonia level greater than 120 μmol/mL in a newborn is considered neurotoxic. Hemodialysis to remove excessive ammonia is more effective than peritoneal or other extracorporeal routes [28,32]. Temporizing empiric therapy with arginine with or without sodium benzoate/phenylacetate can reduce ammonia levels acutely in most urea cycle defects. Table 2 lists specific therapies to consider when suspecting particular IEMs.

Thyroid disorders

Neonatal thyrotoxicosis, also called congenital hyperthyroidism, is usually due to in utero passage of thyroid-stimulating immunoglobulins from the mother to fetus. The incidence is 1 case per 4000 to 50,000 live births [33]. By far, most cases are due to maternal Graves' disease, an autoimmune disorder that produces thyroid-stimulating hormone (TSH) receptor antibodies causing increased thyroid hormone release. The prevalence of Graves' disease in pregnant women is 0.1% to 0.4%, with hyperthyroidism seen in 0.6% to 10% of infants born to these mothers [34]. Euthyroid mothers treated for hyperthyroidism are still at risk for having a newborn with thyrotoxicosis. Diagnosis is made by measuring neonatal levels of serum-free thyroxine (T_4) and TSH shortly after birth. Normal ranges of T_4 and TSH concentrations are higher in neonates than older infants and

Table 2
Specific therapies for inborn errors of metabolism

Drug	Dose	Indication
Arginine HCl 10%[a]	210–600 mg/kg IV	Urea cycle defects
Biotin	10 mg IV or PO	Organic acidemias
Carnitine	50–400 mg/kg IV or PO	Fatty acid defects, organic acidemias
Pyridoxine	100 mg IV	Pyridoxine-dependent seizures
Sodium benzoate[a] and/or phenylacetate[a]	250 mg/kg IV	Urea cycle defects
Thiamine	25–100 mg IV	MSUD, primary lactic acidosis

Abbreviations: IV, intravenous; PO, by mouth; MSUD, maple syrup urine disease.
[a] Can infuse over 1 to 2 hours in dextrose-containing solution.
Data from Refs. [24,27,28,32].

children. Also, thyroid function tests may be unreliable in the first few days of life if the mother was taking antithyroid medications.

Infants with neonatal hyperthyroidism are commonly born preterm with low birth weight, microcephaly, and craniosynostosis. They usually present within a few days of life but can sometimes be delayed 10 days or more. Symptoms are transient and usually last less than 12 weeks, the duration of which is dependent on the persistence of maternally transmitted immunoglobulins. Symptoms include vomiting, diarrhea, poor feeding and weight loss, sweating, and irritability. Most infants will have a goiter, and many will also have exophthalmos, hyperthermia, tachycardia, hepatomegaly, and jaundice. Although transient, neonatal thyrotoxicosis can be life-threatening, with a reported mortality rate of up to 20%, usually from heart failure [33].

Hyperthyroidism in older infants and children is almost always due to Graves' disease. Nearly 5% of all patients with hyperthyroidism are less than 15 years old, with the majority being adolescents. Unlike adults, children with hyperthyroidism usually have an indolent progression of symptoms over months, although it may occur more abruptly. Personality disturbances or motor hyperactivity may be the earliest symptoms, followed by the classic symptoms of weight loss, heat intolerance, diaphoresis, palpitations, diarrhea, and amenorrhea. A goiter is present in nearly 100% of cases, and exophthalmos, tachycardia, and hypertension are common [35]. Thyroid storm can occur in the pediatric population and consists of extreme signs and symptoms of hyperthyroidism combined with a high fever and altered mental status. It is usually precipitated by infection, trauma, or dehydration. Thyroid storm is life-threatening and treatment should be aggressive and similar to adult management.

Neonatal hyperthyroidism and thyroid storm have many therapeutic options. Beta-adrenergic blockade can be achieved with propanolol in a 0.01 mg/kg/dose intravenously and titrated to clinical effect; alternative oral dosing is 2 mg/kg/d in three to four divided doses. Thyroid hormone synthesis can be blocked using propylthiouracil, 5 to 10 mg/kg/d, or methimazole, 0.5 to 1 mg/kg/d, both in three divided oral doses. Iodine can be given in the form of Lugol's solution (8 mg iodine/drop), 1 to 3 drops daily. Iodine should be started at least 1 hour after administering an anti-thyroid drug like propylthiouracil to avoid increasing thyroid gland stores before the anti-thyroid effect occurs. Glucocorticoid treatment with hydrocortisone or prednisone may also be helpful in severe cases, because it inhibits thyroid hormone release and decreases peripheral conversion of T_4 to T_3.

Hypothyroidism does not occur with acute signs or symptoms and is rarely classified as an emergent condition. Congenital hypothyroidism may occasionally be missed due to laboratory errors in newborn screening, and early emergency department detection and treatment within the first few weeks of life are important to prevent irreversible brain damage. The incidence is 1 case per 4000 live births, and it is the most common treatable cause of mental retardation. Classic symptoms include prolonged jaundice, poor feeding, hoarse cry, constipation, somnolence, and hypothermia. Classic signs include coarse puffy facies, large fontanelles, macroglossia, hypotonia, dry skin, jaundice, and a distended abdomen with umbilical hernia.

Emergency department evaluation

Initial emergency department management for a suspected metabolic disorder should begin with the standard ABCs approach. Poorly perfusing or hypotensive infants require standard intravenous fluid replacement, and antibiotics should be administered promptly when sepsis is suspected. If DKA is suspected or confirmed, aggressive fluid resuscitation should be avoided in normotensive infants due to its association with cerebral edema.

A careful history may reveal important clues suggestive of metabolic disease. Questions about prenatal care and maternal medications may elucidate an endocrine disorder. Newborn screening test results are important inquiries when considering an IEM, as is a history of consanguinity or sudden infant death in the immediate family. Feeding difficulties, weight loss, or an association of symptoms with dietary intake or particular types of food are important inquiries, especially in newborns. Vomiting is a prominent feature in most metabolic disorders, both as a primary symptom and a compensatory mechanism by which excess body acid is eliminated via the gastrointestinal tract.

Physical examination should focus on the patient's neurologic and circulatory status. Alterations in consciousness can range from mild lethargy to seizures and coma. Hypotonia with poor suck and Moro reflexes are frequently seen. Dehydration with tachycardia, poor perfusion, or hypotension should be recognized early and treated aggressively. Tachypnea is a characteristic sign in acidotic infants, and the degree of tachypnea frequently correlates with the severity of acidosis. A fruity breath can be seen in DKA or other ketotic diseases, whereas other unusual or peculiar body fluid odors suggest IEMs. Hepatomegaly and jaundice may be prominent, especially in glycogen storage diseases and galactosemia.

Emergent diagnostic testing should begin with bedside glucose testing, which should be verified by standard laboratory testing. Electrolytes with calculation of the anion gap are important for diagnostic classification (see Box 2). Acid-base status can be more precisely measured with an arterial blood gas, although in the absence of hypoxia or poor perfusion, a venous or capillary measurement may be adequate and less invasive in infants. Serum calcium, magnesium, and liver function tests should also be obtained. Urinalysis will reveal the presence or absence of ketones, which can help to differentiate particular metabolic disorders; the lack of an appropriate ketonuric response to metabolic acidosis is indicative of a fatty acid oxidation defect. The pH of urine is normally less than 5 in organic acidemias, whereas the most common urea cycle defect, ornithine transcarbamylase deficiency, may contain urinary orotic acid crystals. The finding of urine reducing substances in the absence of glucosuria is indicative of galactosuria and presumptive galactosemia. Urine reducing substances can also be seen in a few select disorders of amino acid metabolism, such as tyrosinemia. Urine electrolytes and osmolality can better classify a hyponatremic disorder. Serum osmolality, both measured and calculated, is important in managing DKA. Along with drug screens and levels, osmolality can help to exclude a toxicologic cause. Concurrent with these studies should be standard investigations for infection, including a complete blood count, cerebrospinal fluid studies, and body fluid cultures.

The blood ammonia level should be obtained in any altered infant in whom metabolic disease is suspected. Testing for ammonia levels need to be completed within 30 minutes of the blood draw to avoid falsely elevated levels. Ammonia is significantly elevated in urea cycle defects and many of the organic acidemias. Mild transient elevation of ammonia is common in asymptomatic neonates, especially premature infants. Lactate and pyruvate levels can be of use. Although both acids can be elevated in sepsis and IEMs, the lactate-to-pyruvate ratio tends to be increased in sepsis (greater than 10:1), whereas in some IEMs such as primary lactic acidosis the ratio is usually normal. Because stat thyroid function testing is now available in many laboratories, these tests should be initiated in the emergency department when indicated. Although variable studies exist, essential testing should include levels for TSH and free thyroxine (T_4).

Additional archival body fluid samples should be appropriately collected and stored if an undiagnosed metabolic disease is considered in the emergency department and preferably before initiation of any therapy. For adrenal insufficiency and CAH, additional blood studies to consider include cortisol, ACTH, 17-hydroxyprogesterone, aldosterone, renin, insulin, and growth hormone. For organic acidemias and other defects in amino acid and fatty acid metabolism, quantitative blood amino acids and urinary amino and organic acids will aid in definitive diagnosis. Although these tests are nonemergent, the emergency department physician may on occasion be requested to order these studies by a consultant.

Most symptomatic patients with a known or suspected metabolic disorder will require hospitalization, usually in an intensive care setting for frequent monitoring of metabolic parameters and neurologic status. Prompt consultation should be initiated with a pediatric endocrinologist or metabolic specialist. If appropriate resources are unavailable, transfer should be arranged with a pediatric center skilled in managing metabolic disorders. This transfer should be done expeditiously after resuscitation and empiric treatment for likely causes have been started.

In the event of a failed resuscitation or imminent death in a patient with a suspected IEM, permission for autopsy and specimen testing should be thoughtfully discussed with the parents. Perimortem samples to consider obtaining include frozen blood, plasma, and urine specimens, a skin biopsy, and a needle liver biopsy [28,31]. These studies will allow for appropriate genetic counseling for current family members and future siblings.

References

[1] Cornblath M, Hawdon JM, Williams AF, et al. Controversies regarding definition of neonatal hypoglycemia: suggested operational thresholds. Pediatrics 2000;105:1141–5.

[2] Cowett R, Loughead J. Neonatal glucose metabolism: differential diagnoses, evaluation, and treatment of hypoglycemia. Neonatal Netw 2002;21:9–19.

[3] Losek JD. Hypoglycemia and the ABC's (sugar) of pediatric resuscitation. Ann Emerg Med 2000;35:43–6.

[4] Lilien LD, Pildes RS, Srinivasan G, et al. Treatment of neonatal hypoglycemia with minibolus and intravenous glucose infusion. J Pediatr 1980;97:295–8.

[5] Pollack CV Jr. Utility of glucagon in the emergency department. J Emerg Med 1993;11:195–205.

[6] Kappy MS, Bajaj L. Recognition and treatment of endocrine/metabolic emergencies in children: part 1. Adv Pediatr 2002;49:245–72.

[7] von Muhlendahl KE, Herkenhoff H. Long term course of neonatal diabetes. N Engl J Med 1995;333:704–8.

[8] Fosel S. Transient and permanent neonatal diabetes. Eur J Pediatr 1995;154:944–8.

[9] Wolfsdorf J, Glaser N, Sperling M. Diabetic ketoacidosis in infants, children, and adolescents: a consensus statement from the American Diabetes Association. Diabetes Care 2006;29:1150–9.

[10] Iafusco D, Stazi MA, Cotichini R, et al. Permanent diabetes mellitus in the first year of life. Diabetologia 2002;45:798–804.

[11] Quinn M, Fleishman A, Rosner B, et al. Characteristics at diagnosis of type 1 diabetes in children younger than 6 years. J Pediatr 2006;148:366–71.

[12] Shield JPH, Wadsworth EJK, Baum JD. Insulin dependent diabetes in under 5 year olds. Arch Dis Child 1985;60:1144–8.

[13] Glaser N, Barnett P, McCaslin I, et al. Risk factors for cerebral edema in children with diabetic ketoacidosis. N Engl J Med 2001;344:264–9.

[14] Harrison AM, Lynch JM, Dean JM, et al. Comparison of simultaneously obtained arterial and capillary blood gas in pediatric intensive care patients. Crit Care Med 1997;25:1904–8.

[15] McGillivray D, DuCharme FM, Charron Y, et al. Clinical decision making based on venous versus capillary blood gas in the well perfused child. Ann Emerg Med 1999;34:58–63.

[16] Kitabchi AE, Umpierrez GE, Murphy MD, et al. American Diabetes Association. Hyperglycemic crises in diabetes. Diabetes Care 2004;27(Suppl 1):S94–102.

[17] Gruskin AB, Sarnaik A. Hyponatremia: pathophysiology and treatment, a pediatric perspective. Pediatr Nephrol 1992;6:280–6.

[18] Gupta VK, Mishra D, Mathur I, et al. Pyridoxine-dependent seizures: a case report and a critical review of the literature. J Paediatr Child Health 2001;37:592–6.

[19] Lorenz JM, Kleinman LI, Markarian K, et al. Serum anion gap in the differential diagnosis of metabolic acidosis in critically ill newborns. J Pediatr 1999;135:751–5.

[20] Fanconi S, Burger R, Ghelfi D, et al. Hemodynamic effects of sodium bicarbonate in critically ill neonates. Intensive Care Med 1993;19:65–9.

[21] Dixon H, Hawkins K, Stephenson T. Comparison of albumin versus bicarbonate treatment for neonatal metabolic acidosis. Eur J Pediatr 1999;158:414–5.

[22] Merke D, Kabbani M. Congenital adrenal hyperplasia: epidemiology, management and practical drug treatment. Paediatr Drugs 2001;3:599–611.

[23] Greene CL, Goodman SI. Catastrophic metabolic encephalopathies in the newborn period. Clin Perinatol 1997;24:773–86.

[24] Weiner DL. Metabolic emergencies. In: Fleisher GR, Ludwig S, Henretig FM, et al, editors. Textbook of pediatric emergency medicine. Philadelphia: Lippincott Williams and Wilkins; 2006. p. 1193–206.

[25] Calvo M, Artuch R, Macia E, et al. Diagnostic approach to inborn errors of metabolism in an emergency unit. Pediatr Emerg Care 2000;16:405–8.

[26] Henriquez H, el Din A, Ozand PT, et al. Emergency presentations of patients with methyl-malonic acidemia, propionic acidemia and branched chain amino acidemia (MSUD). Brain Dev 1994;16:S86–93.

[27] Ozand PT. Hypoglycemia in association with various organic and amino acid disorders. Semin Perinatol 2000;24:172–93.

[28] Burton BK. Inborn error of metabolism in infancy: a guide to diagnosis. Pediatrics 1998; 102:e69.

[29] Leonard JV, Morris AA. Inborn errors of metabolism around time of birth. Lancet 2000;12: 583–7.

[30] Hazard PB, Griffin JP. Calculation of sodium bicarbonate requirement in metabolic acidosis. Am J Med Sci 1982;283:18–22.

[31] Chakrapani A, Cleary MA, Wraith JE. Detection of inborn errors of metabolism in the newborn. Arch Dis Child Fetal Neonatal Ed 2001;84:F205–10.

[32] de Baulny HO. Management and emergency treatments of neonates with a suspicion of inborn errors of metabolism. Semin Neonatol 2002;7:17–26.

[33] Ogilvy-Stuart AL. Neonatal thyroid disorders. Arch Dis Child Fetal Neonatal Ed 2002;87: F165–71.

[34] Zimmerman D. Fetal and neonatal hyperthyroidism. Thyroid 1999;9:727–33.

[35] Saladino RA. Endocrine and metabolic disorders. In: Barkin RM, Caputo GL, Jaffe DM, et al, editors. Pediatric emergency medicine: concepts and clinical practice. St. Louis (MO): Mosby-Year Book; 1997. p. 755–73.

ELSEVIER
SAUNDERS

Emerg Med Clin N Am
25 (2007) 1061–1086

EMERGENCY
MEDICINE
CLINICS OF
NORTH AMERICA

Childhood Seizures

Michelle D. Blumstein, MD*, Marla J. Friedman, DO

*Division of Emergency Medicine, Miami Children's Hospital,
3100 SW 62nd Avenue, Miami, FL 33155, USA*

A seizure is defined as a paroxysmal electrical discharge of neurons in the brain resulting in an alteration of function or behavior. The area of cortical involvement, the direction and speed of the electrical impulse, and the age of the child all contribute to the clinical manifestations of the seizures [1]. A seizure may be short and self-limited or prolonged and life threatening. Most seizures are followed by a period of confusion, irritability, or fatigue known as the postictal period [2]. The length of this period generally corresponds to the length of the seizure activity. A diagnosis of epilepsy is made only after the occurrence of two or more seizures without evidence of provoking factors. An epileptic syndrome is a cluster of signs and symptoms that is associated with specific neurologic and electroencephalographic (EEG) findings [1]. Continuous seizure activity lasting longer than 30 minutes or two or more seizures without a return to a baseline level of consciousness between events is referred to as status epilepticus [1].

Seizures are the most common neurologic disorder of childhood and one of the most frightening. Seizures occur in approximately 4% to 10% of children and account for 1% of all emergency room visits [3,4]. Children under 3 years of age have the highest incidence of seizures. The incidence decreases with increasing age [5]. Each year, 150,000 children experience an unprovoked, first-time seizure and 30,000 of those children ultimately develop epilepsy [3].

Patients with seizures present frequently to the emergency department, and emergency physicians should be comfortable and proficient in the recognition and acute stabilization of these patients. It is imperative that emergency department physicians differentiate between true seizures and events that mimic seizure activity to provide appropriate treatment, parental reassurance, and safe patient disposition. A thorough knowledge of long-term

---

* Corresponding author.

E-mail address: mblumstein@aol.com (M.D. Blumstein).

seizure management including antiepileptic medications, other therapies, and their various side effects is necessary.

Pathophysiology

A seizure is not a diagnosis itself but rather a symptom of a process that results in a hypersynchrony of neuronal discharges. During a seizure, oxygen and glucose consumption and lactate and carbon dioxide production are all increased. If normal ventilation is maintained, the increase in cerebral blood flow is generally sufficient to compensate for these changes. As a result, brief seizures rarely cause long-term neurologic damage. Seizures with a longer duration may result in permanent sequelae.

During a seizure, sympathetic discharge results in tachycardia, hypertension, and hyperglycemia. Additionally, patients may have difficulty maintaining a patent airway. In patients for whom ventilation is inadequate, hypoxia, hypercarbia, and respiratory acidosis may occur. If seizure activity is prolonged, the risk of lactic acidosis, rhabdomyolysis, hyperkalemia, hyperthermia, and hypoglycemia increases.

Seizure classification

There are many possible etiologies of seizures (Box 1). The determination of a pathologic cause should always be attempted so that the diagnostic and treatment process can begin with the classification of the seizure. Classification systems have been developed to standardize the terminology used to describe seizure activity. Two overall seizure types exist: partial and generalized.

Partial seizures originate in one cerebral hemisphere. This type of seizure has also been referred to as a focal or local seizure. Partial seizures are further subdivided based on whether they result in an altered level of consciousness. A simple partial seizure has no impairment of consciousness, and most commonly manifests as abnormal motor activity. Autonomic, somatosensory, and psychic symptoms can also occur. When an alteration of consciousness is present, the seizure is classified as a complex partial seizure. An "aura" consisting of abnormal perception or hallucination often precedes this type of seizure [1,2]. These seizures may present with lip smacking, a dazed look, or nausea and vomiting [3]. Both simple and complex partial seizures may ultimately become generalized. Generalization occurs in approximately 30% of children [6].

A generalized seizure involves both cerebral hemispheres and may involve a depressed level of consciousness. Generalized seizures are either convulsive, with bilateral motor activity, or nonconvulsive [2]. Various types of generalized seizures can occur, including absence (petit mal), myoclonic, atonic (drop attacks), tonic, clonic, and tonic-clonic (grand mal) seizures

Box 1. Etiology of Seizures

Infectious
Febrile seizure
Meningitis
Encephalitis
Brain abscess
Neurocysticercosis

Neurologic/developmental
Birth injury
Hypoxic-ischemic encephalopathy
Neurocutaneous syndromes
Ventriculoperitoneal shunt malfunction
Congenital anomalies
Degenerative cerebral disease

Metabolic
Hypoglycemia
Hypoxia
Hypomagnesemia
Hypocalcemia
Hypercarbia
Inborn errors of metabolism
Pyridoxine deficiency

Traumatic/vascular
Child abuse
Head trauma
Intracranial hemorrhage
Cerebral contusion
Cerebrovascular accident

Toxicologic
Alcohol, amphetamines, antihistamines, anticholinergics
Cocaine, carbon monoxide
Isoniazid
Lead, lithium, lindane
Oral hypoglycemics, organophosphates
Phencyclidine, phenothiazines
Salicylates, sympathomimetics
Tricyclic antidepressants, theophylline, topical anesthetics
Withdrawals (alcohol, anticonvulsants)
Idiopathic/epilepsy
Obstetric (eclampsia)
Oncologic

Data from Friedman M, Sharieff G. Seizures in children. Pediatr Clin North Am 2006;53:257–77.

[2,6,7]. Absence seizures are characterized by sudden, brief (30 second) staring spells associated with lapses in awareness. Most patients are not aware that a seizure has occurred. Simple (typical) absence seizures are characterized by sudden cessation of activity, a blank stare, and no postictal drowsiness or confusion. Complex (atypical) absence seizures last longer, have a more gradual onset and resolution, and are often associated with myoclonic activity in the face or extremities [5,6,8].

Myoclonic seizures may occur hundreds of times daily and are characterized by a sudden head drop and flexion of the arms ("jackknifing"). Atonic seizures result in a sudden loss of consciousness and muscle tone. Generalized tonic-clonic seizures are the most common seizure type in children. These seizures begin with a tonic phase during which pallor, mydriasis, eye deviation, and muscle contraction occurs. This period is followed by clonic movements including jerking and flexor spasms of the extremities. Bowel or bladder incontinence is common. Tonic-clonic seizures can be preceded by an "aura" in some children but occur suddenly and without warning in most cases [5,6]. Following this type of seizure, the child may experience a transient weakness or paralysis of one area of the body known as Todd's paralysis. This weakness is self-limited and requires only supportive management [2].

Certain epilepsy syndromes are specific to children and are classified by etiology. One fourth of epilepsy is due to an identified preceding neurologic cause and is referred to as symptomatic epilepsy. In cryptogenic epilepsy, the cause is not identified but an occult symptomatic cause is assumed. The term *idiopathic epilepsy* is reserved for syndromes that are presumed to be solely genetic [9].

Infantile spasms (West's syndrome) present with sudden jerking contractions of the extremities, head, neck, and trunk in patients between 4 and 18 months of age. The jerking often occurs in clusters and rarely during sleep. Mental retardation is present in 95% of children with West's syndrome, and 25% of these children have tuberous sclerosis. This syndrome carries a 20% mortality rate. The characteristic pattern of hypsarrhythmia (random high-voltage slow waves with multifocal spikes) is seen on EEG [5,6]. Patients are generally treated with adrenocorticotropic hormone (ACTH) or prednisone [10,11]. Valproic acid, lamotrigine, topiramate, vigabatrin, and zonisamide have been successful as well [10,12–14].

Children with Lennox-Gastaut syndrome present between the ages of 3 and 5 years with intractable mixed type seizures, including tonic, myoclonic, atonic, and absence seizures. An irregular, slow, high-voltage spike pattern is seen on EEG [5,6]. Typically, these children are mentally retarded or have significant behavioral problems. Attainment of seizure control is difficult, although multiple medications have been used. Valproic acid is the most common; however, felbamate, topiramate, lamotrigine, and zonisamide are other alternatives [10,12]. The ketogenic diet has been successful in some children with Lennox-Gastaut syndrome [15].

Benign rolandic epilepsy is a genetic syndrome with an autosomal dominant mode of inheritance. Patients with this syndrome present between the ages of 3 and 13 years with nighttime seizures. They begin with clonic activity of the face (grimacing, vocalizations), and often wake the child from sleep. The EEG shows a characteristic pattern of perisylvian spiking. The syndrome typically resolves spontaneously by early adulthood, and therapy is generally not indicated. If seizures are frequent, carbamazepine is the treatment of choice [3,5,6,10].

Juvenile myoclonic epilepsy of Janz is also inherited in an autosomal dominant fashion and presents with myoclonic jerks, most commonly on awakening. Tonic-clonic and absence seizures occur in 80% and 25% of these patients, respectively. The syndrome most often presents between 12 and 18 years of age and can be provoked by lack of sleep, hormonal changes, alcohol, and stress. EEG findings include a pattern of fast spike-and-wave discharges. Juvenile myoclonic epilepsy of Janz is most commonly treated with valproic acid, but lamotrigine, topiramate, felbamate, and zonisamide can also be used [3,5,6,10].

Special considerations

Neonatal seizures

The immature neonatal brain is more excitable than that of an older child. This excitability allows for synaptogenesis and learning but decreases the threshold for seizure activity [16]. Organized epileptiform activity is difficult to sustain in the immature cortex. The resulting seizures may be subtle and difficult to discern from other normal newborn movements or activities [16]. Lip smacking, eye deviations, or apneic episodes may be the only manifestations of seizure activity in this age group. This presentation contrasts with the more recognizable "shaking" movements in older children. In newborns, apneic episodes, "jitteriness," and autonomic alterations may also occur in the absence of seizure activity. These events must be differentiated from true seizures [16]. True seizures cannot be stopped with passive restraint alone and cannot be elicited by moving or startling the child [17].

In neonates, seizures are the most common neurologic manifestation of impaired brain function. Seizures occur in 1.8 to 3.5 of every 1000 newborns. Although studies have shown that seizure activity causes little direct brain injury in neonates, some data suggest that neonatal seizures may predispose these infants to learning difficulties and increased seizure activity later in life [16]. Low birth weight infants have a higher incidence and worse outcomes following seizure activity. It is not known whether this is due to the seizure activity itself or to an initial cerebral insult [16].

Initial evaluation may include EEG and cerebral imaging studies such as head ultrasound, CT, or MRI. Laboratory evaluation includes glucose, electrolytes, calcium, magnesium, a complete blood count, blood culture, urinalysis, urine culture, and toxicology screens. Cerebrospinal fluid culture, cell counts, and herpes simplex virus (HSV) polymerase chain reaction should be considered. Further testing including blood amino acids, lactate, pyruvate, ammonia, and urine organic acids should be added if the diagnosis of an inborn error of metabolism is considered.

The causes of neonatal seizures are listed in Box 2 [1,18–21]. Perinatal or intrauterine hypoxia accounts for 50% to 65% of neonatal seizures. Intracranial hemorrhage accounts for an additional 15%. Five to ten percent of seizures result from infection, metabolic abnormalities, and toxins [1,19,20].

Benign familial neonatal convulsions and benign idiopathic neonatal convulsions are additional types of seizures that present during the neonatal period. They are considered benign, have no known etiology, and carry

---

Box 2. Causes of neonatal seizures

Perinatal or intrauterine hypoxia/anoxia
Intracranial hemorrhage
Intraventricular
Subdural
Subarachnoid

Infection
Group B streptococcus
Escherichia coli
TORCH
    Toxoplasmosis
    Other (syphilis, hepatitis B, coxsackie virus, Epstein-Barr virus, varicella zoster, parvovirus)
    Rubella
    Cytomegalovirus
    HSV

Metabolic abnormalities
Hypoglycemia
Hypocalcemia
Hypomagnesemia
Pyridoxine deficiency
Inborn errors of metabolism

Other
Toxins/drug withdrawal
Central nervous system abnormalities
Neurocutaneous diseases

a favorable prognosis. Patients with benign familial neonatal convulsions present in the first 3 days of life and usually have a family history of neonatal seizures. This syndrome resolves spontaneously by 6 months of age [1,21]. Benign idiopathic neonatal convulsions are also known as the "fifth day fits" because they present on day 5 of life and generally resolve by day 15 [1,21].

Initial seizure management in neonates is similar to that in older children. Immediate priorities include stabilization of the airway, breathing, and circulation, as well as therapy to abort seizure activity. Phenobarbital is the treatment of choice in these patients. Phenobarbital and phenytoin have shown equal efficacy in many studies, although neither has been particularly successful [16]. Phenytoin exerts a depressive effect on the newborn myocardium and has a variable rate of metabolism in newborns; therefore, it is not often used as a first-line agent [20,21]. Benzodiazepines should be used cautiously due to the risk of hypotension and respiratory depression in this age group [20–22]. In refractory seizures, a trial of pyridoxine is indicated to treat the rare cases of pyridoxine deficiency, an autosomal recessive disorder presenting in the first 1 to 2 days of life. This disease does not respond to conventional therapies [21]. Electrolyte abnormalities should be rapidly corrected, and therapy for underlying infection should be instituted. Long-term anticonvulsant therapy usually includes phenobarbital or fosphenytoin. Both topiramate and zonisamide have been effective as well [17,18].

Febrile seizures

A febrile seizure is defined as a convulsion that occurs in association with a febrile illness in children between the ages of 6 months and 5 years. The peak age of occurrence is between 18 and 24 months. Between 2% to 5% of children will experience at least one febrile seizure before the age of 5 years, making it the most common seizure type in young children [3,23]. Febrile seizures are either simple or complex depending on their clinical features. A simple febrile seizure is brief ($\leq$15 minutes), single, and generalized. A complex febrile seizure lasts longer than 15 minutes, recurs during a single illness, or is focal. Simple febrile seizures are more common and account for 80% of all febrile seizures.

Although the exact pathophysiology is unknown, it is believed that fever lowers the seizure threshold in certain children. It is unclear whether seizure activity is related to the absolute height of the fever or to the rate of rise of the temperature [23–25]. It is evident that some genetic predisposition exists. Between 25% and 40% of children with febrile seizures have a family history of febrile seizures [26].

The vast majority of children who experience a febrile seizure will have no complications and no long-term neurologic effects [23–25]. Recurrence of febrile seizures occurs in approximately 33% of children, with the highest recurrence seen in children who experience their first episode before 1 year of age [27]. Less than 10% of children have more than three seizures [24]. Recurrences tend to occur soon after the first febrile seizure, with 50% occurring within the first 6 months. Seventy-three percent occur in the first year and 90% in the first 2 years [27]. Children with higher temperatures at the time of their febrile seizure are less likely to have a recurrence, but it is unclear whether the type of initial seizure (simple or complex) has any bearing on the risk of recurrence [3,28]. In children with no additional risk factors, the overall risk for nonfebrile seizures in the future (1%–2%) is not statistically greater than for the general population (0.5%–1%) [1,24]. An abnormal neurologic examination before the seizure, a complex febrile seizure, or a family history of epilepsy increases the risk of epilepsy to between 9.6% and 13% [24,27].

A patient who presents to the emergency department during a febrile seizure should be treated in the same fashion as a patient with any other type of seizure. Attention should first be directed at controlling the airway, breathing, and circulation, and then at stopping the seizure activity. As is true for other seizure types, benzodiazepines are the first-line therapy, followed by fosphenytoin and phenobarbital. In addition, treatment to control and reduce the temperature is indicated [24].

Due to the self-limited nature of febrile seizures, children are usually postictal or have returned to baseline by the time they arrive in the emergency department. In these children, a thorough history and physical examination along with an age appropriate search for the source of the fever are appropriate [23,29]. The risk of serious bacterial infections in these children is the same as in children who present with fever alone [25,29,30]. In cases in which a cause of the fever has been identified, viral infections are the most common source. Both influenza A and human herpes virus 6 (roseola infantum) have been linked with an increased incidence of febrile seizures [31,32]. Routine examinations of glucose, electrolytes, calcium, blood urea nitrogen, and creatinine are not necessary in children who have returned to baseline, have no risk factors for epilepsy, and have a normal physical examination [23,27].

The need for routine lumbar puncture in children with a first febrile seizure has generated much controversy. It is universally accepted that a lumbar puncture is required in all children in whom meningeal signs are present. The inability to perform a reliable examination in postictal or very young children has led to considerable variability in the approach to these children. American Academy of Pediatrics guidelines recommend the strong consideration of lumbar puncture in children younger than 12 months of age and consideration in those younger than 18 months of age [23]. Because the incidence of meningitis in children who present with a first febrile seizure is low, recent research recommends that routine lumbar puncture based on age alone is not necessary. These new suggestions rely more strongly on clinical findings in addition to the child's age when making the decision to perform a lumbar puncture. A lumbar puncture should be considered in patients less than 18 months of age who present with a history of irritability, lethargy, or poor oral intake. Additionally, those with an abnormal mental status, slow return from the postictal state, bulging fontanelle, headache, or other meningeal signs should have a lumber puncture performed. Patients whose seizures have complex features, or those who have been pretreated with antibiotics should be considered for lumbar puncture [25].

Emergent EEG is generally not helpful and will be abnormal in approximately 95% of patients shortly after a febrile seizure. It may be useful in patients with an underlying neurologic disorder [27]. Emergent cranial imaging is not necessary in children with a simple febrile seizure and is also not likely to be necessary in well-appearing children with a first complex febrile seizure [28]. Complex febrile seizures may require further neuroimaging on a nonemergent basis.

Prophylactic antipyretic therapy is not effective in the prevention of future febrile seizures, and long-term anticonvulsant medication is generally not indicated in these children. Prophylactic antiepileptic medications may be considered in patients with neurologic deficits, focal or prolonged seizures, or those with a family history of epilepsy. Phenobarbital has been effective in the prevention of future febrile seizures, but its use is limited due to behavioral and cognitive side effects. Furthermore, for it to be effective, phenobarbital must be given continuously and cannot be used only at the onset of fever. Valproic acid is as effective as phenobarbital, but the occurrence of hepatotoxicity and pancreatitis in young children has limited its use. Other antiepileptic medications such as carbamazepine and phenytoin have been evaluated without success. Oral or rectal diazepam (0.5 mg/kg/d) given every 12 hours from the onset of fever has been shown to be as effective as continuous phenobarbital in the prevention of febrile seizures. Side effects include lethargy, irritability, and ataxia [27]. Antiepileptic therapy decreases the recurrence of seizures but does not influence the development of epilepsy.

Most patients who have experienced a febrile seizure may be safely discharged home once sufficient reassurance and parental education has occurred. Patients with features of a complex febrile seizure, those with prolonged seizure activity, or those whose seizure activity fails to stop on its own should be admitted to the hospital for further observation.

Differential diagnosis

Many clinical entities have features that mimic seizure activity (Box 3). Disorders that result in an altered level of consciousness, those with abnormal movements or posturing, psychologic disorders, and some sleep disorders have features in common with seizures. Often, a thorough history and physical examination are all that is necessary to differentiate these entities from true seizure activity. A complete description of the event from a witness is invaluable in making this distinction. Other historical and physical examination findings are also helpful. It is useful to recall that most

---

Box 3. Pediatric conditions often mistaken for seizures

Disorders with altered consciousness
Breath-holding spells
Apnea/syncope
Cardiac dysrhythmias
Migraine

Paroxysmal movement disorders
Tics
Shuddering attacks
Benign myoclonus
Pseudoseizures
Spasmus mutans
Acute dystonia

Sleep disorders
Night terrors
Sleepwalking
Narcolepsy

Psychologic disorders
Attention deficit hyperactivity disorder
Hyperventilation
Hysteria
Panic attacks

Gastroesophageal reflux (Sandifer syndrome)

Data from Friedman M, Sharieff G. Seizures in children. Pediatr Clin North Am 2006;53:257–77.

---

nonepileptic conditions will not be followed by a postictal period. Additionally, seizure activity cannot be stopped by passive restraint alone [17]. The differential diagnosis changes depending on the age of the child.

Breath-holding spells occur in approximately 5% of children between the ages of 6 months and 5 years and resolve spontaneously. In cyanotic breath-holding spells, the child first cries vigorously in response to anger or fear. The child then holds his or her breath, becomes cyanotic, limp, and may experience loss of consciousness and jerking of the extremities. The episode is brief, and the child returns to normal activity rapidly. Pallid breath-holding spells are also brief but generally occur after a minor trauma. In these cases, the child cries, becomes pale, and loses consciousness and motor tone. Neither type is followed by any postictal behavioral changes.

Syncope is defined as a brief sudden loss of consciousness and muscle tone and may result from a variety of causes. Typically, the patient is upright before the event and reports the sensation of lightheadedness or nausea. Signs of increased vagal tone such as pallor, diaphoresis, and dilated pupils are often observed. Syncope is more common in adolescents [5,6,33,34]. Like syncope, narcolepsy presents in adolescence; however, it is significantly less common. It presents with sudden uncontrollable periods of sleep during waking hours. In 50% of cases, it is associated with a sudden loss of muscle tone following an emotional outburst known as cataplexy. These events may be mistaken for atonic type seizures [2,5,6,33,35].

Benign shuddering attacks are characterized by rapid shaking of the head and arms lasting only a few seconds with immediate return to baseline activity. Tics are another movement disorder that may mimic epilepsy. They are brief and repetitive, are partially repressible, and are often induced by stress. Infants with Sandifer's syndrome present with back arching, writhing, and crying associated with vomiting episodes. These manifestations of gastro-esophageal reflux disease may be confused with seizure activity. Spasmus nutans is characterized by head tilting, nodding, and nystagmus and presents between 4 and 12 months of age. Dystonic reactions may be mistaken for a tonic seizure and most often are a side effect of medication. During the reaction, the child experiences sustained contraction of the neck and trunk muscles, abnormal posturing, and facial grimacing. They experience no postictal period [5,6,33,36].

Multiple sleep-related paroxysmal events may be mistaken for seizure activity. Sudden jerking of the extremities, usually on falling asleep, is referred to as benign myoclonus. Night terrors are usually seen in preschool-aged children who wake from sleep crying, confused, and frightened. These episodes are self-limited and last only a few minutes, after which the child has no recollection of the event. School-aged children may also experience somnambulism (sleepwalking). During these events, the child wakes from sleep and wanders around aimlessly for a short period of time before returning to bed [5,6,33,36].

Pseudoseizures are most commonly seen in patients with a known seizure disorder or who have a family member with epilepsy. They are often difficult to differentiate from true seizures. Characteristics of pseudoseizures include suggestibility and moaning or talking during the event. Injury, incontinence, and postictal drowsiness are notably absent. When the diagnosis is unclear, an EEG or video EEG monitoring can be helpful in distinguishing these paroxysmal events from true seizures [5,6,33,36].

Evaluation and management

History and physical examination

The history and physical examination are invaluable elements of the seizure evaluation. Often, they alone can distinguish between true seizure activity and other paroxysmal disorders of childhood. Furthermore, an accurate description of the event can lead to appropriate differentiation between seizure types. The underlying cause of seizure activity may be uncovered during these steps in the evaluation process (see Box 1).

A thorough history of possible precipitating factors should be sought. These factors include fever, current systemic illness or infection, a history of neurologic disease, trauma, possible ingestions, other medications, recent immunizations, and a history of seizures. In patients with a history of seizure disorder, the investigation should include questions specific to previous antiepileptic treatment and seizure type. It is important to determine which, if any, seizure medication the patient is taking, and if there have been recent changes in the medication or dosing. The child's baseline seizure frequency as well as how the current seizure compares with past seizures are crucial historical points. It is helpful to know whether the child has traveled recently or has a family history of seizure disorder. Certain comorbid conditions, such as attention-deficit hyperactivity disorder, mental retardation, and autism, are associated with a higher incidence of seizure disorder, and a history of these conditions should be sought [37].

In addition to these historical features, it is extremely helpful to receive an accurate description of the event from a reliable witness. Events leading up to the seizure, as well as the presence of an aura, are important. The duration of the event, types of movement, eye involvement, loss of consciousness, the presence of incontinence, focal abnormalities following the seizure, and the length of the postictal period should be determined [6].

A thorough physical examination may yield clues to the cause of seizure activity. First, a complete set of vital signs should be obtained and evaluated. The child should be examined for signs of infection, meningeal irritation, signs of elevated intracranial pressure (bulging fontanelle, changes in vital signs), head trauma (bruising, retinal hemorrhages), and focal neurologic deficits. Other less obvious clues to the cause of seizure activity include hepatosplenomegaly associated with glycogen storage diseases and skin manifestations of neurocutaneous diseases (café au lait spots, ash leaf spots, and port wine stains) [6].

Laboratory testing

As in febrile seizures, there is no routine panel of laboratory studies in the evaluation of a first-time unprovoked afebrile seizure. Laboratory testing should be based on the history and physical examination and should attempt to elucidate a treatable cause of seizure activity. A bedside glucose level should be obtained in all patients. Electrolyte abnormalities are more common in actively seizing patients, those younger than 1 month of age, and those with hypothermia ($<36.5°C$) [38]. The presence of hypothermia is the best predictor of hyponatremic seizures in children younger than 6 months [39]. Patients with a history of diabetes or metabolic disease, dehydration or excess free water intake, prolonged seizure, an altered level of consciousness, and those younger than 6 months are also at an increased risk of electrolyte disturbances. Determination of the white blood cell count may be helpful if an infectious cause of the seizure is suspected. Based on the clinical picture, laboratory evaluation may also include toxicology screens, serum ammonia levels, urine amino acids, and serum organic acids [34]. Subtherapeutic anticonvulsant levels are a common cause of seizures in children with known seizure disorders. Serum anticonvulsant levels should be included in the evaluation of these children [7].

A lumbar puncture should be considered in patients with meningeal signs, altered mental status, a prolonged postictal period, or in neonatal seizures. Patients who have returned to their baseline level of activity following a first-time afebrile seizure do not require a cerebrospinal fluid evaluation [34].

Neuroimaging

As is true for laboratory testing, the decision to perform emergent neuroimaging should be made on a case-by-case basis. Although MRI is more sensitive in the detection of certain tumors and vascular malformations, CT is often more readily available [6,7]. Brain CT scan should be performed in patients with a history of trauma, neurocutaneous diseases, ventriculoperitoneal shunt, or exposure to cysticercosis. Those with evidence of increased intracranial pressure, focal seizure activity, focal neurologic deficits, or a prolonged postictal period should also be imaged. Imaging should also be considered in patients with hypercoaguable states (sickle cell disease), bleeding disorders, or immunocompromised states (HIV, malignancy) [40,41]. Following a first-time, unprovoked, nonfebrile seizure, most well-appearing children will have none of the previously mentioned risk factors. These children can be safely discharged home without emergent neuroimaging once follow-up is ensured [34].

Electroencephalography

Emergent EEG should be reserved for patients in whom the diagnosis of nonconvulsive status epilepticus is suspected or in those with refractory seizure activity. Well-appearing children who present to the emergency department with a first-time unprovoked nonfebrile seizure do not require an emergent EEG. These patients can be referred for outpatient EEG analysis including recordings in the sleep and wake states as well as during periods of patient stimulation [6,7]. An EEG during seizure activity is most beneficial. Although positive EEG findings are an important predictor of future seizures, a negative EEG does not rule out a seizure disorder [42].

Initial management

Most seizures are brief and self-limited. As a result, patients generally present to the emergency department after seizure activity has stopped. Patients who are actively seizing on presentation are generally in a prolonged seizure state, and the diagnosis of status epilepticus should be considered. Seizures that last longer than 10 minutes are unlikely to stop on their own and become increasingly refractory to antiepileptic drugs with time [43].

The initial management (Fig. 1) includes evaluation of the airway, breathing, and circulation, with interventions as necessary. Attention may

Time Line   **Intervention**

5 min   Prehospital medications   Lorazepam SL, PR
                                                            Diazepam PR
                                                            Midazolam IN, buccal

                                                      ↓
                                                      ↓
                                                      ↓

10-20 min   ED Arrival:
                                       ABCs, O$_2$, dextrostick,
                                              IV/IO access
                                                      ↓
                                  Consider IV glucose**, naloxone**,
                              pyridoxine** based on clinical situation

                                          ↓ **seizure persists x 3-5 min**
                                                      ↓
                                                      ↓
                         →→→→ Give benzodiazepine   Lorazepam IV, IM*
        repeat 1-2x ↑   ↓   Diazepam IV, PR*
                         ←←←←←←← ↓   Midazolam IV, IM, PR, IN,
buccal*

        seizure persists x 5 min   ↓
                                           ↓
                        Phenytoin or Fosphenytoin 15-20 mg/kg IV
                                           ↓
                                           ↓ **seizure persists x 15 min**
                                           ↓
30 min   Phenobarbital 20mg/kg IV
                                           ↓
        assess airway/consider intubation ↓ **seizure persists x 20 min**
                                           ↓
60 min   intubation / general anesthesia
                             continuous EEG monitoring

Fig. 1. Status epilepticus management algorithm. ABC, airway, breathing, circulation; ED, emergency department; ETT, endotracheal tube; IO, intraosseous; SC, subcutaneous; SL, sublingually; PR, rectally; IM, intramuscularly; IN, intranasally; IV, intravenous. *Lorazepam, 0.05 to 0.1 mg/kg IV/IM (maximum 4 mg/dose). Diazepam, 0.2 to 0.4 mg/kg IV (maximum 10 mg/dose) or 0.5 to 1 mg/kg PR. Midazolam IV: 0.05 to 0.1 mg/kg/dose (maximum 6 mg/dose for <6y, 10 mg/dose >6y), IM: 0.1 to 0.2 mg/kg/dose (maximum 5 mg/dose), IN: 0.2 to 0.3 mg/kg/dose (maximum 7.5 mg/dose), PO: 0.5 to 1 mg/kg/dose (maximum 20 mg/dose). **Dextrose, 2 to 4 mL/kg/dose D25% IV. Naloxone, 0.1 mg/kg/dose IV/IM/SC/ETT if <20 kg, 2 mg/dose if >20 kg. Pyridoxine, 50 to 100 mg/dose IV/IM.

then be focused on the prevention of secondary injuries. Supplemental oxygen should be provided and the airway maintained. Airway positioning is usually sufficient; however, an oral or nasal airway may be required. All necessary medications and equipment should be at the bedside of actively seizing patients because intubation is sometimes required. This access is particularly important after the administration of certain anticonvulsants. If possible, intravenous or intraosseous access should be obtained.

A dextrose bolus (2–4 mL/kg/dose of 25% dextrose intravenously) should be given in all cases of documented hypoglycemia. Empiric dextrose administration should also be given in cases in which rapid glucose testing is unavailable. Empiric dextrose should be avoided in children on the ketogenic diet because administration may interfere with the ketogenic state and worsen seizure activity. In patients with suspected opioid intoxication, naloxone (0.1 mg/kg/dose given intravenous/intramuscular/subcutaneous/ endotracheal tube if <20 kg, 2 mg/dose if >20 kg) should be given. Additionally, pyridoxine (50–100 mg/dose intravenous/intramuscular) should be administered to neonates and in those with isoniazide intoxication [26,43–46].

Benzodiazepines are the initial drug of choice in acute seizure management. They can be administered via multiple routes. Initial medicines may have been given by pre-hospital care providers, and this history should be obtained whenever possible. Lorazepam (Ativan) has an onset of action of 2 to 5 minutes and a half-life of 12 to 24 hours. For these reasons, it is the preferred agent. It can be given either intravenously or intramuscularly at a dose of 0.05 to 0.1 mg/kg (maximum 4 mg/dose) and may be repeated every 5 to 15 minutes; however, its effectiveness decreases with subsequent doses. An alternative medication is diazepam (Valium), whose half-life is less than 30 minutes but with an onset of action similar to lorazepam. Because of its short half-life, an additional agent for long-term seizure control should be added when diazepam is used. It can be administered at a dose of 0.2 to 0.4 mg/kg intravenously (maximum 10 mg/dose) or 0.5 to 1 mg/kg rectally. The rectal dose may be given by instillation of the intravenous formulation or through the use of preformed rectal gel suppositories [26,47,48]. Rectally administered diazepam has a longer onset of action than the intravenous form and is less successful at controlling seizures [49]. Midazolam (Versed) can be administered via various routes including intramuscular, intravenous, intranasal, oral, and buccal forms [26,48,50,51]. The intranasal form has been shown to be more effective than rectal diazepam and as effective as its intravenous form [49]. This preparation may be useful when intravenous access is difficult to obtain or in the pre-hospital setting. Dosing of midazolam varies based on the route of administration (by mouth: 0.25–0.5 mg/kg [maximum 20 mg/dose]; intravenous: 0.05–0.1 mg/kg/dose [maximum 6 mg/dose for <6y, 10 mg/dose >6y]; intramuscular: 0.1–0.2 mg/kg/ dose [maximum 5 mg/dose]; intranasal: 0.2–0.3 mg/kg/dose [maximum 7.5 mg/dose], rectal: 0.5–1 mg/kg/dose [maximum 20 mg/dose]). Benzodiazepines may cause respiratory depression, sedation, and, rarely, hypotension. These effects are more common with multiple doses. Attention to the airway is crucial.

If seizure activity persists despite repeated benzodiazepine dosing, phenytoin or fosphenytoin should be used. These medications are unique in that they do not cause sedation or respiratory depression. Fosphenytoin is a rapidly metabolized prodrug of phenytoin that can be rapidly delivered with fewer systemic and local side effects. The loading dose of phenytoin is 10 to 20 mg/kg intravenously but must be given slower than 50 mg/min. Fosphenytoin is given as phenytoin equivalents at the same dose without the time constraints of phenytoin. It may be infused at rates up to 150 mg/min. Intramuscular fosphenytoin is also available. Patients receiving chronic phenytoin therapy require a smaller loading dose to achieve therapeutic serum levels. In these cases, a typical starting dose is 5 to 10 mg/kg. The serum concentration increases by 1 mg/mL for each mg/kg given. Patients receiving phenytoin should be placed on continuous cardiac monitoring, because the drug may result in hypotension and cardiac dysrhythmias. Phenytoin will precipitate in the intravenous tubing when given with a dextrose-containing solution, but fosphenytoin will not [7,26,43,52].

Phenobarbital is the next antiepileptic drug to be added if seizure activity persists. It is given at a loading dose of 20 mg/kg intravenously over 5 to 10 minutes and requires 15 to 20 minutes to take effect. It has a duration of action lasting between 12 and 24 hours. If intravenous access is unavailable, it may also be given intramuscularly. Phenobarbital is the initial drug of choice in neonatal seizures [43]. Phenobarbital, especially when used in conjunction with benzodiazepines, can lead to significant respiratory depression, sedation, and hypotension. Intubation is frequently necessary at this stage in management [7,26,44–46]. Valproic acid can be substituted for phenytoin or phenobarbital in status epilepticus at a dose of 25 mg/kg/dose. Patients on chronic valproic acid therapy should receive 10 mg/kg/dose to raise serum drug levels [2].

If seizure activity persists longer than 30 to 60 minutes despite these interventions, continuous infusions of pentobarbital, midazolam, or propofol may be necessary. A few patients may require general anesthesia and neuromuscular blockade. These patients require continuous EEG monitoring, and medication doses should be titrated to achieve a flat line or suppression pattern on EEG [6,44–46].

Long-term management

In addition to seizure control, therapeutic goals include improving the quality of life for epileptic patients. Patients with seizure disorders have a high incidence of depression and suicidal ideations [37]. These factors, although not often addressed in the emergency department, may have a role in compliance and may influence treatment decisions.

It is uncommon to begin long-term antiepileptic therapy in the emergency department. Antiepileptic medications may decrease the risk of a second seizure but do not decrease the incidence of epilepsy. For this reason, they are generally not initiated following a first-time afebrile seizure in otherwise well-appearing children. When necessary to begin treatment, these drugs should be given in conjunction with the pediatrician or neurologist who will provide the patient's long-term care. The decision to begin therapy should consider the patient's age, seizure type, comorbid conditions, and risk of seizure recurrence [34,42,53].

Many antiepileptic drugs exist (Table 1), and the decision of which to use can be difficult. A few basic principles can guide proper selection. First, one should choose a drug that is appropriate for the patient's seizure type. If more than one appropriate drug exists, one should choose the one with the least side effects. Second, one should begin with a single agent at the low end of the dosing range. Doses should be titrated up until seizures are controlled or side effects become intolerable. Medications should not be changed until the drug has been allowed to reach a steady state. This level is generally five times the half-life of the medication. A second drug should be added if seizure activity continues. The ultimate goal is to wean to a single drug if possible [6,15,55] When choosing an antiepileptic medication, it is also necessary to consider the patient's comorbid conditions. Certain antiepileptic agents have either beneficial or detrimental effects on other conditions [37]. It is important to inform families that although 75% of patients will achieve seizure control with a single drug [35], dose or medication changes could be necessary before seizure control is obtained.

Carbamazepine (Tegretol) is a first-generation antiepileptic drug recommended for use in the treatment of simple and complex partial seizures and generalized tonic-clonic seizures. Additionally, it is the treatment of choice for benign rolandic epilepsy [5]. Interestingly, carbamazepine induces its own metabolism and decreases its own half-life from 30 to 10 hours. Drug absorption is slow and irregular, resulting in erratic serum drug levels [55]. Dose-related side effects include drowsiness, diplopia, and lethargy. Other side effects include rash, hepatic toxicity, leukopenia, and aplastic anemia. Its use may interfere with the effectiveness of oral contraceptive medications. Carbamazepine exerts some positive effect on mood stabilization [56]. Other medications, including macrolide antibiotics, isoniazide, cimetidine, verapamil, and diltiazam, may interfere with carbamazepine metabolism and result in toxic serum levels. Therapeutic serum levels range from 4 to 12 µg/mL. Dosing begins at 10 mg/kg/d and is increased by 5 mg/kg/d every 3 to 4 days to maintenance dosing (usually 10–40 mg/kg/d divided twice to four times daily) [53,54,57].

Phenytoin (Dilantin) is another first-line antiepileptic drug whose use indicated in the treatment of generalized tonic-clonic seizures and sir and complex partial seizures. It is used in status epilepticus and pos: in neonatal seizures as well. Significant side effects are associated

Table 1
Common anticonvulsant agents

Drug	Indication	Side effects	Maintenance	Miscellaneous
Carbamazepine (Tegretol)	Generalized tonic-clonic, partial, benign rolandic seizures	Rash, hepatitis, diplopia, aplastic anemia, leukopenia	10–40 mg/kg/d	Possible mood stabilization, inexpensive
Clonazepam (Klonopin)	Myoclonic, akinetic, partial seizures, infantile spasms, Lennox-Gastaut	Fatigue, behavioral issues, salivation	0.05–0.3 mg/kg/d	
Ethosuximide (Zarontin)	Absence	GI upset, weight gain, lethargy, SLE, rash	20–40 mg/kg/d	
Felbamate (Felbatol)	Refractory severe epilepsy	Aplastic anemia, hepatotoxicity	15–45 mg/kg/d	
Gabapentin (Neurontin)	Partial and secondarily generalized seizures	Fatigue, dizziness diarrhea, ataxia, weight gain	20–70 mg/kg/d	
Lamotrigine (Lamictal)	Simple/complex partial, atonic, myoclonic, absence, tonic-clonic, Lennox-Gastaut, infantile spasms	Headache, nausea, rash, diplopia, Stevens-Johnson syndrome, GI upset	5–15 mg/kg/d (doses depend on coadministration of medications)	Possible mood stabilization
Levetiracetam (Keppra)	Adjunctive therapy for refractory partial seizures	Headache, anorexia, fatigue, infection, behavioral problems	10–60 mg/kg/d	
Oxcarbazepine (Trileptal)	Adjunctive therapy for partial seizures	Fatigue, low Na, nausea, ataxia, rash	5–45 mg/kg/d	Possible mood stabilization
Phenobarbital (Luminol)	Generalized tonic-clonic, partial, myoclonic	Sedation, behavioral issues, sleep abnormalities, rash, hypersensitivity	2–6 mg/kg/d	Inexpensive, readily available

Drug	Indications	Side effects	Dose	Comments
Phenytoin (Dilantin)	Generalized tonic-clonic, partial, atonic, myoclonic, neonatal	Gum hyperplasia, hirsutism, ataxia, Stevens-Johnson syndrome, lymphoma	4–8 mg/kg/d	Inexpensive, readily available
Primidone (Mysoline)	Generalized tonic-clonic, partial	Rash, ataxia, behavioral issues, sedation, anemia	10–25 mg/kg/d	
Tiagabine (Gabitril)	Adjunctive therapy for refractory complex partial (focal) seizures	Fatigue, headache, tremor, dizziness, anorexia	0.5–1 mg/kg/d	
Topiramate (Topamax)	Refractory complex partial seizures, adjunctive therapy for temporal lobe epilepsy	Fatigue, nephrolithiasis, ataxia, headache, weight loss, tremor, GI upset	1–9 mg/kg/d	Weight loss, migraine prevention
Valproic acid (Depakote)	Generalized tonic-clonic, absence, myoclonic, partial, akinetic, infantile spasms	GI upset, liver involvement, tremor, alopecia, sedation, weight gain, menstrual irregularities, thrombocytopenia	10–60 mg/kg/d	Inexpensive, readily available, possible mood stabilization, migraine prevention
Vigabatrin (Sabril)	Infantile spasms, adjunctive therapy for refractory seizures	Weight gain, behavior changes, visual field constriction	50–150 mg/kg/d	
Zonisamide (Zonegran)	Adjunctive therapy for partial seizures, atonic, infantile spasms	Fatigue, ataxia, anorexia, GI upset, headache, rash, weight loss	2–8 mg/kg/d	Weight loss

Abbreviations: GI, gastrointestinal; SLE, systemic lupus erythematosus.
Data from Friedman M, Sharieff G. Seizures in children. Pediatr Clin North Am 2006;53:257–77.

its use. Dose-related side effects that usually occur at supratherapeutic levels include nausea, vomiting, drowsiness, ataxia, and nystagmus. Cosmetic effects include acne, gingival hyperplasia, and hirsuitism. Blood and liver toxicity and drug-induced rashes (Stevens-Johnson syndrome) can also occur. Therapeutic levels range from 10 to 20 µg/mL, but higher levels may be necessary in some patients. Dosing ranges from 4 to 8 mg/kg/d divided once to three times daily. Changes between generic and trade forms of the drug as well as small changes in dosing may significantly alter serum drug levels. Like carbamazepine, phenytoin has multiple drug interactions. Its levels may be increased with concomitant use of cimetidine, isoniazide, anticoagulants, estrogens, chlorpromazine, and chloramphenicol. Phenytoin also alters drug levels of other antiseizure medications. Carbamazepine, clonazepam, and primidone levels are lowered, whereas phenobarbital levels may be increased with concurrent use of phenytoin [9,26,53,54,57].

Phenobarbital (Luminal) is effective against generalized tonic-clonic and partial seizures, both simple and complex. It is used in the treatment of status epilepticus and is the treatment of choice in neonatal seizures. A significant proportion (30%–50%) of children experience side effects including hyperactivity, lethargy, sleep and behavioral disorders, rash, and hypersensitivity reactions. Due to its low cost, it is often tried initially and discontinued if side effects are problematic. Therapeutic levels range between 10 to 40 µg/mL. The phenobarbital dose ranges from 2 to 6 mg/kg/d divided once or twice a day [9,26,53,57].

Primidone (Mysoline) is metabolized into phenobarbital and is useful in partial (simple and complex) and generalized tonic-clonic seizures as well. The side effect profiles are similar. Serum drug levels of phenobarbital are followed for monitoring and should range between 5 and 12 µg/mL. The usual maintenance dose is 10 to 25 mg/kg/d divided between two and four times per day [53,54,57].

Valproate (Depakote) is primarily used to treat absence or myoclonic seizures but is also effective in the treatment of generalized tonic-clonic seizures and both simple and complex partial seizures. It is occasionally used in the treatment of Lennox-Gastaut syndrome, juvenile myoclonic epilepsy of Janz, and infantile spasms [5,12]. Side effects include nausea, vomiting, drowsiness, alopecia, weight gain, and menstrual irregularities. Idiosyncratic pancreatitis and hepatic failure may occur, especially in children less than 2 years old. Additional dose-related effects include thrombocytopenia, platelet dysfunction, and tremors. Beneficial effects include migraine prevention and mood stabilization. Administration of valproate may increase serum drug levels of phenobarbital, phenytoin, carbamazepine, diazepam, clonazepam, and ethosuximide. Doses are started at 10 mg/kg and increased weekly by 10 mg/kg. The usual maintenance dose is between 10 and 60 mg/kg/d and is given in two to four divided doses. Therapeutic serum concentrations range from 50 to 100 µg/mL [53,54,56,57].

Ethosuximide (Zarontin) is the last of the first-generation antiepileptic drugs. It is most effective in absence seizure therapy. Side effects include nausea, vomiting, hiccups, and headache. Erythema multiforme, Stevens-Johnson syndrome, and a lupus-like syndrome have been reported on rare occasions. Its dose is from 20 to 40 mg/kg/d given in two divided doses with therapeutic levels ranging from 40 to100 µg/mL [53,54,56].

Clonazepam (Klonopin) can be used to treat myoclonic and atonic seizures as well as absence type seizures. Side effects include ataxia, drowsiness, and drooling. Therapeutic drug levels range from 0.02 to 0.08 µg/mL and are generally achieved with doses of 0.05 to 0.3 mg/kg/d divided from two to four times per day [54,57].

Lamotrigine (Lamictal) is indicated as adjunctive therapy in partial seizures, atonic, tonic, and myoclonic seizures in addition to Lennox-Gastaut syndrome. Lamotrigine monotherapy may be effective for generalized tonic-clonic and partial seizures, but further studies are required [56]. Lamotrigine dosing ranges from 5 to 15 mg/kg/d given once or twice daily. Because it interferes with other anticonvulsant medications, its dosage must be adjusted when given concurrently. Side effects include insomnia, gastrointestinal upset, headache, dizziness, and diplopia and are more pronounced in patients also receiving valproate. Lamotrigine has mood stabilizing effects and may be beneficial in patients with depression or bipolar disorder [10,14,26,37,53,56,58,59].

Felbamate (Felbatol) is most often used to treat refractory seizures, especially those associated with Lennox-Gastaut syndrome. Its use results in increased levels of phenytoin and valproate and decreased levels of carbamazepine, and its side effects are intensified when used with other medications. As a result, it is generally used as monotherapy. Side effects include insomnia, somnolence, anorexia, and vomiting. Its use has decreased secondary to the incidence of aplastic anemia and hepatic failure. Children on felbamate should have liver function tests and blood counts monitored frequently. Dosing should start at the low end of the dosing range and be increased every 1 to 2 weeks if tolerated. The usual dose is 15 to 45 mg/kg/d divided three to four times daily [10,14,37,53,58].

Gabapentin (Neurontin) has been used as adjunctive therapy in patients with refractory partial and secondary tonic-clonic seizures. It is relatively well tolerated with side effects including weight gain, fatigue, dizziness, ataxia, and diarrhea. Maintenance dosing ranges from 20 to 70 mg/kg/d divided in three to four doses daily. It can be rapidly titrated if necessary and has no interaction with other antiepileptic drugs [10,14,26,53,56,58].

Vigabatrin (Sabril) is indicated for the management of refractory partial seizures and infantile spasms. In some children with infantile spasms, treatment results in the replacement of infantile spasms with partial seizures. This effect is considered by most experts to be an improvement. In infants with tuberous sclerosis and infantile spasms, vigabatrin has been shown to be equally as effective as ACTH therapy [14]. Side effects include rash, sedation, ataxia, behavioral changes, and visual field constriction. Generally, dosing is started at 50 mg/kg/d given once daily or divided in two doses. It is increased to a goal of 75 to 150 mg/kg/d if some response is seen with the initial dose. Patients who do not respond or who worsen with treatment are considered resistant to the drug [10,14,26,53].

Zonisamide (Zonegran) is an effective adjunctive therapy for partial seizures in patients over 16 years of age. It has also been used effectively in generalized tonic-clonic, myoclonic and atonic seizures, infantile spasms, and Lennox-Gastaut syndrome. Some recent evidence shows that it may be useful as monotherapy in multiple seizure types including absence seizures [60–62]. Side effects are more common early in treatment and include nausea, vomiting, anorexia, fatigue, ataxia, and rash. Dosing begins at 2 to 4 mg/kg/d divided two to three times daily. It is titrated to maintenance dosing between 4 and 8 mg/kg/d [10,58].

Oxcarbazepine (Trileptal) is indicated in partial seizures as an adjunctive therapy. Side effects may include nausea, ataxia, diplopia, somnolence, rash, and hypersensitivity reactions. Twenty-five percent of children allergic to carbamazepine are also sensitive to oxcarbazepine. It is better tolerated than phenytoin and may have mood stabilizing benefits. Use of this medication may increase serum levels of phenobarbital and phenytoin. Dosing is started at 5 mg/kg/d and increased to 45 mg/kg/d divided in two doses [6,10,56].

Levetiracetam (Keppra) is a useful adjunct in the treatment of partial seizures in children between the ages of 6 and 12 years. Side effects include behavioral problems, somnolence, vomiting, anorexia, rhinitis, pharyngitis, otitis media, and gastroenteritis. Leukopenia has been reported in adults but has not been observed in children. The usual maintenance dose is between 10 and 60 mg/kg/d [10,56,58,63].

Tiagabine (Gabitril) is an adjunctive medication useful for refractory partial seizures. Side effects include headache, mood disturbances, inability to concentrate, fatigue, and dizziness. They are accentuated with multidrug therapy. Maintenance doses range from 0.5 to 1 mg/kg/d titrated from a starting dose of 0.1 mg/kg/d [10,14,26,53,58].

Topiramate (Topamax) is an adjunctive therapy in partial or generalized tonic-clonic seizures, refractory complex partial seizures, Lennox-Gastaut syndrome, and infantile spasms. Its side effects include anorexia, weight loss, renal stones, headache, fatigue, diplopia, and metabolic acidosis. Sleep disturbances, behavioral and cognitive effects, confusion, and speech problems can also occur. A few recent studies have documented hypohydrosis and intermittent hyperthermia occurring as a result of topiramate administration. The effects were reversible and resolved shortly after the medication was discontinued [37,64]. Topiramate may be beneficial in patients with migraine headaches [37]. Dosing begins at 1 mg/kg/d and is titrated to a maintenance dose of 3 to 9 mg/kg/d divided twice daily [10,14,26,53,58].

The ketogenic diet has been used with success in patients with refractory seizure types who have failed standard medical therapy. It has been used in multiple seizure types, including tonic-clonic, myoclonic, atonic, atypical absence, infantile spasms, and Lennox-Gastaut syndrome. A seizure reduction rate of 50% to 70% has been achieved in some studies [10,15]. Although it has traditionally been reserved for patients with refractory seizures, some evidence suggests that it may be a valuable treatment option early in therapy as well [65]. The diet, which is low in protein and carbohydrates and high in fat, induces a ketogenic state that results in a reduction in seizure frequency. At the start of the diet, patients are admitted to the hospital for approximately 4 days to educate the family and closely monitor for side effects. During the initial 48-hour fasting phase, these patients are at risk for hypoglycemia, vomiting, and dehydration and must be monitored closely. Long-term side effects include renal tubular acidosis, nephrolithiasis, constipation, growth retardation, weight loss, hyperlipidemia, hypoproteinemia, and an increase in hepatic and pancreatic enzymes. An increased risk of infection and prolonged QT intervals are other potential risks. An EKG and a thorough metabolic evaluation should be performed before initiation of the diet. Routine laboratory monitoring and vitamin supplementation are necessary [6,10,26,66]. Some recent evidence suggests that a modification of the popular Atkins' diet may be as effective as and better tolerated than the traditional ketogenic diet. This therapy eliminates the need for initial admission and has fewer dietary restrictions than the traditional diet [66].

In addition to the ketogenic diet, other nonmedical therapies are available in certain cases. These therapies include anterior temporal lobectomy, corpus callostomy, and vagal nerve stimulation therapy. These methods have considerable risks and side effects but are useful in carefully selected patients [37].

Patients, especially adolescents, should be educated about lifestyle modifications that may decrease their seizure activity. Alcohol consumption should be kept to a minimum, and patients should be encouraged to maintain regular sleep-wake cycles because disruption to their circadian rhythm can lead to increased seizures [37].

Disposition

Following a first-time afebrile seizure, well-appearing children can be safely managed on an outpatient basis. Adequate follow-up should be ensured, and sufficient parental education and reassurance should be provided. Additional work-up, including EEG, can be performed on an outpatient basis [6]. Very young infants, those with prolonged seizure activity, a prolonged postictal state, and who require anticonvulsant medications warrant hospital admission and further inpatient evaluation. EEG, whether performed in the hospital or after discharge, can help predict future seizure recurrence. Patients with a normal EEG have a 2-year recurrence rate of 28%, whereas the rate of recurrence in those with abnormal findings rises to 58% [67].

Acknowledgments

The authors thank Ghazala Q. Sharieff, MD, of Children's Hospital and Health Center, University of California, San Diego, for her assistance on this project.

References

[1] Fuchs S. Seizures. In: Barkin R, Caputo G, Jaffe D, et al, editors. Pediatric emergency medicine. 2nd edition. St. Louis (MO): Mosby; 1997. p. 1009–17.

[2] Gorelick M, Blackwell C. Neurologic emergencies. In: Fleisher G, Ludwig S, Henretig F, et al, editors. Textbook of pediatric emergency medicine. 5th edition. Philadelphia: Lippincott Williams and Wilkins; 2006. p. 759–79.

[3] McAbee GN, Wark JE. A practical approach to uncomplicated seizures in children. Am Fam Physician 2000;62(5):1109–16.

[4] Roth H, Drislane F. Seizures. Neurol Clin 1998;16:257–84.

[5] Vining EP. Pediatric seizures. Emerg Med Clin North Am 1994;12(4):973–88.

[6] Shneker BF, Fountain NB. Epilepsy. Dis Mon 2003;49:426–78.

[7] Reuter D, Brownstein D. Common emergent pediatric neurologic problems. Emerg Med Clin North Am 2002;20(1):155–76.

[8] Pellock J. Seizures and epilepsy in infancy and childhood. Neurol Clin 1993;11:755–75.

[9] Tang-Wai R, Oskoui M, Webster R, et al. Outcomes in pediatric epilepsy: seeing through the fog. Pediatr Neurol 2005;33:244–50.

[10] Jarrar RG, Buchhalter JR. Therapeutics in pediatric epilepsy, part 1: the new antiepileptic drugs and the ketogenic diet. Mayo Clin Proc 2003;78:359–70.

[11] Cossette P, Riviello J, Carmant L. ACTH versus vigabatrin therapy in infantile spasms: a retrospective study. Neurology 1999;52(8):1691–4.

[12] Trevathan E. Infantile spasms and Lennox-Gastaut syndrome. J Child Neurol 2002; 17(Suppl 2):2S9–2S22.

[13] Elterman RD, Shields WD, Mansfield KA, et al. Randomized trial of vigabatrin in patients with infantile spasms. Neurology 2001;57(8):1416–21.

[14] Marks WJ, Garcia PA. Management of seizures and epilepsy. Am Fam Physician 1998;57(7): 1589–600.

[15] Vining EP, Freeman JM, Ballaban-Gil K, et al. A multi-center study of the efficacy of the ketogenic diet. Arch Neurol 1998;55(11):1433–7.

[16] Wirrell E. Neonatal seizures: to treat or not to treat? Semin Pediatr Neurol 2005;12:97–105.

[17] Zupance ML. Neonatal seizures. Pediatr Clin North Am 2004;51:961–78.

[18] Stafstrom C. Neonatal seizures. Pediatr Rev 1995;16:248–55.

[19] Bernes S, Kaplan AM. Evolution of neonatal seizures. Pediatr Clin North Am 1994;41: 1069–104.

[20] Rennie JM, Boylan GB. Neonatal seizures and their treatment. Curr Opin Neurol 2003;16: 177–81.

[21] Evans D, Levene M. Neonatal seizures. Arch Dis Child Fetal Neonatal Ed 1998;78:F70–5.

[22] Ng E, Klinger G, Shah V, et al. Safety of benzodiazepines in newborns. Ann Pharmacother 2002;36:1150–5.

[23] Bergman D, Baltz R, Cooley J, et al. Provisional Committee on Quality Improvement, Subcommittee on Febrile Seizures. Practice parameter: the neurodiagnostic evaluation of the child with a first simple febrile seizure. Pediatrics 1996;97:769–72.

[24] Bergman D, Baltz R, Cooley J, et al. Committee on Quality Improvement, Subcommittee on Febrile Seizures. Practice parameter: long-term treatment of the child with simple febrile seizures. Pediatrics 1999;103:1307–9.

[25] Warden CR, Zibulewsky J, Mace S, et al. Evaluation and management of febrile seizures in the out of hospital and emergency department settings. Ann Emerg Med 2003;41:215–22.

[26] Wolf SM, Ochoa JG, Conway EE. Seizure management in pediatric patients for the nineties. Pediatr Ann 1998;27:653–64.

[27] Gonzalez Del Rey J. Febrile seizures. In: Barkin R, Caputo G, Jaffe D, et al, editors. Pediatric emergency medicine. 2nd edition. St. Louis (MO): Mosby; 1997. p. 1017–9.

[28] Teng D, Dayan P, Tyler S, et al. Risk of intracranial pathologic conditions requiring emergency intervention after a first complex febrile seizure episode among children. Pediatrics 2006;117:304–8.

[29] Chamberlain JM, Gorman RL. Occult bacteremia in children with simple febrile seizures. Am J Dis Child 1988;142:1073–6.

[30] Trainor JL, Hampers LC, Krug SE, et al. Children with first-time simple febrile seizures are at low risk of serious bacterial illness. Acad Emerg Med 2001;8:781–7.

[31] Chiu SS, Tse CYC, Lau YL, et al. Influenza A infection is an important cause of febrile seizures. Pediatrics 2001;108:e63.

[32] Barone SR, Kaplan MH, Krilov LR. Human herpesvirus-6 infection in children with first febrile seizures. J Pediatr 1995;127:95–7.

[33] Barron T. The child with spells. Pediatr Clin North Am 1991;38(3):711–24.

[34] Hirtz D, Ashwal S, Berg A, et al. Practice parameter: evaluating a first nonfebrile seizure in children. Neurology 2000;55:616–23.

[35] Arunkumar G, Morris H. Epilepsy update: new medical and surgical treatment options. Cleve Clin J Med 1998;65:527–37.

[36] Selbst SM, Clancy R. Pseudoseizures in the pediatric emergency department. Pediatr Emerg Care 1996;12(3):185–8.

[37] Nadkarni S, LaJoie J, Devinsky O. Current treatments of epilepsy. Neurology 2005;64: S2–11.

[38] Scarfone RJ, Pond K, Thompson K, et al. Utility of laboratory testing for infants with seizures. Pediatr Emerg Care 2000;16:309–12.

[39] Farrar HC, Chande VT, Fitzpatrick DF, et al. Hyponatremia as the cause of seizures in infants: a retrospective analysis of incidence, severity, and clinical predictors. Ann Emerg Med 1995;26:42–8.

[40] Warden C, Browenstein D, Del Beccaro M. Predictors of abnormal findings of computed tomography of the head in pediatric patients presenting with seizures. Ann Emerg Med 1997; 29:518–23.

[41] Sharma S, Riviello JJ, Harper MB, et al. The role of emergent neuroimaging in children with new-onset afebrile seizures. Pediatrics 2003;111:1–6.

[42] Scheuer ML, Pedley TA. The evaluation and treatment of seizures. N Engl J Med 1990;323: 1468–74.

[43] Prasad A, Seshia S. Status epilepticus in pediatric practice: neonate to adolescent. Adv Neurol 2006;97:229–43.

[44] Lowenstein DH, Alldredge BK. Status epilepticus. N Engl J Med 1998;338:970–6.

[45] Haafiz A, Kissoon N. Status epilepticus: current concepts. Pediatr Emerg Care 1999;15: 119–29.

[46] Hanhan UA, Fiallos MR, Orlowski JP. Status epilepticus. Pediatr Clin North Am 2001;48: 683–94.

[47] Fitzgerald BJ, Okos AJ, Miller JW. Treatment of out of hospital status epilepticus with diazepam rectal gel. Seizure 2003;12:52–5.

[48] Scott RC, Besag FM, Neville BG. Buccal midazolam and rectal diazepam for treatment of prolonged seizures in childhood and adolescence: a randomized trial. Lancet 1999;353: 623–6.

[49] Wolfe T, Macfarlane T. Intranasal midazolam therapy for pediatric status epilepticus. Am J Emerg Med 2006;24:343–6.

[50] Chamberlain JM, Altiere MA, Futterman C, et al. A prospective, randomized study comparing intramuscular midazolam with intravenous diazepam for the treatment of seizures in children. Pediatr Emerg Care 1997;13:92–4.

[51] Vilke GM, Sharieff GQ, Marino A, et al. Midazolam for the treatment of out of hospital pediatric seizures. Prehosp Emerg Care 2002;6:215–7.

[52] Wheless J. Treatment of acute seizures and status epilepticus in children. J Child Neurol 1999;20:S47–51.

[53] Russell RJ, Parks B. Anticonvulsant medications. Pediatr Ann 1999;28:238–45.

[54] Vining EP, Freeman JM. Where, why, and what type of therapy. Pediatr Ann 1985;14:741–5.

[55] Sobaniec W, Kulak W, Strzelecka J, et al. A comparative study of vigabatrin vs. carbamazepine in monotherapy of newly diagnosed partial seizures in children. Pharmacol Rep 2005; 57:646–53.

[56] Sullivan J, Dlugos D. Antiepileptic drug monotherapy: pediatric concerns. Semin Pediatr Neurol 2005;12:88–96.

[57] Abramowicz M. Drugs for epilepsy. Med Lett Drugs Ther 1995;37:37–40.

[58] Bergin AM. Pharmacotherapy of pediatric epilepsy. Expert Opin Pharmacother 2003;4: 421–31.

[59] Verdru P. Epilepsy in children: the evidence for new antiepileptic drugs. Acta Neurol Scand 2005;112:17–20.

[60] Wilfong A. Zonisamide monotherapy for epilepsy in children and young adults. Pediatr Neurol 2005;32:77–80.

[61] Santos C, Brotherton T. Use of zonisamide in pediatric patients. Pediatr Neurol 2005;33: 12–4.

[62] Wilfong A, Schultz R. Zonisamide for absence seizures. Epilepsy Res 2005;64:31–4.

[63] Glauser TA, Ayala R, Elterman R, et al. Double-blind placebo-controlled trial of adjunctive levetiracetam in pediatric partial seizures. Neurology 2006;66:1654–60.

[64] Cerminara C, Seri S, Bombardieri R, et al. Hypohydrosis during topiramate: a rare and reversible side effect. Pediatr Neurol 2006;34:392–4.

[65] Rubenstein J, Kossoff E, Pyzik P, et al. Experience in the use of the ketogenic diet as early therapy. J Child Neurol 2005;20:31–4.

[66] Kossoff E, McGrogan J, Bluml R, et al. A modified Atkins diet is effective for the treatment of intractable pediatric epilepsy. Epilepsia 2006;47(2):421–4.

[67] Shinnar S, Berg AT, Moshe SL, et al. The risk of seizure recurrence after a first unprovoked afebrile seizure in childhood: an extended follow-up. Pediatrics 1996;98:216–25.

ELSEVIER
SAUNDERS

Emerg Med Clin N Am
25 (2007) 1087–1115

EMERGENCY
MEDICINE
CLINICS OF
NORTH AMERICA

The Evolving Approach to the Young Child Who Has Fever and No Obvious Source

Paul Ishimine, MD[a,b,c,*]

[a]Departments of Medicine and Pediatrics, University of California,
San Diego School of Medicine, San Diego, CA, USA
[b]Department of Emergency Medicine, University of California, San Diego Medical Center,
200 West Arbor Drive, San Diego, CA 92103–8676, USA
[c]Division of Emergency Medicine, Rady Children's Hospital and Health Center,
3020 Children's Way, MC 5075, San Diego, CA 92123, USA

Although fever is one of the most common presenting complaints to emergency departments [1], the approach to the febrile young child remains controversial. Despite attempts to simplify and unify the approach to febrile children, the evaluation and treatment of these patients varies considerably [2–4]. Furthermore, recent advances, such as vaccination with the heptavalent pneumococcal conjugate vaccine, warrant the need to reevaluate previously used strategies in the evaluation of the young child who has fever.

The presence of fever worries clinicians and parents alike. Although the differential diagnosis of fever is broad and includes both infectious and noninfectious causes [5], the majority of febrile children have viral infections as sources of their fevers. Febrile young children present a particularly vexing group; when compared with older children, young children are less articulate and less able to localize signs and symptoms, and this age group is the most likely group of children to sustain occult bacterial infections.

Attempts have been made to standardize the approach to the young febrile child. Several algorithmic approaches apply to the evaluation of the young child who has a fever without source (FWS) [6–8]. These patients have traditionally been divided into three subgroups: neonates (birth to 28 days old), young infants (commonly defined as infants between 1 to 3 months of age, although some define this group as children between 1 month and 2 months of

* Department of Emergency Medicine, University of California, San Diego Medical Center, 200 West Arbor Drive, San Diego, CA 92103–8676.
E-mail address: pishimin@ucsd.edu

0733-8627/07/$ - see front matter © 2007 Elsevier Inc. All rights reserved.
doi:10.1016/j.emc.2007.07.012

age), and the older infant or toddler (commonly defined as 3 to 36 months of age, although some studies include patients only up to 24 months old).

Limitations of current approaches

The approach to the young child who has a FWS has traditionally emphasized the detection of serious bacterial infections such as meningitis, pneumonia, urinary tract infection (UTI), bacterial gastroenteritis, osteomyelitis, and bacteremia. Most viral infections cause self-limited illnesses that do not cause significant morbidity or mortality. Conversely, bacterial infections are more likely to be associated with worse outcomes, a characteristic that has led many to ignore the role of viral infections, especially in the young patient. The role of rapid viral testing in the emergency department, which is becoming increasingly available to emergency clinicians, remains unclear.

Further confusing the approach to these patients is the changing epidemiology of invasive bacterial infections. *Haemophilus influenzae* type b (Hib) previously presented a substantial burden of disease resulting in considerable morbidity and mortality in young children, but, since the early 1990s, universal Hib vaccination has nearly eliminated this organism as a significant cause of disease [9–12].

With the eradication of *Haemophilus influenzae* type b, *Streptococcus pneumoniae* emerged as the predominant bacterial pathogen. In the late 1990s, *S pneumoniae* represented 83% to 92% of positive blood cultures taken from young febrile children presenting to emergency departments, and the overall prevalence of occult bacteremia was 1.6% to 1.9% [9,11]. An effective, 23-valent polysaccharide pneumococcal vaccine has been licensed since 1983, but this vaccine is insufficiently immunogenic in young children and is not recommended for children younger than 2 years of age (the age group at greatest risk for invasive pneumococcal infection).

The heptavalent pneumococcal conjugate vaccine (PCV7), licensed in 2000, covers the seven most common pneumococcal serotypes and has changed the landscape of invasive bacterial disease in young children. The seven serotypes included in this vaccine caused approximately 82% of cases of invasive pneumococcal disease [13]. This vaccine is recommended for universal administration to children younger than 2 years old in a four-dose regimen (doses are given at 2, 4, 6, and 12 to 15 months), as well as to high-risk older children (eg, children who have sickle cell disease, HIV infection, cochlear implants, and other causes of immunocompromise) [14].

This vaccine has been shown to be safe [15,16] and highly effective in preventing invasive pneumococcal disease. In a post licensure surveillance of the Northern California Kaiser Permanente study cohort, the incidence of invasive pneumococcal disease caused by vaccine and cross-reactive vaccine serotypes declined from 51.5 to 98.2 cases of invasive disease per 100,000 person-years in children less than 1 year old to zero cases per 100,000 person-years 4 years after licensure [17]. There was also a reduction of invasive pneumococcal disease in children less than 2 years old, declining from 81.7 to 113.8 cases of invasive disease per 100,000 person-years to zero cases per 100,000 person-years 4 years after the vaccine was licensed [17]. Additionally, there was a decline in invasive pneumococcal disease for all serotypes, not just the seven covered by PCV7, and a significant decline in drug-resistant pneumococci. Moreover, there was a 25% decrease in invasive pneumococcal disease in persons older than 5 years, suggesting herd immunity because these patients were not themselves immunized. These reductions have been replicated in other settings [18–25]. This success has also been reflected in changes in the epidemiology from blood cultures obtained from the emergency department. The incidence of positive blood cultures for all pathogens from emergency department patients is less than 1% [21,25,26].

History and physical examination

The history and physical examination are invaluable in the assessment of the febrile child. A fever is defined as temperature of 38.0°C (100.4°F). Rectal thermometry is considered the gold standard for temperature measurement, because this route is thought to most closely represent the core temperature and is more accurate than oral, axillary, tympanic membrane, and temporal artery thermometry [27–32]. Bundling a young child may increase the skin temperature but probably does not increase the core temperature [33]. Subjective determination of fever by parents at home is moderately accurate [34–36], but further evaluation should be considered in this population because a subjective fever at home may be the only indicator of a potentially serious bacterial infection in a child who is afebrile in the emergency department [37]. Patients who have fevers measured rectally at home should undergo the same evaluation as if these measurements were obtained in the emergency department.

The characteristics of a patient's fever may provide useful information. There is an increase in the rate of pneumococcal bacteremia with an increase in temperature, and this increase is more pronounced in young children [38]. Other studies suggest that the incidence of serious bacterial infections is higher in patients who have hyperpyrexia [39,40]. The duration of the fever at the time of emergency department presentation does not predict whether a child has occult bacteremia [41]. The use of antipyretics should be noted; however, a response (or lack thereof) to antipyretic medications does not predict whether the underlying cause is bacterial or viral [42–46]. Additional important data include associated signs and symptoms, underlying medical conditions, exposure to ill contacts, and immunization status.

An assessment of the child's overall appearance is critical. Although there is an imperfect correlation between physical examination findings and serious bacterial illness, ill-appearing children are more likely than well-appearing children to have serious bacterial infection, and most well-appearing children do not have serious bacterial infection [47–50]. In the child who has a toxic appearance, an aggressive work-up, antibiotic treatment, and hospitalization are mandated regardless of age or risk factors. The physical examination may reveal obvious sources of infection, and the identification of a focal infection may decrease the need for additional testing. For example, febrile patients who have clinically recognizable viral conditions (eg, croup, chicken pox, and stomatitis) have lower rates of bacteremia than patients who have no obvious source of infection [51].

With the exception of neonates and young infants, if a child has a non-toxic appearance, a more selective approach can be undertaken. When a child who has a febrile illness has an obviously identifiable cause, the treatment and disposition should generally be tailored to this specific infection. The approach to the young child who has a FWS is discussed in the following sections.

Neonates: birth to 28 days old

Neonates are at particularly high risk for serious bacterial infection (Fig. 1). Although most febrile neonates presenting to the emergency department are diagnosed ultimately as having a nonspecific viral illness, approximately 12% to 28% of all febrile neonates presenting to a pediatric emergency department have serious bacterial illness [52–54]. Neonates are infected typically by more virulent bacteria such as group B *Streptococcus*, *Escherichia coli*, and *Listeria monocytogenes*. Group B *Streptococcus*, a common bacterial pathogen in this age group, is associated with high rates of meningitis (39%), non-meningeal foci of infection (10%), and sepsis (7%) [55]. Although only a small percentage of neonates are infected by *S pneumoniae*, these neonates have a mortality rate of 14% [56]. The most common bacterial infections in this are group are UTIs and occult bacteremia [52,54]. Neonates are more likely to experience serious sequelae from viral infections (eg, herpes simplex virus [HSV] meningitis).

Evaluation of the febrile neonate

Traditional risk stratification strategies have used ancillary testing to supplement the limited information available from the history and physical examination. Unfortunately, it is difficult to predict accurately which neonates have invasive disease, even when laboratory testing is used. Initial studies by Dagan and colleagues [57,58] appeared promising. The "Rochester criteria" were applied to infants less than 90 days old, and neonates were included. Using these criteria, Jaskiewicz and colleagues [59] found that 2 of 227 children younger than 30 days old who met low-risk criteria had serious bacterial infection. Ferrera and colleagues [60] found that 6% of neonates who were retrospectively classified as low risk by the Rochester criteria had serious bacterial infection.

Baker and colleagues retrospectively stratified neonates into high- and low-risk patients based on the "Philadelphia criteria" [61] they had derived for older infants. The neonates who were placed in the high-risk category had a higher incidence of bacterial disease (18.6%), but 4.6% of neonates who were classified as low-risk patients had serious bacterial infections. Additionally, 11 different bacterial pathogens were identified in 32 patients who had serious bacterial infections, and only 1 of these 32 patients was infected with *S pneumoniae*. Kadish and colleagues [54] found a similar rate of serious bacterial infections in neonates whom they categorized as low risk when they retrospectively applied both the Philadelphia criteria and similar criteria created by Baskin and colleagues (the "Boston criteria"). They also found a wide range of bacterial pathogens, but only two cultures in 55 patients who had serious bacterial infection were positive for *S pneumoniae*. Chiu and colleagues [53,62] have also demonstrated low but significant rates of serious bacterial infections in neonates initially classified as low risk.

Because of the inability of the physical examination to accurately predict serious infections in neonates, recommendations for these patients include obtaining blood cultures, urine for rapid urine testing, urine cultures, and cerebrospinal fluid (CSF) studies [6]. A peripheral white blood cell (WBC) count is often ordered in the evaluation of febrile neonates, but the discriminatory value of the WBC count is insufficient to differentiate between patients who have serious bacterial infections and those who do not [63,64]. Because of the inability of the WBC count to predict bacteremia, blood cultures should be ordered for all patients. Although various options for rapidly testing for UTI exist (eg, urine dipstick, standard urinalysis, and enhanced urinalysis), no rapid test detects all cases of UTI; therefore, urine cultures must be ordered for all of these patients [65,66]. Urine should be collected by bladder catheterization or suprapubic aspiration because bag urine specimens are associated with high rates of contamination [67–70]. Because the peripheral WBC is a poor screening test for meningitis [71], a lumbar puncture should be performed in all febrile neonates. Chest radiographs are indicated only in the presence of respiratory symptoms, and stool analyses are indicated only in the presence of diarrhea. In neonates, the presence of signs suggestive of viral illness does not negate the need for a full diagnostic evaluation. Unlike in older children, in whom documented respiratory syncytial virus (RSV) infections decrease the likelihood of serious bacterial illness, RSV-infected neonates have the same rate of serious bacterial infection when compared with RSV-negative neonates [72].

Treatment and disposition of the febrile neonate

Because of the high rates of serious bacterial infections, all febrile neonates should receive antibiotics. Typically, these patients are treated with a third-generation cephalosporin or gentamicin. Ceftriaxone is not recommended for neonates who are jaundiced because of the concern for inducing

unconjugated hyperbilirubinemia [73,74]. Other third-generation cephalosporins, such as cefotaxime, 50 mg/kg intravenously (75–100 mg/kg if there
is a concern for meningitis based on CSF results), or gentamicin, 2.5 mg/kg
intravenously, are used in this age group. Additionally, although the incidence of *L monocytogenes* is low [75], ampicillin, 50 mg/kg intravenously
(100 mg/kg intravenously if there is a concern for meningitis) is still recommended in the empiric treatment of these patients [76].

Neonatal HSV infections occur in approximately 1 in 3200 deliveries in
the United States [77]. Neonates who have HSV infections usually present
within the first 2 weeks of life, and only a minority of infected children
have fever [78]. Rates of morbidity and mortality are high with neonatal

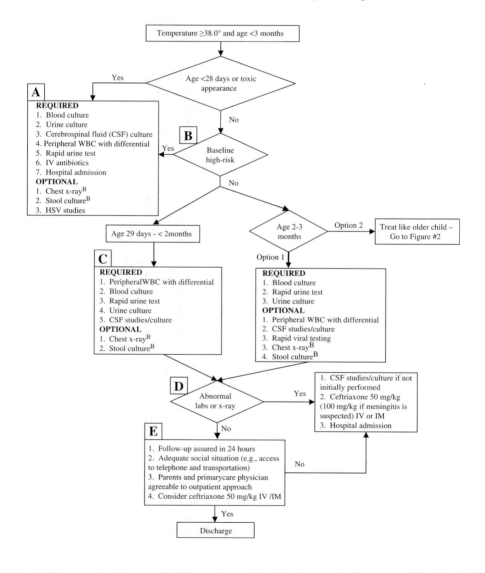

HSV, but treatment with high-dose acyclovir (20 mg/kg intravenously) improves outcomes in patients [79]. Acyclovir is not recommended routinely for empiric treatment in addition to standard antibiotics in febrile neonates [78] but should be considered in febrile neonates with risk factors for neonatal HSV. Risk factors include primary maternal infection, especially for neonates delivered vaginally, prolonged rupture of membranes at delivery, the use of fetal scalp electrodes, skin, eye, or mouth lesions, seizures, and CSF pleocytosis [77,80,81].

Febrile neonates should be hospitalized regardless of the results of laboratory studies. Outpatient management of these patients has been suggested and occurs frequently when patients present to pediatricians' offices [37]; however, given the lack of prospective studies addressing this approach as well as the limitations inherent in the screening evaluation in the emergency department and the difficulties in arranging follow-up evaluation, hospitalization is strongly recommended.

Young infants: 1 to 2 or 3 months old

The approach to febrile young infants, defined most commonly as children less than 2 or 3 months old, changed dramatically in the 1980s and early 1990s (see Fig. 1). Before this time, most febrile young infants presenting to academic medical centers were hospitalized and frequently started on antibiotic therapy [82]. This aggressive approach was based, in part, on the

Fig. 1. Fever without an apparent source in children less than 3 months of age. (*A*) Urine testing can be accomplished by microscopy, Gram stain, or urine dipstick. Chest radiographs are indicated in patients who have hypoxia, tachypnea, abnormal lung sounds, or respiratory distress. Stool studies are indicated in patients who have diarrhea. HSV testing should be considered in the presence of risk factors (see text for details). HSV testing is best accomplished by polymerase chain reaction or viral culture. Neonates should receive both ampicillin (50 mg/kg intravenously; 100 mg/kg intravenously if concern for meningitis) and cefotaxime (50 mg/kg; 100 mg/kg intravenously if concern for meningitis) or gentamicin (2.5 mg/kg intravenously). Older children should receive ceftriaxone (50 mg/kg intravenously; 100 mg/kg intravenously if concern for meningitis). (*B*) Young patients who have increased underlying risk include children who were premature, who had prolonged hospital stays after birth, those who have underlying medical conditions, patients who have indwelling medical devices, patients who have a fever greater than 5 days, and patients already on antibiotics. (*C*) Urine testing can be accomplished by microscopy, Gram stain, or urine dipstick. Chest radiographs are indicated in patients who have hypoxia, tachypnea, abnormal lung sounds, or respiratory distress. Stool studies are indicated in patients who have diarrhea. (*D*) Abnormal laboratory values are as follows: peripheral WBC count, $<5000/mm^3$ or $>15,000/mm^3$ or band-to-neutrophil ratio >0.2; urine testing, ≥ 5 WBC/hpf, bacteria on Gram stain, or positive leukocyte esterase or nitrite; CSF, ≥ 8 WBC/mm^3 or bacteria on Gram stain; stool specimen, ≥ 5 WBC/hpf; chest radiograph, infiltrate on chest film. (*E*) Administering ceftriaxone (50 mg/kg intravenously or intramuscularly) is optional but should be considered in patients who have undergone lumbar puncture. Patients who have not undergone lumbar puncture should not be given ceftriaxone. (*Adapted in part from* Ishimine P. Fever without source in children 0 to 36 months of age. Pediatr Clin N Am 2006;53:184; with permission.)

relatively limited amount of information obtainable from the examination of young infants [83] and the high morbidity rate observed with *H influenzae* type b infection. Several decision rules were developed in an attempt to identify febrile young children who were believed to be at low risk for serious bacterial infection and who could be treated on an outpatient basis.

The Rochester criteria stratified children less than 60 days old into high- and low-risk groups. The children who met the low-risk criteria appeared well, had been previously healthy, and had no evidence of skin, soft tissue, bone, joint, or ear infections. Additionally, these children had normal peripheral WBC counts (5000–15,000/mm^3), normal absolute band counts ($\leq$1500/mm^3), $\leq$10 WBC/high-power field (hpf) of centrifuged urine sediment, and, for those patients who have diarrhea, $\leq$5 WBC/hpf on stool smear [57,58]. The low-risk group identified children who were unlikely to have serious bacterial infections, with a negative predictive value of 98.9% [59].

Baskin and colleagues [84] described the Boston criteria for febrile children between 1 and 3 months of age who presented to the emergency department with temperatures $\geq$38.0°C. Infants were discharged after an intramuscular injection of ceftriaxone, 50 mg/kg, if they generally appeared to be well (not strictly defined) and had no ear, soft tissue, joint, or bone infections on physical examination. Furthermore, these patients had to have CSF with $\leq$10 WBC/hpf, microscopic urinalysis with $\leq$10 WBC/hpf or a urine dipstick negative for leukocyte esterase, a peripheral WBC count of $\leq$20,000/mm^3, and normal findings when a chest radiograph was obtained (all tests except the chest radiograph were performed on all patients). Twenty-seven of 503 children (5.4%) were later found to have serious bacterial infection (bacterial gastroenteritis, UTI, and occult bacteremia).

Baker and colleagues [85] developed the Philadelphia criteria and similarly sought to identify low-risk patients between 29 and 56 days old with temperatures of $\geq$38.2°C. Patients who appeared to be well (as defined by an Infant Observation Score of 10 or less) had a peripheral WBC count of $\leq$15,000/mm^3, a band-to-neutrophil ratio of $\leq$0.2, a urinalysis with fewer than 10 WBC/hpf, few or no bacteria on a centrifuged urine specimen, CSF with fewer than 8 WBC/mm^3, a gram-negative stain, negative results on chest radiographs (obtained on all patients), negative stool findings for blood, and few or no WBCs on microscopy (ordered for patients who had watery diarrhea). These patients were considered to have a negative screen and were not treated with antibiotics. Of the 747 consecutively enrolled patients, 65 (8.7%) had serious bacterial infections. All 65 patients who had serious bacterial infections were identified using these screening criteria. In a follow-up study (in which fever was defined as $\geq$38.0°C rectally) of 422 consecutively enrolled febrile young infants, 43 (10%) had serious bacterial infections, and all 101 patients who were identified as low risk had no serious bacterial infections. All 43 patients who had serious bacterial infections were identified prospectively as high risk using the Philadelphia criteria [86].

The most common bacterial infections in this age group are UTIs; correspondingly, the most common bacterial pathogen identified is *E coli* [61,84,86]. In the large studies by Baskin and Baker and colleagues [84], only a minority of patients who had serious bacterial infection had pneumococcal infection; therefore, children in this age group are unlikely to benefit directly from the PCV7 vaccine. In the Baskin study, only one of nine patients who had occult bacteremia in this study was infected with *S pneumoniae*. Four of 70 bacterial infections were caused by *S pneumoniae* in Baker's original study [61].

Evaluation of the febrile young infant

Because relying solely on the clinical examination results in a substantial number of missed serious bacterial infections, laboratory testing is required in this age group. A catheterized urinalysis and blood and urine cultures should be obtained in all patients. Although an abnormally high or low WBC count increases the concern for bacteremia or meningitis, it is an imperfect screening tool for bacteremia and meningitis, and the decision to obtain blood cultures and spinal fluid should not depend on the results of the WBC count [63,64,71]. Stool studies for WBC counts and stool cultures should be ordered in patients who have diarrhea. Chest radiographs should be obtained only in young febrile infants who have signs of pulmonary disease (tachypnea ≥ 50 breaths/min, rales, rhonchi, retractions, wheezing, coryza, grunting, nasal flaring, or cough) [87,88].

The results of these tests help to risk stratify these young children. The WBC count is considered abnormal if it is greater than $15,000/mm^3$ or less than $5000/mm^3$, or if the band-to-neutrophil ratio is greater than 0.2. There should be fewer than 8 WBC/mm^3 and no organisms on Gram stain of the CSF. The urine is considered abnormal if the urine dipstick is positive for nitrite or leukocyte esterase, if there are ≥ 5 WBC/hpf on microscopy, or if organisms are seen on a Gram-stained sample of uncentrifuged urine. If obtained, there should be fewer than 5 WBC/hpf in the stool specimen and no evidence of pneumonia on a chest radiograph [6].

The need for lumbar puncture is controversial in this age group. Although the Boston and Philadelphia criteria require CSF analysis, the Rochester criteria do not mandate lumbar puncture. The rarity of bacterial meningitis contributes to the controversy surrounding the utility of the lumbar puncture. The prevalence of bacterial meningitis in febrile infants less than 3 months old is 4.1 cases per 1000 patients, and neither the clinical examination nor the peripheral WBC count is reliable in diagnosing meningitis in this age group [63,71]; therefore, lumbar puncture should be strongly considered. Additional controversy surrounds the need for antibiotics in patients who are identified as low risk. Patients identified as low risk by the Philadelphia protocol were not given antibiotics, whereas patients enrolled in the Boston study were given intramuscular ceftriaxone.

There is some concern that performing a lumbar puncture in a bacteremic patient may lead to meningitis [89,90]. Four of 8300 children 3 months of age or less who underwent CSF analysis had bacterial meningitis and ≤ 8 WBC/mm^3 in the CSF [91], and clinical decision rules to determine which children who have CSF pleocytosis have bacterial infection are less accurate in this young age group [92]. Published recommendations state that parenteral antibiotics should be "considered" if a lumbar puncture is performed [6].

The presence of a documented viral infection lowers but does not eliminate the likelihood of a serious bacterial infection in this age group. Young infants classified as high-risk patients using the Rochester criteria who had test-proven viral infection (enterovirus, respiratory virus, rotavirus, and herpes virus) were at lower risk for serious bacterial infection when compared with patients who did not have an identified source (4.2% versus 12.3%) [93]. A subgroup analysis of 187 febrile infants 28 to 60 days old from the largest prospective multicenter study of RSV infection in young infants showed a significantly lower rate of serious bacterial infection in RSV-positive patients when compared with RSV-negative patients (5.5% versus 11.7%) [72], confirming the results of similar studies in young infants who had bronchiolitis. Most of these bacterial infections were UTIs [94,95]. These studies were underpowered to detect differences in rates of bacteremia and meningitis between RSV-positive and RSV-negative patients. Based on available data, it remains unclear whether the clinician can forgo blood and spinal fluid testing in RSV-positive infants. Patients less than 90 days old who have enteroviral infections have a similar rate of concurrent serious bacterial infections (mostly UTI) of 7% [96].

Treatment and disposition of the febrile young infant

Most infants who have a FWS who are otherwise healthy and born at full term, who are well appearing, and who have normal laboratory values can be managed on an outpatient basis. If the patient undergoes a reliable follow-up within 24 hours, if the parents have a way of immediately accessing health care if there is a change in the patient's condition, and if the parents and the primary care physician understand and agree with this plan of care, the patient may be discharged home. Ceftriaxone, 50 mg/kg intravenously or intramuscularly, can be given before discharge, but withholding antibiotics in these low-risk patients is acceptable as well. Patients who do not undergo lumbar puncture in the emergency department should not receive antibiotics because this will confound the evaluation for meningitis if the patient is still febrile on follow-up examination. Close follow-up reevaluation must be ensured before discharge.

For patients who have abnormal test results or who appear to be ill, antibiotic therapy and hospitalization are warranted. Ceftriaxone, 50 mg/kg intramuscularly or intravenously (100 mg/kg if meningitis is suspected), is commonly used for these patients. Additional antibiotics should be considered in select circumstances (eg, ampicillin or vancomycin for suspected infection by *Listeria*, gram-positive cocci, or *Enterococcus*). Some studies suggest that patients in this age group who have UTIs may be treated on an outpatient basis [97,98]; however, no large prospective studies provide evidence as to the safety of outpatient management in this age range. Young infants who are RSV positive are at higher risk of serious complications, such as apnea [99], and the clinician must evaluate this concern in addition to the risks of serious bacterial infection when making a disposition decision.

Older infants and toddlers: 3 months and older

A temperature of 38.0°C defines a fever and is the usual threshold at which diagnostic testing is initiated in the young infant; however, in febrile children 3 months and older (some studies extend this group to include 2-month-old infants), a temperature of 39.0°C is commonly used as the temperature for initiating further evaluation (Fig. 2). This higher temperature cutoff is used because of the increasing risk of occult pneumococcal bacteremia with increasing temperatures [38] and because large studies of occult bacteremia, widely referenced in the medical literature, use this temperature as the study entry criteria [9,11,100]. No systematic studies have been conducted in the post-PCV7 era to determine whether an increasing height of fever is still correlated with increasing rates of bacterial infection. Although the rates of serious bacterial infection may be higher in children who have temperatures $\geq 39.0°C$, these patients may still have occult infections with lower heights of fever.

Evaluation of the child 3 months and older

The history is often helpful in this age group. Patients are more likely to be able to communicate complaints, and the physical examination is more informative. Clinical assessment as to whether a child appears to be well, ill, or toxic is important. A well appearance does not completely exclude bacteremia [101], but children who appear toxic are much more likely to have serious illness when compared with ill- or well-appearing children (92% versus 26% versus 3%, respectively) [102]. Many bacterial infections can be identified by history and physical examination alone, but some infections may be occult. The most common serious bacterial infections in this age group that may not be clinically apparent are bacteremia, UTI, and pneumonia. Rapid influenza testing may result in a decreased need for diagnostic testing [103]; febrile children between 3 and 36 months who are influenza A positive are less likely to have serious bacterial infections than children who are influenza A negative [104]. If no focal infection is identified and the cause is not believed to be viral, diagnostic testing in this age group is undertaken for the purposes of identifying occult bacterial infections.

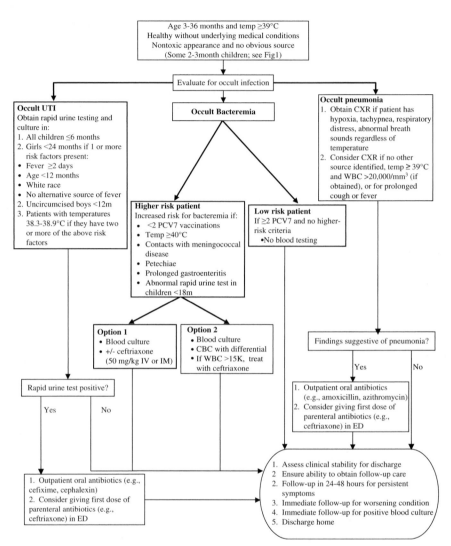

Fig. 2. Fever without apparent source in children 3 to 36 months of age. CBC, complete blood count; CXR, chest radiography; ED, emergency department. (*Adapted in part from* Ishimine P. Fever without source in children 0 to 36 months of age. Pediatr Clin N Am 2006;53:186.)

Occult bacteremia

In the pre-PCV7 era, the children at greatest risk for occult bacteremia were 6 to 24 months old, and the most common pathogen was *S pneumoniae* [9,11]. In the era of universal PCV7 vaccination, the overall incidence of pneumococcal bacteremia (and, accordingly, the total overall incidence of bacteremia) has dropped substantially. In a population immunized with PCV7, *E coli* bacteremia is at least as common as pneumococcal bacteremia.

This changing epidemiology has added to the confusion regarding the utility of blood testing in the evaluation of the febrile child, specifically regarding the value of blood testing in the identification of occult bacteremia. Although there is an increased risk of bacteremia with an increasing WBC count, the sensitivity and specificity of a WBC count $\geq 15,000/mm^3$ is only 74% to 86% and 55% to 77%, respectively [11,21,105,106]. Similarly, patients who had *E coli* bacteremia were more likely to have elevated WBC counts when compared with control subjects without bacteremia; however, the WBC counts in patients who have *Salmonella* [21], *Staphylococcus aureus* [21], and *Neisseria meningitidis* [107] bacteremia do not differ from that in control patients without bacteremia. Using an elevated WBC or absolute neutrophil count as a surrogate marker for occult bacteremia means that many patients will unnecessarily receive antibiotics and a substantial number of patients who have bacteremia will be untreated.

The shifting epidemiology of bacteremia has prompted cost-effectiveness analyses of various management strategies. Using pre-PCV7 data, Lee and colleagues analyzed five strategies for the 3- to 36-month-old febrile child who did not have an identifiable source of infection. In their sensitivity analysis, they found that when the prevalence rate of pneumococcal bacteremia dropped to 0.5%, which is essentially the current rate of pneumococcal bacteremia in emergency departments [21,25,26,108], clinical judgment (eg, patients who were deemed to be at low risk clinically for occult pneumococcal bacteremia received no testing or antibiotics) was the most cost-effective strategy [109].

The role of antibiotics in children believed to be at high risk for bacteremia is controversial as well. Currently, there is no way of prospectively identifying bacteremic patients. Practically, this means that, at the time of the emergency department visit, many febrile children who are at risk for bacteremia must be treated to prevent a single serious bacterial infection. Before PCV7, the use of amoxicillin [110] and ceftriaxone [100,105] appeared to shorten the duration of fever in bacteremic febrile children. Nevertheless, there is a paucity of randomized, placebo-controlled data demonstrating that the use of either oral or parenteral antibiotics prevents significant adverse infectious sequelae in these children. One study compared amoxicillin with placebo for the treatment of febrile children and showed no difference in the rates of subsequent focal infection [110], but another retrospective study demonstrated that, in patients ultimately found to have bacteremia, treatment with oral or parenteral antibiotics reduced persistent fever, persistent bacteremia, and hospital admission [111]. A subsequent meta-analysis has shown that, although ceftriaxone prevents serious bacterial infection in patients who had proven occult bacteremia, 284 patients at risk for bacteremia would need to be treated with antibiotics to prevent one case of meningitis [112]. Complicating this analysis is the fact that in a majority of patients who have pneumococcal bacteremia, the bacteremia will resolve spontaneously [9]. Focal infections develop in 15% of bacteremic children [9], and meningitis develops in 2.7% to 5.8% of patients who have occult pneumococcal bacteremia [112,113]. These analyses were conducted on data obtained in the pre-PCV7 era, and similar risk-benefit analyses have not been conducted after the introduction of PCV7. Nonetheless, it is clear that with the significant decrease in invasive pneumococcal disease [17,24,114], many more children will be treated unnecessarily with antibiotics to prevent a single serious outcome.

PCV7 has led to remarkable declines in the rates of invasive pneumococcal disease. Declines in the rate of invasive disease occur even when the four-dose regimen is incomplete, and even one dose of PCV7 offers some protection, although one dose given before 6 months of age did not seem to protect against illness occurring after 6 months or more [115]. Although maximum individual protection against the seven serotypes covered by this vaccine occurs after completion of the four-dose immunization regimen (the standard immunization regimen entails doses at age 2 months, 4 months, 6 months, and 12 to 15 months) [116], similarly high rates of vaccine efficacy in protecting against serotype disease were noted in two- and three-dose immunization regimens as well [115]. Among the seven serotypes, the amount of disease reduction is variable [18,20,117]. Although the overall rate of invasive pneumococcal disease is declining, the rates of invasive disease caused by nonvaccine serotypes appear to be stable and may be increasing [24,27,118–120]. The clinical implications of this serotype replacement are unclear.

In addition to pneumococcus, another common cause of bacteremia is *E coli*. *E coli* bacteremia is more common in children aged less than 12 months and is most common in children 3 to 6 months of age. *E coli* bacteremia is commonly associated with a concomitant UTI [121]; in one recent study, all 27 patients identified with *E coli* bacteremia had UTIs [21]. *Salmonella* causes 4% to 8% of occult bacteremia, occurring in 0.1% of all children 3 to 36 months old who have temperatures $\geq 39.0°C$ [9,11,21,100]. Although the majority of patients who have *Salmonella* bacteremia have gastroenteritis, 5% will have primary bacteremia [122]. One large retrospective study of children who have non-typhi *Salmonella* bacteremia showed that 54% of bacteremic children had temperatures less than 39.0°C (29% of patients were afebrile) and a median WBC count of 10,000/mm^3. These children had a 41% rate of persistent bacteremia on follow-up cultures, and the rates of persistent bacteremia were the same in patients who were treated with antibiotics at the initial visit and those who were not. Among immunocompetent patients, 2.5% of patients who had *Salmonella* bacteremia had focal infections, and no differences in rates of focal infection were noted in children older and younger than 3 months of age [123].

Meningococcal infections are infrequent causes of bacteremia but are associated with high rates of morbidity and mortality [124]. *Neisseria meningitidis* is a leading cause of bacterial meningitis [125]. Combining the data from Boston and Philadelphia occult bacteremia studies, 0.02% of children who appeared to be nontoxic and who had temperatures $\geq 39.0°C$ had meningococcal disease [9,11]. Usually, these patients are overtly sick; however,

12% to 16% of patients who have meningococcal disease have unsuspected infection [107,126]. Although there is an association between younger age and elevated band count with meningococcal disease, the positive predictive values of these variables are low given the low prevalence of this disease, and the researchers in one large meningococcal disease study believe that routine screening for all young febrile children who have complete blood counts for meningococcal bacteremia is not useful [107]. Patients who had unsuspected meningococcal disease who were treated empirically with antibiotics had fewer complications than patients who were untreated, but there were no differences in rates of permanent sequelae or death [127]. Nevertheless, testing and empiric treatment may be warranted for children at higher risk for meningococcal disease. Risk factors for meningococcal bacteremia include contact with patients who have meningococcal disease, periods of meningococcal disease outbreaks, and the presence of fever and petechiae (although most children who have fever and petechiae do not have invasive bacterial disease) [128–130]. A new tetravalent meningococcal conjugate vaccine was licensed for use in the United States in 2005. Although clinical trials in infants and young children are in progress, this vaccine has been licensed and recommended for routine administration in children 11 years old and older [131].

Children who have positive blood cultures need to be reexamined. A child who has a positive blood culture with any pathogen who appears ill needs a repeat blood culture, lumbar puncture, intravenous antibiotics, and hospital admission. Because the rates of spontaneous clearance of pneumococcal bacteremia are high, patients who have pneumococcal bacteremia who are afebrile on repeat evaluation can be observed on an outpatient basis [132] after repeat blood cultures are obtained and these patients are given antibiotics. Children who have pneumococcal bacteremia and who are persistently febrile need repeat blood cultures and generally should undergo lumbar puncture and require hospital admission. The treatment and disposition for well-appearing children who have *Salmonella* bacteremia are less clear, but patients with meningococcal bacteremia should be hospitalized for parenteral antibiotics [106]. Furthermore, the approach to the patient who has an *E coli* UTI who later grows *E coli* in a blood culture is unclear, although repeat assessment and blood culture should be performed, and consideration should be given to lumbar puncture and admission.

Contaminated blood cultures are common, and in younger children, the rate of contaminated cultures frequently exceeds the rate of true positive cultures [9,11,21,25,108,133]. False-positive blood cultures lead to further testing and unnecessary use of antibiotics and hospitalizations [134], along with the attendant iatrogenic complications [135].

Given the observed decline in invasive pneumococcal disease, the inconsistent relationship between the height of a fever and rates of bacteremia, the strong association between *E coli* UTIs and *E coli* bacteremia, the relative infrequency of meningococcemia and *Salmonella* bacteremia, and the limited value of the WBC count in predicting the latter two diseases, the need for a routine complete blood count, blood cultures, and empiric anti-biotics has been called into question in fully immunized children [21,25,136,137]. If the clinician decides to obtain blood testing, the most important test is the blood culture, because this is the gold standard test for bacteremia. At best, the WBC count is a limited screening tool, and an abnormality is a relatively poor surrogate marker for bacteremia. It is reasonable to address parental preferences when devising a "risk-minimizing" versus a "test-minimizing" [138] approach to these children, because parental perceptions and preferences regarding risk may differ from those of the treating clinician [139–141].

Occult urinary tract infection

UTIs are common sources of fever in young children, and these children are at risk for permanent renal damage from such infections. In older children, historical and examination features such as dysuria, urinary frequency, and abdominal and flank pain may suggest UTI; however, in young children, symptoms are usually nonspecific. Although the overall prevalence in children is 2% to 5% [142–144], certain subgroups of children are at higher risk for UTIs. White race, girls, uncircumcised boys, children who have no alternative source of fever, and temperatures $\geq 39.0°C$ are associated with a higher risk of UTI. Sixteen percent of white girls less than 2 years old with temperatures $\geq 39.0°C$ and a FWS had UTI [143,144]. UTIs were found in 2.7% to 3.5% of febrile children, even when there were other potential sources of fever (eg, gastroenteritis, otitis media, upper respiratory tract infection, and nonspecific rash) [143,144].

Gorelick and Shaw [145] derived a clinical decision rule which has been subsequently validated for febrile girls with temperatures $\geq 38.3°C$ who are less than 24 months of age. Urine testing is indicated if two or more of the following risk factors are present: age less than 12 months, fever for 2 or more days, temperature $\geq 39.0°C$, white race, and no alternative source of fever. This rule has a sensitivity of 95% to 99% and a false-positive rate of 69% to 90% in detecting girls with UTI [145,146]. No similar clinical decision rules exist for boys, but, because the prevalence in boys less than 6 months old is 2.7% [144], urine should be collected in all boys in this age group. The prevalence of UTIs in uncircumcised boys is eight to nine times higher than in circumcised boys; therefore, uncircumcised boys younger than 12 months should also undergo urine testing [144,147,148].

Several rapid urine tests have good sensitivity for detecting UTIs. Enhanced urinalysis (≥ 10 WBC/hpf or bacteria on Gram-stained, uncentrifuged urine) [65,149] and a combination of ≥ 10 WBC/hpf and bacteriuria (on either centrifuged or uncentrifuged urine) [150] are both excellent screening tests. The more readily available urine dipstick (positive for either leukocyte esterase or nitrites) has a sensitivity of 88% [65]. Because no rapid screening test detects all UTIs, urine cultures should be ordered for all of these patients [68]. Any positive test results from a rapid test should lead to a presumptive diagnosis of a UTI, and antibiotic treatment should be initiated. Most patients who have UTIs and appear well can be treated on an outpatient basis. Empiric antibiotic therapy should be tailored to local bacterial epidemiology, but reasonable outpatient medications include cefixime (8 mg/kg twice on the first day of treatment, then 8 mg/kg/d starting from the second day) or cephalexin (25–100 mg/kg/d divided into four doses). The duration of therapy should be from 7 to 14 days.

Occult pneumonia

Young children commonly develop pneumonia, and the most common pathogens are viruses and (based on pre-PCV7 data) *S pneumoniae* [151]. The diagnosis of pneumonia based on clinical examination can be difficult [152]. Multiple attempts have been made at deriving clinical decision rules for the accurate diagnosis of pneumonia, but none has been successfully validated [153–155]. The presence of any pulmonary findings on examination (eg, tachypnea, crackles, respiratory distress, or decreased breath sounds) increases the likelihood of pneumonia, and, conversely, the absence of these findings decreases the likelihood of pneumonia [156–158]. The role of pulse oximetry in detecting pneumonia is unclear [159,160]. Although the chest radiograph is often believed to be the gold standard, there is variability in the interpretation of radiographs even by pediatric radiologists [161]. Furthermore, radiographic findings cannot be used to reliably distinguish between bacterial and nonbacterial causes [162,163].

Some cases of pneumonia are likely to be clinically occult. In the pre-PCV7 era, Bachur and colleagues found that 19% to 26% of children younger than 5 years old who had a temperature of $\geq 39.0°C$, a WBC count $\geq 20,000/mm^3$, and no other source or only a "minor" bacterial source on examination had a pneumonia infection as seen on a chest radiograph [164]. This study has been criticized because of a high degree of interobserver variability in chest radiograph interpretation, because of the failure to perform a WBC count on over half the infants who had a temperature $\geq 38°C$, and because the majority of clinical assessments were preformed by residents. Furthermore, a retrospective study at the same institution after universal PCV7 vaccination showed a 5% "occult" (ie, no respiratory distress, no tachypnea or hypoxia, and no lower respiratory tract abnormalities on examination) pneumonia rate in patients selected to undergo chest radiography [165]. A clinical policy guideline from the American College of Emergency Physicians states that, although there is insufficient evidence to determine when a chest radiograph is required, the clinician is advised to "consider" a chest radiograph in children older than 3 months who have a temperature $\geq 39°C$ and a WBC count $\geq 20,000/mm^3$. Furthermore, a chest radiograph is usually not indicated in febrile children older than 3 months who have a temperature $< 39°C$ without clinical evidence of acute pulmonary disease [87]. The British Thoracic Society similarly recommends that a chest radiograph should be considered in children younger than 5 years old who have a temperature $\geq 39°C$ caused by an unclear source of infection [166]. These recommendations may change based on the decline of the prevalence of pneumococcal pneumonia [167]. A chest radiograph should be obtained in all febrile children regardless of fever height if there are physical examination findings suggestive of pneumonia, such as tachypnea, increased work of breathing, asymmetric or abnormal breath sounds, or hypoxia.

No decision rules exist for pediatric pneumonia that help with disposition decisions in children who have pneumonia, but the majority of patients are treated on an outpatient basis. Both amoxicillin (80 mg/kg/d divided twice or three times daily) and macrolide antibiotics (eg, azithromycin, 10 mg/kg by mouth on the first day, then 5 mg/kg/d for 4 more days) are acceptable. Treatment duration is usually from 7 to 10 days (with the exception of azithromycin), but no definitive evidence supports a specific duration of therapy [166].

Future directions and questions

The pneumococcal vaccine has already had a significant impact on the epidemiology of bacterial infection in young children, and this vaccine seems to have had some impact on the practice patterns of pediatricians. Pediatricians who were surveyed ordered fewer blood and urine tests and were less likely to prescribe antibiotics in a hypothetical scenario of an 8-month-old febrile but otherwise healthy infant when the child had been fully immunized with PCV7 versus when they had not been immunized [168]. The number of blood cultures ordered by pediatricians (but not by emergency physicians) has fallen by 35% in the Northern California Kaiser Permanente system [21].

Although the decline in invasive pneumococcal disease has been dramatic, the rise in nonvaccine serotype pneumococcal disease raises concerns [118,169]. Likewise, there is an increase in antibiotic resistance in nonvaccine serotype pneumococci [19,120,170]. Newer pneumococcal conjugate vaccines with increased serotype coverage are in development [171].

Despite the use of the PCV7 vaccine, bacteremia will still develop in patients; therefore, there remains a need for better tests to diagnose invasive bacterial disease. Several additional tests are being studied as potential surrogate markers for bacterial disease in young children: procalcitonin, C-reactive protein, and interleukin-6 [172–180].

Summary

Most children aged 0 to 36 months who have a FWS have viral infections, but certain subsets of febrile children are at higher risk for more serious bacterial disease. The child who appears to be toxic, regardless of age, needs a comprehensive work-up, antibiotic coverage, and admission to the hospital. Generally, this work-up entails a complete blood count with differential, blood culture, urinalysis and urine culture, lumbar puncture with CSF analysis, Gram stain and culture, and, when indicated, chest radiographs and stool studies. These patients should receive broad-spectrum parenteral antibiotics before hospital admission. Additionally, the approach to patients who are immunocompromised (eg, sickle cell disease, cancer, or long-term steroid use), who have indwelling medical devices (eg, ventriculoperitoneal shunts and indwelling venous access catheters), who are currently taking antibiotics, or who have prolonged fevers should be individualized.

The febrile neonate (0–28 days old) is at high risk for serious bacterial infection, even with a benign examination and normal screening laboratory results; therefore, these patients also need a complete blood count with differential, blood culture, urinalysis and urine culture, lumbar puncture with CSF analysis, Gram stain and culture, and, when indicated, chest radiographs and stool studies. Febrile neonates should receive empiric antibiotic coverage, typically with ampicillin (50 mg/kg intravenously, or 100 mg/kg if meningitis is suspected) and cefotaxime (50 mg/kg intravenously, or 100 mg/kg if meningitis is suspected) or gentamicin (2.5 mg/kg intravenously).

The febrile young infant (1–3 months old) is also at significant risk for bacterial infection. These patients need complete blood counts, blood cultures, urinalyses, and urine cultures. A lumbar puncture with CSF analysis, Gram stain, and culture should be strongly considered because other laboratory tests such as the WBC count are inaccurate in predicting which patients have meningitis. When clinically indicated, chest radiographs and stool studies should be obtained as well. If any of these test findings are abnormal (including a peripheral WBC $\geq 15,000/mm^3$ or $\leq 5000/mm^3$, a band-to-neutrophil ratio ≥ 0.2, a urine dipstick test positive for nitrite or leukocyte esterase or a finding of ≥ 5 WBCs/hpf or organisms seen on Gram stain, CSF fluid with ≥ 8 WBC/mm^3 or organisms on Gram stain, ≥ 5 WBC/hpf in the stool specimen, or evidence of pneumonia on a chest radiograph), the patient should receive ceftriaxone (50 mg/kg intravenously or intramuscularly, or 100 mg/kg intravenously if meningitis is suspected) and should be admitted to the hospital. If these initial laboratory results are normal, the patient can be discharged if follow-up within 24 hours can be ensured. The administration of ceftriaxone, 50 mg/kg intravenously or intramuscularly, should be considered if a lumbar puncture is performed; if a lumbar puncture is not performed, antibiotics should be withheld. If a patient is 2 to 3 months old and the practitioner is comfortable with his or her pediatric assessment skills, these children can be treated similarly to older febrile children.

The older infant or toddler (3–36 months old) who has a temperature of $\geq 39.0°C$ may be treated more selectively. In this age group, if no febrile source is identified definitively, a catheterized urine specimen for evaluation (dipstick, urinalysis, microscopy, or Gram stain) and urine culture should be obtained in girls less than 2 years old if one or more of the following risk factors are present: age less than 12 months, fever for 2 or more days, white race, and no alternative source of fever. Urine testing should also be considered in girls who have temperatures of 38.3°C to 39.0°C if they meet two of the previous risk factors. All boys younger than 6 months and all uncircumcised boys younger than 12 months should also have catheterized urine sent for rapid urine testing and culture. Chest radiographs should be considered in children who have physical examination findings suggestive of pneumonia. Additionally, a chest film should be considered in a child with an unexplained peripheral WBC count ≥ 20,000 (if obtained), or with prolonged fever or cough.

Patients who have not received at least two PCV7 vaccinations should still be considered to be susceptible to pneumococcal bacteremia, but these children benefit to some degree from herd immunity conferred by the population as a whole. Based on pre-PCV7 data, the most cost-effective approach to the child who has had fewer than three PCV7 doses is to obtain a peripheral WBC count. If the WBC count is ≥ 15,000/mm³, a blood culture should be ordered, and the administration of ceftriaxone should be considered [109]; however, other options (eg, blood culture with or without empiric antibiotic administration, or a WBC count and blood culture with selective antibiotic administration) are also reasonable. This approach should also be considered when parents are unsure of their child's immunization status, because parental recall of immunization status is relatively inaccurate [181].

Blood testing should be considered optional in patients who have received two or more PCV7 vaccinations, because the rate of bacteremia in this population is less than 1%. This approach is acceptable because of the low overall rates of bacteremia, the limited accuracy of the WBC count in predicting bacteremia, and the high rate of spontaneous resolution of pneumococcal bacteremia. Additional benefits of this approach include forgoing the discomfort and expense of testing, as well as the complications associated with false-positive results (which are more likely than true-positive results). This approach presumes that the clinician and the parents accept the risk of missing some cases of occult bacteremia with the attendant risk of morbidity. Although an elevated complete blood count can be suggestive of pneumococcal and E coli bacteremia, this is neither a sensitive nor specific test. Furthermore, the complete blood count is unhelpful as a screen for other types of occult bacteremia. Empiric antibiotic therapy is generally not indicated for these patients; however, if the clinician chooses to obtain a complete blood count and this is elevated, or if there is any other concern for an increased risk of bacteremia (eg, hyperpyrexia [40]), blood cultures and antibiotics should be considered.

No combination of clinical assessment and diagnostic testing will successfully identify all patients who have serious infection at the time of initial presentation; therefore, the importance of timely reassessment (even for the child with initially normal test results or the child who has received antibiotic therapy) cannot be overemphasized, and caretakers must be instructed to return to the emergency department or primary care provider's office immediately for any deterioration in the child's condition. A systematic plan for the evaluation and treatment of the febrile child may help reduce unnecessary testing and morbidity associated with serious infection; however, no single strategy can capture the nuances of all febrile young patients. Any standardized approach to the febrile young child should serve as an adjunct to, and not a replacement for, the judgment of the treating clinician.

References

[1] McCaig LF, Nawar EW. National hospital ambulatory medical care survey: 2004 emergency department summary. Adv Data 2006;372:1–29.

[2] Belfer RA, Gittelman MA, Muniz AE. Management of febrile infants and children by pediatric emergency medicine and emergency medicine: comparison with practice guidelines. Pediatr Emerg Care 2001;17(2):83–7.

[3] Isaacman DJ, Kaminer K, Veligeti H, et al. Comparative practice patterns of emergency medicine physicians and pediatric emergency medicine physicians managing fever in young children. Pediatrics 2001;108(2):354–8.

[4] Wittler RR, Cain KK, Bass JW. A survey about management of febrile children without source by primary care physicians. Pediatr Infect Dis J 1998;17(4):271–7 [discussion: 7–9].

[5] Alpern E, Henretig F. Fever. In: Fleisher G, Ludwig S, Henretig F, et al, editors. Textbook of pediatric emergency medicine. 5th edition. Philadelphia: Lippincott Williams & Wilkins; 2006. p. 295–306.

[6] Baraff L. Management of fever without source in infants and children. Ann Emerg Med 2000;36(6):602–14.

[7] Steere M, Sharieff GQ, Stenklyft PH. Fever in children less than 36 months of age: questions and strategies for management in the emergency department. J Emerg Med 2003;25(2):149–57.

[8] Ishimine P. Fever without source in children 0 to 36 months of age. Pediatr Clin North Am 2006;53:167–94.

[9] Alpern ER, Alessandrini EA, Bell LM, et al. Occult bacteremia from a pediatric emergency department: current prevalence, time to detection, and outcome. Pediatrics 2000;106(3):505–11.

[10] Bisgard KM, Kao A, Leake J, et al. *Haemophilus influenzae* invasive disease in the United States, 1994–1995: near disappearance of a vaccine-preventable childhood disease. Emerg Infect Dis 1998;4(2):229–37.

[11] Lee GM, Harper MB. Risk of bacteremia for febrile young children in the post-*Haemophilus influenzae* type b era. Arch Pediatr Adolesc Med 1998;152(7):624–8.

[12] Wenger JD. Epidemiology of *Haemophilus influenzae* type B disease and impact of *Haemophilus influenzae* type b conjugate vaccines in the United States and Canada. Pediatr Infect Dis J 1998;17(Suppl 9):S132–6.

[13] Robinson KA, Baughman W, Rothrock G, et al. Epidemiology of invasive *Streptococcus pneumoniae* infections in the United States, 1995–1998: opportunities for prevention in the conjugate vaccine era. JAMA 2001;285(13):1729–35.

[14] American Academy of Pediatrics. Pneumococcal infections. In: Red Book: 2006 Report of the Committee on Infectious Diseases. 27th edition. Elk Grove Village (IL): American Academy of Pediatrics; 2006. p. 525–37.

[15] Wise RP, Iskander J, Pratt RD, et al. Postlicensure safety surveillance for 7-valent pneumococcal conjugate vaccine. JAMA 2004;292(14):1702–10.

[16] Black S, Shinefield H, Fireman B, et al. Efficacy, safety and immunogenicity of heptavalent pneumococcal conjugate vaccine in children: Northern California Kaiser Permanente vaccine study center group. Pediatr Infect Dis J 2000;19(3):187–95.

[17] Black S, Shinefield H, Baxter R, et al. Postlicensure surveillance for pneumococcal invasive disease after use of heptavalent pneumococcal conjugate vaccine in Northern California Kaiser Permanente. Pediatr Infect Dis J 2004;23(6):485–9.

[18] Hsu K, Pelton S, Karumuri S, et al. Population-based surveillance for childhood invasive pneumococcal disease in the era of conjugate vaccine. Pediatr Infect Dis J 2005;24(1):17–23.

[19] Kaplan SL, Mason EO Jr, Wald ER, et al. Decrease of invasive pneumococcal infections in children among 8 children's hospitals in the United States after the introduction of the 7-valent pneumococcal conjugate vaccine. Pediatrics 2004;113(3):443–9.

[20] Whitney CG, Farley MM, Hadler J, et al. Decline in invasive pneumococcal disease after the introduction of protein-polysaccharide conjugate vaccine. N Engl J Med 2003; 348(18):1737–46.

[21] Herz AM, Greenhow TL, Alcantara J, et al. Changing epidemiology of outpatient bacteremia in 3- to 36-month-old children after the introduction of the heptavalent-conjugated pneumococcal vaccine. Pediatr Infect Dis J 2006;25(4):293–300.

[22] Poehling KA, Lafleur BJ, Szilagyi PG, et al. Population-based impact of pneumococcal conjugate vaccine in young children. Pediatrics 2004;114(3):755–61.

[23] Poehling KA, Szilagyi PG, Edwards K, et al. Streptococcus pneumoniae-related illnesses in young children: secular trends and regional variation. Pediatr Infect Dis J 2003;22(5): 413–8.

[24] Poehling KA, Talbot TR, Griffin MR, et al. Invasive pneumococcal disease among infants before and after introduction of pneumococcal conjugate vaccine. JAMA 2006;295(14): 1668–74.

[25] Stoll ML, Rubin LG. Incidence of occult bacteremia among highly febrile young children in the era of the pneumococcal conjugate vaccine: a study from a Children's Hospital Emergency Department and Urgent Care Center. Arch Pediatr Adolesc Med 2004;158(7): 671–5.

[26] Carstairs KL, Tanen DA, Johnson AS, et al. Pneumococcal bacteremia in febrile infants presenting to the emergency department before and after the introduction of the heptavalent pneumococcal vaccine. Ann Emerg Med 2007;49(6):772–7.

[27] Centers for Disease Control and Prevention. Recommended childhood and adolescent immunization schedule—United States, July-December 2004. MMWR Morb Mortal Wkly Rep 2004;53(13):Q1–3.

[28] Craig JV, Lancaster GA, Taylor S, et al. Infrared ear thermometry compared with rectal thermometry in children: a systematic review. Lancet 2002;360(9333):603–9.

[29] Craig JV, Lancaster GA, Williamson PR, et al. Temperature measured at the axilla compared with rectum in children and young people: systematic review. BMJ 2000; 320(7243):1174–8.

[30] Greenes DS, Fleisher GR. When body temperature changes, does rectal temperature lag? J Pediatr 2004;144(6):824–6.

[31] Greenes DS, Fleisher GR. Accuracy of a noninvasive temporal artery thermometer for use in infants. Arch Pediatr Adolesc Med 2001;155(3):376–81.

[32] Jean-Mary MB, Dicanzio J, Shaw J, et al. Limited accuracy and reliability of infrared axillary and aural thermometers in a pediatric outpatient population. J Pediatr 2002;141(5): 671–6.

[33] Grover G, Berkowitz CD, Thompson M, et al. The effects of bundling on infant temperature. Pediatrics 1994;94(5):669–73.

[34] Banco L, Veltri D. Ability of mothers to subjectively assess the presence of fever in their children. Am J Dis Child 1984;138(10):976–8.

[35] Graneto JW, Soglin DF. Maternal screening of childhood fever by palpation. Pediatr Emerg Care 1996;12(3):183–4.

[36] Hooker EA, Smith SW, Miles T, et al. Subjective assessment of fever by parents: comparison with measurement by noncontact tympanic thermometer and calibrated rectal glass mercury thermometer. Ann Emerg Med 1996;28(3):313–7.

[37] Pantell RH, Newman TB, Bernzweig J, et al. Management and outcomes of care of fever in early infancy. JAMA 2004;291(10):1203–12.

[38] Kuppermann N, Fleisher G, Jaffe D. Predictors of occult pneumococcal bacteremia in young febrile children. Ann Emerg Med 1998;31(6):679–87.

[39] Stanley R, Pagon Z, Bachur R. Hyperpyrexia among infants younger than 3 months. Pediatr Emerg Care 2005;21(5):291–4.

[40] Trautner BW, Caviness AC, Gerlacher GR, et al. Prospective evaluation of the risk of serious bacterial infection in children who present to the emergency department with hyperpyrexia (temperature of 106°F or higher). Pediatrics 2006;118(1):34–40.

[41] Teach SJ, Fleisher GR. Duration of fever and its relationship to bacteremia in febrile outpatients 3 to 36 months old: the occult bacteremia study group. Pediatr Emerg Care 1997; 13(5):317–9.

[42] Baker MD, Fosarelli PD, Carpenter RO. Childhood fever: correlation of diagnosis with temperature response to acetaminophen. Pediatrics 1987;80(3):315–8.

[43] Baker RC, Tiller T, Bausher JC, et al. Severity of disease correlated with fever reduction in febrile infants. Pediatrics 1989;83(6):1016–9.

[44] Huang SY, Greenes DS. Effect of recent antipyretic use on measured fever in the pediatric emergency department. Arch Pediatr Adolesc Med 2004;158(10):972–6.

[45] Torrey SB, Henretig F, Fleisher G, et al. Temperature response to antipyretic therapy in children: relationship to occult bacteremia. Am J Emerg Med 1985;3(3):190–2.

[46] Yamamoto LT, Wigder HN, Fligner DJ, et al. Relationship of bacteremia to antipyretic therapy in febrile children. Pediatr Emerg Care 1987;3(4):223–7.

[47] Bonadio WA. The history and physical assessments of the febrile infant. Pediatr Clin North Am 1998;45(1):65–77.

[48] Bonadio WA, Hennes H, Smith D, et al. Reliability of observation variables in distinguishing infectious outcome of febrile young infants. Pediatr Infect Dis J 1993;12(2):111–4.

[49] McCarthy PL, Lembo RM, Fink HD, et al. Observation, history, and physical examination in diagnosis of serious illnesses in febrile children less than or equal to 24 months. J Pediatr 1987;110(1):26–30.

[50] McCarthy PL, Lembo RM, Baron MA, et al. Predictive value of abnormal physical examination findings in ill-appearing and well-appearing febrile children. Pediatrics 1985;76(2): 167–71.

[51] Greenes DS, Harper MB. Low risk of bacteremia in febrile children with recognizable viral syndromes. Pediatr Infect Dis J 1999;18(3):258–61.

[52] Baker MD, Bell LM. Unpredictability of serious bacterial illness in febrile infants from birth to 1 month of age. Arch Pediatr Adolesc Med 1999;153(5):508–11.

[53] Chiu CH, Lin TY, Bullard MJ. Identification of febrile neonates unlikely to have bacterial infections. Pediatr Infect Dis J 1997;16(1):59–63.

[54] Kadish HA, Loveridge B, Tobey J, et al. Applying outpatient protocols in febrile infants 1-28 days of age: can the threshold be lowered? Clin Pediatr (Phila) 2000;39(2):81–8.

[55] Pena BM, Harper MB, Fleisher GR. Occult bacteremia with group B streptococci in an outpatient setting. Pediatrics 1998;102(1 Pt 1):67–72.

[56] Hoffman JA, Mason EO, Schutze GE, et al. Streptococcus pneumoniae infections in the neonate. Pediatrics 2003;112(5):1095–102.

[57] Dagan R, Powell KR, Hall CB, et al. Identification of infants unlikely to have serious bacterial infection although hospitalized for suspected sepsis. J Pediatr 1985;107(6): 855–60.

[58] Dagan R, Sofer S, Phillip M, et al. Ambulatory care of febrile infants younger than 2 months of age classified as being at low risk for having serious bacterial infections. J Pediatr 1988; 112(3):355–60.

[59] Jaskiewicz JA, McCarthy CA, Richardson AC, et al. Febrile infants at low risk for serious bacterial infection: an appraisal of the Rochester criteria and implications for management. Pediatrics 1994;94(3):390–6.

[60] Ferrera PC, Bartfield JM, Snyder HS. Neonatal fever: utility of the Rochester criteria in determining low risk for serious bacterial infections. Am J Emerg Med 1997;15(3):299–302.

[61] Baker MD, Bell LM, Avner JR. Outpatient management without antibiotics of fever in selected infants. N Engl J Med 1993;329(20):1437–41.

[62] Chiu CH, Lin TY, Bullard MJ. Application of criteria identifying febrile outpatient neonates at low risk for bacterial infections. Pediatr Infect Dis J 1994;13(11):946–9.

[63] Bonsu BK, Harper MB. A low peripheral blood white blood cell count in infants younger than 90 days increases the odds of acute bacterial meningitis relative to bacteremia. Acad Emerg Med 2004;11(12):1297–301.

[64] Bonsu BK, Harper MB. Identifying febrile young infants with bacteremia: is the peripheral white blood cell count an accurate screen? Ann Emerg Med 2003;42(2):216–25.

[65] Gorelick MH, Shaw KN. Screening tests for urinary tract infection in children: a meta-analysis. Pediatrics 1999;104(5):e54.

[66] Shaw KN, McGowan KL, Gorelick MH, et al. Screening for urinary tract infection in infants in the emergency department: which test is best? Pediatrics 1998;101(6):e1.

[67] Al-Orifi F, McGillivray D, Tange S, et al. Urine culture from bag specimens in young children: are the risks too high? J Pediatr 2000;137(2):221–6.

[68] Committee on Quality Improvement, Subcommittee on Urinary Tract Infection. Practice Parameter. The diagnosis, treatment, and evaluation of the initial urinary tract infection in febrile infants and young children. Pediatrics 1999;103(4):843–52.

[69] McGillivray D, Mok E, Mulrooney E, et al. A head-to-head comparison: "clean-void" bag versus catheter urinalysis in the diagnosis of urinary tract infection in young children. J Pediatr 2005;147(4):451–6.

[70] Schroeder AR, Newman TB, Wasserman RC, et al. Choice of urine collection methods for the diagnosis of urinary tract infection in young, febrile infants. Arch Pediatr Adolesc Med 2005;159(10):915–22.

[71] Bonsu BK, Harper MB. Utility of the peripheral blood white blood cell count for identifying sick young infants who need lumbar puncture. Ann Emerg Med 2003;41(2):206–14.

[72] Levine DA, Platt SL, Dayan PS, et al. Risk of serious bacterial infection in young febrile infants with respiratory syncytial virus infections. Pediatrics 2004;113(6):1728–34.

[73] Martin E, Fanconi S, Kalin P, et al. Ceftriaxone–bilirubin-albumin interactions in the neonate: an in vivo study. Eur J Pediatr 1993;152(6):530–4.

[74] Robertson A, Fink S, Karp W. Effect of cephalosporins on bilirubin-albumin binding. J Pediatr 1988;112(2):291–4.

[75] Sadow KB, Derr R, Teach SJ. Bacterial infections in infants 60 days and younger: epidemiology, resistance, and implications for treatment. Arch Pediatr Adolesc Med 1999;153(6):611–4.

[76] Brown JC, Burns JL, Cummings P. Ampicillin use in infant fever: a systematic review. Arch Pediatr Adolesc Med 2002;156(1):27–32.

[77] Brown ZA, Wald A, Morrow RA, et al. Effect of serologic status and cesarean delivery on transmission rates of herpes simplex virus from mother to infant. JAMA 2003;289(2):203–9.

[78] Kimberlin DW, Lin CY, Jacobs RF, et al. Natural history of neonatal herpes simplex virus infections in the acyclovir era. Pediatrics 2001;108(2):223–9.

[79] Kimberlin DW, Lin CY, Jacobs RF, et al. Safety and efficacy of high-dose intravenous acyclovir in the management of neonatal herpes simplex virus infections. Pediatrics 2001;108(2):230–8.

[80] Kimberlin D. Herpes simplex virus, meningitis and encephalitis in neonates. Herpes 2004;11(Suppl 2):65A–76A.

[81] Kimberlin DW. Neonatal herpes simplex infection. Clin Microbiol Rev 2004;17(1):1–13.

[82] DeAngelis C, Joffe A, Willis E, et al. Hospitalization vs outpatient treatment of young, febrile infants. Am J Dis Child 1983;137(12):1150–2.

[83] Baker MD, Avner JR, Bell LM. Failure of infant observation scales in detecting serious illness in febrile, 4- to 8-week-old infants. Pediatrics 1990;85(6):1040–3.

[84] Baskin MN, O'Rourke EJ, Fleisher GR. Outpatient treatment of febrile infants 28 to 89 days of age with intramuscular administration of ceftriaxone. J Pediatr 1992;120(1):22–7.

[85] Baker MD, Bell LM, Avner JR. The efficacy of routine outpatient management without antibiotics of fever in selected infants. Pediatrics 1999;103(3):627–31.

[86] Byington CL, Rittichier KK, Bassett KE, et al. Serious bacterial infections in febrile infants younger than 90 days of age: the importance of ampicillin-resistant pathogens. Pediatrics 2003;111(5 Pt 1):964–8.

[87] American College of Emergency Physicians Clinical Policies Committee, Clinical Policies Subcommittee on Pediatric Fever. Clinical policy for children younger than three years presenting to the emergency department with fever. Ann Emerg Med 2003;42(4):530–45.

[88] Bramson RT, Meyer TL, Silbiger ML, et al. The futility of the chest radiograph in the febrile infant without respiratory symptoms. Pediatrics 1993;92(4):524–6.

[89] Shapiro ED, Aaron NH, Wald ER, et al. Risk factors for development of bacterial meningitis among children with occult bacteremia. J Pediatr 1986;109(1):15–9.

[90] Teele DW, Dashefsky B, Rakusan T, et al. Meningitis after lumbar puncture in children with bacteremia. N Engl J Med 1981;305(18):1079–81.

[91] Bonsu BK, Harper MB. Accuracy and test characteristics of ancillary tests of cerebrospinal fluid for predicting acute bacterial meningitis in children with low white blood cell counts in cerebrospinal fluid. Acad Emerg Med 2005;12(4):303–9.

[92] Nigrovic LE, Kuppermann N, Malley R. Development and validation of a multivariable predictive model to distinguish bacterial from aseptic meningitis in children in the post-*Haemophilus influenzae* era. Pediatrics 2002;110(4):712–9.

[93] Byington CL, Enriquez FR, Hoff C, et al. Serious bacterial infections in febrile infants 1 to 90 days old with and without viral infections. Pediatrics 2004;113(6):1662–6.

[94] Liebelt EL, Qi K, Harvey K. Diagnostic testing for serious bacterial infections in infants aged 90 days or younger with bronchiolitis. Arch Pediatr Adolesc Med 1999;153(5):525–30.

[95] Titus MO, Wright SW. Prevalence of serious bacterial infections in febrile infants with respiratory syncytial virus infection. Pediatrics 2003;112(2):282–4.

[96] Rittichier KR, Bryan PA, Bassett KE, et al. Diagnosis and outcomes of enterovirus infections in young infants. Pediatr Infect Dis J 2005;24(6):546–50.

[97] Dayan PS, Hanson E, Bennett JE, et al. Clinical course of urinary tract infections in infants younger than 60 days of age. Pediatr Emerg Care 2004;20(2):85–8.

[98] Hoberman A, Wald ER, Hickey RW, et al. Oral versus initial intravenous therapy for urinary tract infections in young febrile children. Pediatrics 1999;104(1 Pt 1):79–86.

[99] American Academy of Pediatrics Subcommittee on the Diagnosis and Management of Bronchiolitis. Diagnosis and management of bronchiolitis. Pediatrics 2006;118(4):1774–93.

[100] Fleisher GR, Rosenberg N, Vinci R, et al. Intramuscular versus oral antibiotic therapy for the prevention of meningitis and other bacterial sequelae in young, febrile children at risk for occult bacteremia. J Pediatr 1994;124(4):504–12.

[101] Teach SJ, Fleisher GR. Efficacy of an observation scale in detecting bacteremia in febrile children three to thirty-six months of age, treated as outpatients: Occult Bacteremia Study Group. J Pediatr 1995;126(6):877–81.

[102] McCarthy PL, Sharpe MR, Spiesel SZ, et al. Observation scales to identify serious illness in febrile children. Pediatrics 1982;70(5):802–9.

[103] Abanses JC, Dowd MD, Simon SD, et al. Impact of rapid influenza testing at triage on management of febrile infants and young children. Pediatr Emerg Care 2006;22(3):145–9.

[104] Smitherman HF, Caviness AC, Macias CG. Retrospective review of serious bacterial infections in infants who are 0 to 36 months of age and have influenza A infection. Pediatrics 2005;115(3):710–8.

[105] Bass JW, Steele RW, Wittler RR, et al. Antimicrobial treatment of occult bacteremia: a multicenter cooperative study. Pediatr Infect Dis J 1993;12(6):466–73.

[106] Kuppermann N. Occult bacteremia in young febrile children. Pediatr Clin North Am 1999; 46(6):1073–109.

[107] Kuppermann N, Malley R, Inkelis SH, et al. Clinical and hematologic features do not reliably identify children with unsuspected meningococcal disease. Pediatrics 1999;103(2): e20.

[108] Sard B, Bailey MC, Vinci R. An analysis of pediatric blood cultures in the postpneumococcal conjugate vaccine era in a community hospital emergency department. Pediatr Emerg Care 2006;22(5):295–300.

[109] Lee GM, Fleisher GR, Harper MB. Management of febrile children in the age of the conjugate pneumococcal vaccine: a cost-effectiveness analysis. Pediatrics 2001;108(4):835–44.

[110] Jaffe DM, Tanz RR, Davis AT, et al. Antibiotic administration to treat possible occult bacteremia in febrile children. N Engl J Med 1987;317(19):1175–80.

[111] Harper MB, Bachur R, Fleisher GR. Effect of antibiotic therapy on the outcome of outpatients with unsuspected bacteremia. Pediatr Infect Dis J 1995;14(9):760–7.

[112] Bulloch B, Craig WR, Klassen TP. The use of antibiotics to prevent serious sequelae in children at risk for occult bacteremia: a meta-analysis. Acad Emerg Med 1997;4(7):679–83.

[113] Baraff LJ, Oslund S, Prather M. Effect of antibiotic therapy and etiologic microorganism on the risk of bacterial meningitis in children with occult bacteremia. Pediatrics 1993; 92(1):140–3.

[114] Haddy RI, Perry K, Chacko CE, et al. Comparison of incidence of invasive *Streptococcus pneumoniae* disease among children before and after introduction of conjugated pneumococcal vaccine. Pediatr Infect Dis J 2005;24(4):320–3.

[115] Whitney CG, Pilishvili T, Farley MM, et al. Effectiveness of seven-valent pneumococcal conjugate vaccine against invasive pneumococcal disease: a matched case-control study. Lancet 2006;368(9546):1495–502.

[116] CDC. Recommended immunization schedules for persons aged 0–18 years—United States, 2007. MMWR 2006;55(51 & 52):Q1–4.

[117] Kaplan SL, Mason EO Jr, Wald E, et al. Six year multicenter surveillance of invasive pneumococcal infections in children. Pediatr Infect Dis J 2002;21(2):141–7.

[118] Kyaw MH, Lynfield R, Schaffner W, et al. Effect of introduction of the pneumococcal conjugate vaccine on drug-resistant *Streptococcus pneumoniae*. N Engl J Med 2006;354(14): 1455–63.

[119] Singleton RJ, Hennessy TW, Bulkow LR, et al. Invasive pneumococcal disease caused by nonvaccine serotypes among Alaska native children with high levels of 7-valent pneumococcal conjugate vaccine coverage. JAMA 2007;297(16):1784–92.

[120] Steenhoff AP, Shah SS, Ratner AJ, et al. Emergence of vaccine-related pneumococcal serotypes as a cause of bacteremia. Clin Infect Dis 2006;42(7):907–14.

[121] Bonadio WA, Smith DS, Madagame E, et al. *Escherichia coli* bacteremia in children: a review of 91 cases in 10 years. Am J Dis Child 1991;145(6):671–4.

[122] Yang YJ, Huang MC, Wang SM, et al. Analysis of risk factors for bacteremia in children with nontyphoidal *Salmonella* gastroenteritis. Eur J Clin Microbiol Infect Dis 2002;21(4): 290–3.

[123] Zaidi E, Bachur R, Harper M. Non-typhi *Salmonella* bacteremia in children. Pediatr Infect Dis J 1999;18(12):1073–7.

[124] Kaplan SL, Schutze GE, Leake JA, et al. Multicenter surveillance of invasive meningococcal infections in children. Pediatrics 2006;118(4):e979–84.

[125] Nigrovic LE, Kuppermann N, Macias CG, et al. Clinical prediction rule for identifying children with cerebrospinal fluid pleocytosis at very low risk of bacterial meningitis. JAMA 2007;297(1):52–60.

[126] Wang VJ, Kuppermann N, Malley R, et al. Meningococcal disease among children who live in a large metropolitan area, 1981–1996. Clin Infect Dis 2001;32(7):1004–9.

[127] Wang VJ, Malley R, Fleisher GR, et al. Antibiotic treatment of children with unsuspected meningococcal disease. Arch Pediatr Adolesc Med 2000;154(6):556–60.

[128] Mandl K, Stack A, Fleisher G. Incidence of bacteremia in infants and children with fever and petechiae. J Pediatr 1997;131(3):398.

[129] Nelson DG, Leake J, Bradley J, et al. Evaluation of febrile children with petechial rashes: is there consensus among pediatricians? Pediatr Infect Dis J 1998;17(12):1135–40.

[130] Wells LC, Smith JC, Weston VC, et al. The child with a non-blanching rash: how likely is meningococcal disease? Arch Dis Child 2001;85(3):218–22.

[131] Committee on Infectious Diseases. Prevention and control of meningococcal disease: recommendations for use of meningococcal vaccines in pediatric patients. Pediatrics 2005; 116(2):496–505.

[132] Bachur R, Harper MB. Reevaluation of outpatients with *Streptococcus pneumoniae* bacteremia. Pediatrics 2000;105(3 Pt 1):502–9.

[133] Bandyopadhyay S, Bergholte J, Blackwell CD, et al. Risk of serious bacterial infection in children with fever without a source in the post-*Haemophilus influenzae* era when antibiotics are reserved for culture-proven bacteremia. Arch Pediatr Adolesc Med 2002;156(5): 512–7.

[134] Thuler LC, Jenicek M, Turgeon JP, et al. Impact of a false-positive blood culture result on the management of febrile children. Pediatr Infect Dis J 1997;16(9):846–51.

[135] DeAngelis C, Joffe A, Wilson M, et al. Iatrogenic risks and financial costs of hospitalizing febrile infants. Am J Dis Child 1983;137(12):1146–9.

[136] Baraff LJ. Editorial: clinical policy for children younger than three years presenting to the emergency department with fever. Ann Emerg Med 2003;42(4):546–9.

[137] Kuppermann N. The evaluation of young febrile children for occult bacteremia: time to reevaluate our approach? Arch Pediatr Adolesc Med 2002;156(9):855–7.

[138] Green S, Rothrock S. Evaluation styles for well-appearing febrile children: are you a "Risk-Minimizer" or a "Test-Minimizer?". Ann Emerg Med 1999;33(2):211–4.

[139] Madsen KA, Bennett JE, Downs SM. The role of parental preferences in the management of fever without source among 3- to 36-month-old children: a decision analysis. Pediatrics 2006;117(4):1067–76.

[140] Bennett JE, Sumner Ii W, Downs SM, et al. Parents' utilities for outcomes of occult bacteremia. Arch Pediatr Adolesc Med 2000;154(1):43–8.

[141] Oppenheim PI, Sotiropoulos G, Baraff LJ. Incorporating patient preferences into practice guidelines: management of children with fever without source. Ann Emerg Med 1994;24(5): 836–41.

[142] Bachur R, Harper MB. Reliability of the urinalysis for predicting urinary tract infections in young febrile children. Arch Pediatr Adolesc Med 2001;155(1):60–5.

[143] Hoberman A, Chao HP, Keller DM, et al. Prevalence of urinary tract infection in febrile infants. J Pediatr 1993;123(1):17–23.

[144] Shaw KN, Gorelick M, McGowan KL, et al. Prevalence of urinary tract infection in febrile young children in the emergency department. Pediatrics 1998;102(2):e16.

[145] Gorelick MH, Shaw KN. Clinical decision rule to identify febrile young girls at risk for urinary tract infection. Arch Pediatr Adolesc Med 2000;154(4):386–90.

[146] Gorelick MH, Hoberman A, Kearney D, et al. Validation of a decision rule identifying febrile young girls at high risk for urinary tract infection. Pediatr Emerg Care 2003;19(3): 162–4.

[147] Schoen EJ, Colby CJ, Ray GT. Newborn circumcision decreases incidence and costs of urinary tract infections during the first year of life. Pediatrics 2000;105(4 Pt 1): 789–93.

[148] Task Force on Circumcision. Circumcision policy statement. Pediatrics 1999;103(3): 686–93.

[149] Zorc JJ, Kiddoo DA, Shaw KN. Diagnosis and management of pediatric urinary tract infections. Clin Microbiol Rev 2005;18(2):417–22.

[150] Huicho L, Campos-Sanchez M, Alamo C. Meta-analysis of urine screening tests for determining the risk of urinary tract infection in children. Pediatr Infect Dis J 2002;21(1):1–11, 88.

[151] Wubbel L, Muniz L, Ahmed A, et al. Etiology and treatment of community-acquired pneumonia in ambulatory children. Pediatr Infect Dis J 1999;18(2):98–104.

[152] Margolis P, Gadomski A. Does this infant have pneumonia? JAMA 1998;279(4):308–13.

[153] Jadavji T, Law B, Lebel MH, et al. A practical guide for the diagnosis and treatment of pediatric pneumonia. CMAJ 1997;156(5):S703–11.

[154] Lynch T, Platt R, Gouin S, et al. Can we predict which children with clinically suspected pneumonia will have the presence of focal infiltrates on chest radiographs? Pediatrics 2004;113(3 Pt 1):e186–9.

[155] Rothrock SG, Green SM, Fanelli JM, et al. Do published guidelines predict pneumonia in children presenting to an urban ED? Pediatr Emerg Care 2001;17(4):240–3.

[156] Leventhal JM. Clinical predictors of pneumonia as a guide to ordering chest roentgenograms. Clin Pediatr (Phila) 1982;21(12):730–4.

[157] Taylor JA, Del Beccaro M, Done S, et al. Establishing clinically relevant standards for tachypnea in febrile children younger than 2 years. Arch Pediatr Adolesc Med 1995; 149(3):283–7.

[158] Zukin DD, Hoffman JR, Cleveland RH, et al. Correlation of pulmonary signs and symptoms with chest radiographs in the pediatric age group. Ann Emerg Med 1986;15(7):792–6.

[159] Mower WR, Sachs C, Nicklin EL, et al. Pulse doximetry as a fifth pediatric vital sign. Pediatrics 1997;99(5):681–6.

[160] Tanen DA, Trocinski DR. The use of pulse oximetry to exclude pneumonia in children. Am J Emerg Med 2002;20(6):521–3.

[161] Davies HD, Wang EE, Manson D, et al. Reliability of the chest radiograph in the diagnosis of lower respiratory infections in young children. Pediatr Infect Dis J 1996;15(7):600–4.

[162] Courtoy I, Lande AE, Turner RB. Accuracy of radiographic differentiation of bacterial from nonbacterial pneumonia. Clin Pediatr (Phila) 1989;28(6):261–4.

[163] McCarthy PL, Spiesel SZ, Stashwick CA, et al. Radiographic findings and etiologic diagnosis in ambulatory childhood pneumonias. Clin Pediatr (Phila) 1981;20(11):686–91.

[164] Bachur R, Perry H, Harper MB. Occult pneumonias: empiric chest radiographs in febrile children with leukocytosis. Ann Emerg Med 1999;33(2):166–73.

[165] Murphy CG, van de Pol AC, Harper MB, et al. Clinical predictors of occult pneumonia in the febrile child. Acad Emerg Med 2007;14(3):243–9.

[166] British Thoracic Society of Standards of Care. BTS guidelines for the management of community acquired pneumonia in childhood. Thorax 2002;57(90001):1i–24i.

[167] Black SB, Shinefield HR, Ling S, et al. Effectiveness of heptavalent pneumococcal conjugate vaccine in children younger than five years of age for prevention of pneumonia. Pediatr Infect Dis J 2002;21(9):810–5.

[168] Lee KC, Finkelstein JA, Miroshnik IL, et al. Pediatricians' self-reported clinical practices and adherence to national immunization guidelines after the introduction of pneumococcal conjugate vaccine. Arch Pediatr Adolesc Med 2004;158(7):695–701.

[169] Peters TR, Poehling KA. Invasive pneumococcal disease: the target is moving. JAMA 2007; 297(16):1825–6.

[170] Farrell DJ, Klugman KP, Pichichero M. Increased antimicrobial resistance among nonvaccine serotypes of Streptococcus pneumoniae in the pediatric population after the introduction of 7-valent pneumococcal vaccine in the United States. Pediatr Infect Dis J 2007;26(2): 123–8.

[171] Oosterhuis-Kafeja F, Beutels P, Van Damme P. Immunogenicity, efficacy, safety and effectiveness of pneumococcal conjugate vaccines (1998–2006). Vaccine 2007;25(12):2194–212.

[172] Carrol ED, Newland P, Riordan FA, et al. Procalcitonin as a diagnostic marker of meningococcal disease in children presenting with fever and a rash. Arch Dis Child 2002;86(4): 282–5.

[173] Fernandez Lopez A, Luaces Cubells C, Garcia Garcia JJ, et al. Procalcitonin in pediatric emergency departments for the early diagnosis of invasive bacterial infections in febrile infants: results of a multicenter study and utility of a rapid qualitative test for this marker. Pediatr Infect Dis J 2003;22(10):895–903.

[174] Galetto-Lacour A, Zamora SA, Gervaix A. Bedside procalcitonin and C-reactive protein tests in children with fever without localizing signs of infection seen in a referral center. Pediatrics 2003;112(5):1054–60.

[175] Gendrel D, Raymond J, Coste J, et al. Comparison of procalcitonin with C-reactive protein, interleukin 6 and interferon-alpha for differentiation of bacterial vs. viral infections. Pediatr Infect Dis J 1999;18(10):875–81.

[176] Hsiao AL, Baker MD. Fever in the new millennium: a review of recent studies of markers of serious bacterial infection in febrile children. Curr Opin Pediatr 2005;17(1):56–61.

[177] Isaacman DJ, Burke BL. Utility of the serum C-reactive protein for detection of occult bacterial infection in children. Arch Pediatr Adolesc Med 2002;156(9):905–9.

[178] Pulliam PN, Attia MW, Cronan KM. C-reactive protein in febrile children 1 to 36 months of age with clinically undetectable serious bacterial infection. Pediatrics 2001;108(6):1275–9.

[179] van Rossum AM, Wulkan RW, Oudesluys-Murphy AM. Procalcitonin as an early marker of infection in neonates and children. Lancet Infect Dis 2004;4(10):620–30.

[180] Hsiao AL, Chen L, Baker MD. Incidence and predictors of serious bacterial infections among 57- to 180-day-old infants. Pediatrics 2006;117(5):1695–701.

[181] Czaja C, Crossette L, Metlay JP. Accuracy of adult reported pneumococcal vaccination status of children. Ann Epidemiol 2005;15(4):253–6.

ELSEVIER
SAUNDERS

Emerg Med Clin N Am
25 (2007) 1117–1135

EMERGENCY
MEDICINE
CLINICS OF
NORTH AMERICA

An Emergency Medicine Approach to Neonatal Hyperbilirubinemia

James E. Colletti, MD, FAAEM, FAAP[a],*,
Samip Kothori, MD[b], Danielle M. Jackson, MD[c],
Kevin P. Kilgore, MD[c], Kelly Barringer, MD[c]

[a]Department of Emergency Medicine, Mayo Clinic College of Medicine,
200 First St. SW, Rochester, MN 55905, USA
[b]Department of Pediatrics, University of Arizona,
150 N. Campbell Avenue, Tucson, AZ 85724, USA
[c]Department of Emergency Medicine, Regions Hospital, 640 Jackson Street,
Mail Stop 11102F, St. Paul, MN 55101, USA

Jaundice, also known as hyperbilirubinemia, is a yellowish-greenish pigmentation of the sclera and skin caused by an increase in bilirubin production or a defect in bilirubin elimination. Jaundice is defined by a serum bilirubin concentration greater than 5 mg/dL. Neonatal jaundice is estimated to occur in the majority of term infants (60%) in the first week of life, and approximately 2% of infants reach total serum bilirubin (TSB) levels in excess of 20 mg/dL [1–4]. The TSB normally rises during the first 3 to 5 days of life and then begins to decline [3]. As such, it is important that bilirubin levels are interpreted based on the neonate's age in hours [5].

The feared complication of neonatal jaundice is bilirubin encephalopathy, the result of prolonged unconjugated hyperbilirubinemia. Acute bilirubin encephalopathy can eventually develop into chronic bilirubin encephalopathy (kernicterus). Kernicterus has been called the ultimate adverse manifestation of severe hyperbilirubinemia [6] and was rarely seen in the decades following the introduction of phototherapy and exchange transfusion; however, recent reports suggest it is reemerging [6]. A concerning number of cases have been reported in healthy term and near-term neonates [7]. Since 1990, the Pilot Kernicterus Registry has identified kernicterus in greater than 120 near-term and term infants who had been discharged as healthy from the hospital [7–10]. In 2001, the Joint Commission on Accreditation of Health Care Organizations issued a sentinel event alert notifying

* Corresponding author.
E-mail address: jamesecolletti@gmail.com (J.E. Colletti).

0733-8627/07/$ - see front matter © 2007 Elsevier Inc. All rights reserved.
doi:10.1016/j.emc.2007.07.007   *emed.theclinics.com*

health care providers and hospitals that kernicterus is a threat to otherwise healthy newborns. The reemergence of kernicterus has been attributed in part to earlier hospital discharge, before the natural peak of bilirubin in the neonate, as well as a result of relaxation of treatment criteria [4,9,11,12].

Newborns are often discharged from the hospital within 48 hours of birth; as a result, hyperbilirubinemia is not as often detected before discharge as it had been previously [13]. The practice of early newborn discharge has transformed neonatal hyperbilirubinemia from an inpatient issue to an outpatient one [14,15]. Currently, hyperbilirubinemia is one of the most common reasons for readmission of a newborn [16,17]. As such, emergency physicians should be comfortable with the diagnosis, evaluation, and management of the jaundiced newborn [2,18]. Vales eloquently stated in a commentary that, in an ideal world, "the issue of dangerous hyperbilirubinemia should have been solved before embarking in a drastic cut on the in-hospital observation" of newborns [19].

Epidemiology

Hyperbilirubinemia is one of the most common reasons for the presentation of neonates to the emergency department and one of the major causes for hospital readmission. Overall, jaundice is observed in the first week of life in 60% of term infants and 80% of preterm infants [1,20]. In a case-control review, Maisels and Kring [17] concluded that hyperbilirubinemia is the major reason for hospital readmission in the first 2 weeks of life (incidence of 4.2 cases per 1000 discharges). Although the percentage of jaundiced newborns is higher among preterm newborns, the majority of data on the assessment, evaluation, and management of jaundice have been collected on term newborns with birth weights of 2500 g or greater.

Pathophysiology

Bilirubin is produced from the breakdown of hemoglobin (Fig. 1). Hemoglobin is degraded by heme oxygenase, resulting in the release of iron and the formation of carbon monoxide and biliverdin. Biliverdin is then converted to bilirubin by biliverdin reductase.

Unconjugated bilirubin (also known as indirect bilirubin) is initially only soluble in lipids, not water, and is subsequently bound by albumin in the blood stream. Any substance competing for binding sites, such as organic acids or drugs, can increase the levels of free bilirubin. In this unconjugated state, bilirubin is difficult to excrete (because it is lipid soluble), and it can easily pass into the central nervous system where it is neurotoxic and can produce kernicterus [11]. Unconjugated bilirubin is taken up by the liver, where it is conjugated by uridine diphosphate glucuronosyltransferase (UDPGT) to a conjugated form.

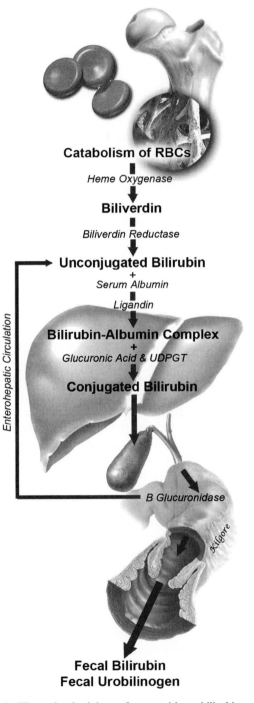

Fig. 1. The pathophysiology of neonatal hyperbilirubinemia.

Conjugated bilirubin (direct bilirubin) is water soluble, non-toxic, and unable to cross the blood-brain barrier. It also binds to albumin and can compete with unconjugated bilirubin for binding sites. It is excretable into the biliary or intestinal tract. Once conjugated bilirubin enters the intestinal tract, it is either excreted in stool or deconjugated by bacteria, where it may reenter the circulation (enterohepatic circulation). Total bilirubin is bound to protein (mainly albumin) in the blood and is a combination of unconjugated and conjugated bilirubin.

There are three main causes of hyperbilirubinemia in the neonate, which generally manifests as elevated levels of unconjugated bilirubin: (1) an increase in hemolysis, (2) a delay in maturation or inhibition of conjugating mechanisms in the liver, and (3) interference with hepatic uptake of unconjugated bilirubin. Neonates are especially prone to hyperbilirubinemia secondary to increased hemoglobin from high red blood cell volume, shortened red blood cell survival (and therefore increased breakdown), and relative immaturity of UDPGT in the liver.

Clinical presentation

The emergency physician should be familiar with historical clues that put the neonate at increased risk for severe hyperbilirubinemia. Risk factors to consider are jaundice in the first 24 hours, visible jaundice before hospital discharge, fetal-maternal blood type incompatibility (ABO incompatibility as well as Rh incompatibility), prematurity, exclusive breastfeeding as well as significant weight loss associated with breastfeeding, maternal age greater than or equal to 25 years, male sex, delayed meconium passage, and excessive birth trauma such as bruising or cephalohematomas [6,21,22]. The parents should be asked specifically about poor feeding, urine output (including dark urine), stooling (delayed passage of meconium or light-colored stool), vomiting, or any changes in behavior (lethargy, changes in cry pattern, cries becoming more shrill, arching of the body) [18].

Pertinent family history includes ethnicity, as well as siblings with hyperbilirubinemia, anemia, liver disease, or splenectomy. Ethnicity is a factor in determining the likelihood of hyperbilirubinemia. Individuals of East Asian descent, certain tribes of Native Americans such as the Navajo, and those of Greek ancestry have a higher incidence of hyperbilirubinemia [3,15,23]. It is important to inquire about siblings with jaundice, because there is a 12.5 times greater risk for severe jaundice in newborns who have one or more siblings affected with severe neonatal hyperbilirubinemia when compared with newborns who have prior siblings without severe neonatal hyperbilirubinemia [24].

Physical assessment begins with the clinical appearance of the infant. Jaundice is assessed through blanching the skin with digital pressure, revealing the underlying color of the skin and subcutaneous tissue. The clinical assessment of jaundice is best undertaken in a well-lit room to maximize the ability to determine true skin color [21]. Jaundice in term and preterm infants follows a cephalocaudal progression [25]. Visual estimation of the severity of jaundice is unpredictably and imprecisely related to the actual serum bilirubin level, especially in infants with dark skin pigmentation and once the jaundice has extended to the lower legs and feet [5,9,26–28]. Moyer and colleagues [28] evaluated 122 healthy infants who underwent examination by two observers followed by measurements of serum bilirubin. The investigation concluded that visual estimation of infantile jaundice was not reliable, and that prediction of serum bilirubin concentration by clinical examination is not accurate [28]. After assessing the skin, it is important to look for other signs indicative of pathologic jaundice, such as pallor, petechiae, hydration, and weight status. Signs of blood loss or blood sequestration such as excessive bruising, hepatosplenomegaly, or cephalohematoma should be sought out as well [22].

A review of the birth history should be performed. First, it is important to establish whether the child was large for gestational age (LGA), within normal range, or small for gestational age (SGA). Infants that are SGA have associated complications such as hypoglycemia, polycythemia, and abnormal neurologic symptoms. Although hyperbilirubinemia is not directly linked to SGA infants, polycythemia can lead to an increased bilirubin level secondary to increased red cell destruction [29,30]. Infants that are LGA have an increased incidence of birth trauma due to their size. Excessive bruising and cephalohematomas can be acquired from birth trauma. One study determined that over a 10-year period, 2.5% of all breech births had an associated cephalohematoma [31]. Forceps and vacuum extraction deliveries can also cause bruising and cephalohematomas to occur [30]. Other injuries such as clavicle fractures and brachial plexus injuries are also associated with hyperbilirubinemia. Clavicle fractures are often secondary to shoulder dystocia. These injuries are linked to hyperbilirubinemia secondary to the extravasation of blood from the associated trauma [32]. Information regarding medications administered to the mother before and during delivery should be obtained, because certain medications, such as oxytocin, can result in an increased incidence of hyperbilirubinemia [30,33].

On initial inspection of a jaundiced neonate, the clinician should have an increased index of suspicion for underlying disease entities. Among these entities are sepsis and galactosemia. A diagnosis of sepsis should be considered in the infant presenting with apnea or temperature instability. Galactosemia presents as feeding intolerance manifested by persistent vomiting, an enlarged liver, seizures, and lethargy [34].

Differential diagnosis

There are two different classifications of jaundice to consider—physiologic and pathologic. Physiologic jaundice is the transient elevation of serum bilirubin during the first week of life. Pathologic jaundice occurs in the first 24 hours of life and is often associated with anemia or hepatosplenomegaly. Furthermore, pathologic jaundice can be characterized by a rapidly rising serum bilirubin (>5 mg/dL per day), prolonged jaundice (>7 to 10 days in a full-term infant), and an elevated conjugated bilirubin concentration (>2 mg/dL or more than 20% of TSB).

Two main categories of hyperbilirubinemia are unconjugated or conjugated, also known, respectively, as indirect or direct. One may further breakdown the etiology of unconjugated hyperbilirubinemia into an increased bilirubin load, decreased bilirubin excretion, or bilirubin increase due to breastfeeding. One of the major causes of increased bilirubin load is blood group incompatibility.

ABO blood group incompatibility is the leading cause of hemolytic disease of the newborn. One of the primary clinical features of ABO blood group incompatibility is hyperbilirubinemia. Approximately one third of infants with ABO incompatibility have a positive direct antiglobulin test (DAT or Coombs' test), indicating that they have anti-A or anti-B antibodies attached to their red cells [35]. Of this third, 20% will have a peak TSB of greater than 12.8 mg/dL [35]. Although ABO-incompatible, DAT-positive infants are more likely to develop moderate hyperbilirubinemia, severe jaundice is uncommon [35]. Overall, ABO hemolytic disease is a common cause of early hyperbilirubinemia before the infant leaves the nursery; it is a rare cause of hyperbilirubinemia in infants who are discharged and return for evaluation [35]. A mechanism similar to that of ABO incompatibility exists for Rh incompatibility. Of note, 15% of all births are a set-up for ABO incompatibility, but only 0.33% to 2.2% of all neonates will have some manifestation of the disease [36,37]. Several other minor blood group types, such as Kell and Duffy, can also cause hemolytic disease.

Enzyme deficiencies in the glycolysis pathway, such as glucose-6-phosphate dehydrogenase (G6PD) deficiency and pyruvate kinase deficiency, also increase the indirect bilirubin load. G6PD deficiency mainly affects the red blood cells and can cause acute hemolysis. Many infants, although not all, with this disease present with hyperbilirubinemia. The exact mechanism as to how G6PD deficiency causes hyperbilirubinemia is unknown; however, the leading explanation is a decrease in bilirubin elimination [38]. G6PD deficiency affects between 200 and 400 million people worldwide and is the leading cause of hyperbilirubinemia in certain population subtypes such as African Americans, those of Mediterranean descent, and some Far East populations [39,40]. Multiple studies have shown that infants who are affected by hyperbilirubinemia and who have G6PD deficiency have the same clinical course and clinical indicators as infants with hyperbilirubinemia who do not have G6PD deficiency; therefore, it is prudent to include G6PD deficiency in the differential diagnosis if there is a family history of G6PD deficiency or if the patient fits into an at-risk demographic group [39,41].

Pyruvate kinase deficiency is the second leading cause of red blood cell enzyme deficiency in North America and overall is an uncommon cause of hyperbilirubinemia. The clinician should have a higher index of suspicion for pyruvate kinase deficiency as a cause of hyperbilirubinemia in populations in which pyruvate kinase deficiency is more common, such as neonates of Indian descent [42,43]. An investigation by Kedar and colleagues determined the prevalence of pyruvate kinase deficiency in jaundiced neonates in India to be 3.21% [43].

Abnormalities in the red blood cell membrane, such as hereditary spherocytosis and elliptocytosis/ovalocytosis, may also result in an increase in indirect bilirubin levels. In hereditary spherocytosis, there is a defect in the red cell membrane causing an increase in red cell breakdown and abnormal red blood cells. Fifty percent of individuals with hereditary spherocytosis state they had significant jaundice as newborns. Trucco and Brown [44] suggest that the clinical findings of hereditary spherocytosis can include early onset of jaundice or a marked increase in bilirubin beyond what is expected with physiologic jaundice. An osmotic fragility test is considered to be the gold standard to confirm a diagnosis of hereditary spherocytosis [45,46]. Elliptocytosis/ovalocytosis is an autosomal dominant disease affecting predominantly Southeast Asian and Mediterranean populations. Several case studies have reported that it results in an elevation of indirect bilirubin [47,48].

It is important to exclude hemolytic disease as the cause of increased indirect bilirubin levels. The diseases discussed previously can cause hemolysis, and it is important to identify factors that will help diagnosis hemolytic disease early. A family history of significant hemolytic disease, a high-risk ethnic background, early or severe jaundice, or the development of jaundice in the newborn before 24 hours of life suggest the possibility of hemolytic disease in the newborn. In addition, a bilirubin level in a neonate that does not respond to phototherapy may indicate that breakdown is ongoing from an underlying disease process that requires further evaluation. A rapid rate of rise in the bilirubin level should cause concern for hemolytic disease [1,13].

Increased indirect bilirubin can also be caused by decreased bilirubin excretion. One of the main causes of decreased bilirubin excretion is that neonates have a decrease in bowel motility which results in an increase in the enterohepatic circulation, in turn, leading to increased indirect bilirubin [22,49]. One of the more life-threatening causes of hyperbilirubinemia by impaired bilirubin excretion is Crigler-Najjar syndrome. There are two types, both of which are due to defects in bilirubin-UDP-glucuronosyltransferase (B-UGT). Type I is characterized by an absence of enzyme activity and is the more severe type which can lead to kernicterus and death by the age of 1 to 2 years of age without treatment. Type II has some enzyme activity and is therefore less fatal. Without B-UGT, unconjugated bilirubin accumulates in the body. Once the threshold of albumin and other tissue phospholipids is reached, the brain becomes stained and kernicterus develops. The disease is rare and inherited in an autosomal recessive fashion. The clinical presentation includes elevated bilirubin levels and symptoms of kernicterus despite phototherapy treatment [50,51]. Congenital hypothyroidism is another disease that can cause hyperbilirubinemia through decreased bilirubin excretion. It presents with prolonged jaundice, lethargy, constipation, poor feeding, hypotonia, and enlarged fontanelles. It is extremely important to follow-up on thyroid levels in the newborn genetic screening of neonates who have hyperbilirubinemia with concerns of hypothyroidism [52].

Increased indirect bilirubin levels can also result from breastfeeding. When compared with formula feeding, breastfeeding has been associated with neonatal jaundice that is more severe and longer in duration [53,54]. This type of hyperbilirubinemia can present in two ways. The first is a delayed course in which the bilirubin level rises on the fourth to seventh day of life after physiologic jaundice is resolving. The bilirubin then peaks at about 2 weeks of life (to a level of 15–25 mg/dL) and stays in this range for another 2 weeks before a decrease is observed [55]. The second type has also been described as an exaggerated physiologic jaundice. It occurs earlier than the first type, typically on the third or fourth day of life, with bilirubin levels above 10 mg/dL [54]. The exact mechanism of action is unknown. There is evidence to suggest that caloric deprivation results in hyperbilirubinemia. Because it may take anywhere from 2 to 5 days for the production of breast milk, a breastfed infant may experience a calorie deficiency [56]. Furthermore, it has been shown that human breast milk has a substance within it that inhibits hepatic B-UGT, which, in turn, leads to hyperbilirubinemia [57,58]. It is recommended by the American Academy of Pediatrics that, even with this risk, it is still better to breastfeed than to switch to formula when breastfeeding jaundice is suspected [1]. Human milk jaundice syndrome, also know as breastfeeding-associated jaundice, should be distinguished from breastfeeding jaundice. Human milk jaundice appears later than breastfeeding jaundice, typically on the fourth to seventh day of life, and is more prolonged than breastfeeding jaundice [35].

Important clues to the etiology of jaundice are the time of onset and the duration [59,60]. Jaundice in the first 24 hours may be secondary to blood type incompatibilities such as ABO and Rh. Sepsis should also be considered, because several investigations have described as association between proven bacterial infection and neonatal jaundice [60–66]. Arthur and Williams [62], Seeler [65], and Littlewood [64] demonstrated an association between hyperbilirubinemia and urinary tract infections in neonates. A few investigations have concluded that jaundice as the only symptom of sepsis is rare, especially in a well-appearing neonates [67–69].

Jaundice appearing during the second to third day of life is most likely physiologic and will dissipate by the fifth or sixth day. If the newborn is breastfed, he or she may develop breastfeeding jaundice that can be present for 2 weeks. The clinician should consider a pathologic etiology of jaundice if it persists for longer than 2 weeks. A prospective investigation by Maisels and Kring [69] demonstrated that most newborns admitted for indirect hyperbilirubinemia are healthy breastfed infants. Newborns who warrant careful screening are those presenting with late-onset jaundice, direct hyperbilirubinemia, or signs of sepsis.

Conjugated hyperbilirubinemia is concerning because, although it is nontoxic, it is a marker for serious underlying disease. Etiologies of conjugated hyperbilirubinemia are summarized in Table 1. Associated findings of conjugated hyperbilirubinemia are pale acholic stools, dark urine, or the presence of bilirubin in the urine [1].

Emergency department evaluation

Evaluation should be guided by the clinical appearance of the neonate and the timing of jaundice. A full-term, well-appearing, asymptomatic infant is at low risk of complications, especially in the absence of danger signs (Box 1) and when presenting within a time frame that is consistent with physiologic jaundice [70]. To aid in the assessment of the jaundiced neonate, several laboratory investigations may be obtained, including TSB, a direct Coombs' test, blood group testing, hemoglobin, urinalysis, as well as a full sepsis work-up (white blood cell count, cerebral spinal fluid for analysis and culture, and blood and urine cultures).

A serum bilirubin and hemoglobin measurement should be routinely ordered for the jaundiced infant. Inaccuracy between the physician's clinical estimation and actual serum bilirubin levels is well documented, as is poor interrater reliability; therefore, physical examination alone should not be relied upon. Measurements of total and direct serum bilirubin should be obtained to differentiate conjugated from unconjugated hyperbilirubinemia. Unfortunately, measurement of bilirubin has a notorious wide range, is inaccurate, and is associated with a tremendous amount of interlaboratory variability [70–78]. In a well-appearing, afebrile infant with unconjugated hyperbilirubinemia and normal hemoglobin, no further tests are needed (although some practitioners would obtain a urinalysis and urine culture) [2].

Table 1
Etiology of conjugated hyperbilirubinemia

Infectious	Anatomic	Metabolic
TORCH	Biliary atresia	Inborn errors of metabolism
Hepatitis	Choledochal cyst	Cystic fibrosis
Sepsis (usually presents with other signs of sepsis, ie, vomiting, abdominal distention, respiratory distress, and poor feeding)	Alagille syndrome (arteriohepatic dysplasia) Cholestasis Mass lesion	Alpha-1-antitrypsin deficiency

---

Box 1. Danger signs

1. Family history of significant hemolytic disease
2. Vomiting
3. Lethargy
4. Poor feeding
5. Fever
6. Onset of jaundice after the third day of life
7. High-pitched cry
8. Dark urine
9. Light stools

As alluded to earlier in this manuscript, obtaining a urinalysis may prove helpful in the infant with physiologic jaundice. Several investigations have indicated an association between jaundice and asymptomatic urinary tract infections [2,62,64,67,79–82]. A series of articles by Seeler indicate that jaundice may be one of the earliest signs of a urinary tract infection [64,79,81]. Ng and Rawstron described a case series of six neonates in whom jaundice was the prominent feature in acute urinary tract infection [80]. Chavalitdhamrong and colleagues [68] prospectively identified two urinary tract infections in 69 infants with unexplained jaundice. Rooney and colleagues [62] found urinary tract infections in 40% (9 of 22) of infants with documented bacterial infections. Garcia and Nager [82] prospectively evaluated asymptomatic, afebrile, jaundiced infants for evidence of a urinary tract infection, which they found in 7.5% of infants less than 8 weeks of age. Furthermore, neonates presenting with an onset of jaundice after 8 days of age or those with an elevated conjugated bilirubin fraction were more likely to have a urinary tract infection. Garcia and Nager recommend testing for a urinary tract infection as part of the evaluation of the asymptomatic jaundiced infant presenting to the emergency department [82].

In cases in which anemia is present, a complete blood count with peripheral smear, Coombs' test, and maternal and fetal blood types should be analyzed (ABO and Rh(D) typing) [2]. Neonates who are Coombs' positive are approximately twice as likely as their comparable peers to have a serum bilirubin level of more than 12 mg/dL [70]. In the presence of a positive Coombs' test, ABO or Rh incompatibility is the most likely cause of jaundice, because the majority of neonates with other causes of hemolysis will be Coombs' negative [2]. Furthermore, a G6PD level has been recommended for any infant undergoing phototherapy with an appropriate genetic or geographic background, and for any neonate who does not respond well to phototherapy [2].

In cases of conjugated hyperbilirubinemia, evaluation efforts should be directed to determining the underlying etiology [2]. Most commonly, conjugated hyperbilirubinemia is infectious in origin, and these causes should be assessed with a TORCH infection panel (toxoplasmosis, others, rubella, cytomegalovirus, and herpes simplex), hepatitis B serology, and urinalysis for cytomegalovirus. Although less common, jaundice may be the presenting complaint in neonates with inborn errors of metabolism, cystic fibrosis, alpha-1-antitrypsin deficiency, and iron storage deficiencies. When any of these processes are suspected, investigative studies should be broad and include liver function tests, ammonia, albumin and total protein levels, and a complete chemistry panel. Examination of urine for reducing substances, sweat chloride testing, and red blood cell galactose-1-phosphate uridyltransferase activity may be required.

Obstructive causes may be more difficult to identify owing to their insidious and often intermittent presentation. Abdominal ultrasound and hepatobiliary scintigraphy to assess for biliary atresia or a choledochal cyst may provide a diagnosis that, when reached promptly, improves outcomes due to early surgical intervention.

In cases of significant hyperbilirubinemia (serum bilirubin level > 15 mg/dL) with or without symptoms of illness, the following laboratory values should be obtained: direct and indirect bilirubin, complete blood cell count, peripheral blood smear for hemolysis, reticulocyte count, liver function tests, thyroid function tests, as well as an evaluation for sepsis. If an exchange transfusion is anticipated, a type and cross must be obtained. Indirect hyperbilirubinemia, reticulocytosis, and a smear consistent with red blood cell destruction are suggestive of hemolysis [58]. Infants with hemolysis as a cause of their hyperbilirubinemia are at greater risk for kernicterus [83] and should be admitted.

Kernicterus

Kernicterus (bilirubin encephalopathy) is a rare but catastrophic bilirubin-induced brain injury that is one of the known causes of cerebral palsy [7,35,84,85]. It is one of the few causes of brain damage in the neonatal period that, with current diagnostic and treatment regimens, is preventable [11]. The link between hyperbilirubinemia and brain damage was first established in the early 1950s when Mollison and Hsia and colleagues demonstrated that the risk of kernicterus in infants with hemolytic disease of the newborn dramatically increased with the bilirubin level and that an exchange transfusion could dramatically decrease that risk [70,86,87]. The likelihood of kernicterus depends on the bilirubin level, as well as the age of the child and comorbidities.

A schema for grading the severity of acute bilirubin encephalopathy has been described [10,88]. The earliest signs are often subtle and may be missed but include early alterations in tone of the extensor muscles (hypotonia or hypertonia), retrocollis (backward arching of the neck), opisthotonus (backward arching of the trunk), as well as a poor suck response [10,13,89]. The hypertonia and retrocollis will often increase in severity and may be by accompanied by a shrill cry as well as unexplained irritability alternating with lethargy and fever [89]. Prompt and effective therapy during the early phase of bilirubin-induced neurologic dysfunction can prevent chronic kernicteric sequelae [10].

Advanced signs of bilirubin encephalopathy are cessation of feeding, bicycling movements, irritability, seizures, fever, and altered mental status. These late findings are predictors of severe kernicteric sequelae. The final stage is chronic irreversible bilirubin encephalopathy, also known as kernicterus [10]. The classic tetrad [11] of chronic irreversible bilirubin encephalopathy are athetoid cerebral palsy, deafness or hearing loss, impairment of upward gaze, and enamel dysplasia of the primary teeth.

Kernicterus was rarely seen in the decades following the introduction of phototherapy and exchange transfusion, but recent reports suggest it is reemerging despite virtual elimination of Rh disease [4,11]. The majority of cases reported in the last decade have not occurred in infants with ABO, Rh, other hemolytic disease but in apparently healthy near-term and term infants with significantly elevated bilirubin levels (well above 30 mg/dL) [90].

Bhutani and colleagues [6] preformed a review in which steps were designed to facilitate a safer experience with newborn jaundice and prevent the feared manifestation of severe hyperbilirubinemia—kernicterus. A root cause analysis of cases of kernicterus was also performed by the American Academy of Pediatrics Subcommittee on Neonatal Hyperbilirubinemia who identified several potentially correctable factors that are associated with the development of kernicterus [89]. Based on Bhutani's review and the recommendations of the subcommittee, the principles that are most applicable to the practice of emergency medicine include an increased level of concern by the clinician, an objective assessment of the presence or absence of jaundice, the identification of risk factors of potential severe disease, careful attention to parental concern regarding jaundice, the identification of poor feeding and lethargy, and timely intervention for infants with TSB greater than the 95th percentile [6,89].

Emergency department management and disposition

Emergency department management of the jaundiced neonate depends on several factors. Management of jaundice in the term newborn is challenging because the clinician must balance the risks of aggressive versus conservative management [70]. Careful consideration must be given to the risks and benefits of each therapeutic intervention. Clinical decision making is aided by weighing variables such as the infant's age, clinical appearance, bilirubin level, the etiology, and the timing of jaundice.

In unconjugated hyperbilirubinemia, the ultimate goal is the prevention of kernicterus and its potentially devastating effects. The full-term, well-appearing, and afebrile neonate without significant risk factors and a bilirubin level less than 17 mg/dL may be simply observed, monitoring closely for increasing jaundice. Any dehydration should be corrected according to weight with normal saline boluses, and the frequency of feeding may be increased to aid in the excretion of bilirubin. Frequent feeding and frequent stools aid in bilirubin excretion and should be encouraged. The issue of continuing breastfeeding often arises. The American Academy of Pediatrics does not recommend the discontinuation of breastfeeding in healthy term newborns and encourages frequent breastfeeding of at least eight to ten times per 24-hour time period [1,2]. The major risk of interrupting breastfeeding is that the interruption may result in permanent discontinuation, losing its considerable benefits; however, a temporary cessation may be considered to augment phototherapy [70]. After bilirubin has fallen to a safe level, breastfeeding should be reinstated and the adequacy of this intake monitored to ensure proper hydration. Supplemental feedings in the form of water or dextrose solutions have not been found to precipitate the resolution of serum bilirubin levels to normal, nor are they preventative against the development of jaundice; therefore, they are not routinely recommended for healthy breastfed neonates. Depending on the preferences of the newborn's parents and physician, several options for feeding exist (with or without phototherapy) [2]. A candid conversation should be entered with the newborn's parents outlining the risks and benefits of the continuation of breastfeeding with close monitoring, supplementation with formula, or a brief substitution of breastfeeding with formula, each of which may be implemented with or without phototherapy. Ultimately, feeding options for jaundiced newborns sufficiently healthy to be monitored on an outpatient basis depend on both the parents' and physician's preferences [2]. In cases of breast milk jaundice, one consideration is the temporary cessation of breast milk with reintroduction after the bilirubin has fallen to a safe level.

Phototherapy, one of the mainstays of therapy for the jaundiced neonate, is carried out with a blue light that causes photoconversion of the bilirubin molecule to a water-soluble product that is excreted in the urine and stool. The use of phototherapy may lead to greater water loss; therefore, fluid intake must be increased by 20%. Breastfeeding may be continued. A general rule of thumb regarding when to initiate phototherapy for a full-term healthy infant is to begin the therapy at a bilirubin level of 17 mg/dL or higher and to discontinue therapy once the bilirubin level is less than 12 mg/dL. Table 2 lists further recommendations based on age in hours and risk. Phototherapy should be started at lower bilirubin levels (15 mg/dL) for neonates with a rapid rise in bilirubin, when ABO incompatibility exists, and in the preterm and near-term infant [1].

"Near-term" is a phrase used to describe newborns who do not meet the World Health Organization's definition of 38 to 42 weeks' gestation but are

Table 2
American Academy of Pediatrics recommendations for phototherapy

| | Total serum bilirubin (mg/dL) | | | | |
| | Age (h) | | | | |
Risk category	24	36	48	72	96
High risk (35–37 weeks + risk factors[a])	8	9	11	13	14
Medium risk (≥38 weeks + risk factors or 35–37 weeks and well)	10	12	13	15	17 ·
Low risk (>38 weeks and well)	12	13	15	18	20

[a] Risk factors are defined as isoimmune hemolytic disease, G6PD deficiency, asphyxia, significant lethargy, temperature instability, sepsis, acidosis.

Data from the American Academy of Pediatrics Clinical Practice Guidelines Subcommittee on Hyperbilirubinemia. Management of hyperbilirubinemia in the newborn infant 35 or more weeks of gestation. Pediatrics 2004;114:297–316.

over 2500 g in birth weight [35,89,91]. A commentary by the American Academy of Pediatrics Subcommittee on Neonatal Hyperbilirubinemia concluded that newborns who are near-term are at significant risk of severe hyperbilirubinemia [89]. A prospective investigation by Sarici and colleagues [91] determined that neonates between 35 and 37 weeks' gestation (near-term newborns) were 2.4 times more likely than those at 38 to 42 weeks to develop significant hyperbilirubinemia. These investigators stated near-term infants should be considered to be a high-risk group because one of four of these infants requires phototherapy for jaundice.

Exchange transfusion should be initiated emergently for markedly elevated serum bilirubin levels (Table 3). A body of literature suggests that exchange transfusion to maintain a bilirubin level below 20 mg/dL prevents kernicterus in infants with severe hemolytic disease of the newborn [86,87,92,93]. An exchange transfusion is recommended for term infants with hemolysis, if phototherapy is unable to maintain the total bilirubin

Table 3
American Academy of Pediatrics recommendations for exchange transfusion

| | Total serum bilirubin (mg/dL) | | | | |
| | Age (h) | | | | |
Risk category	24	36	48	72	96
High risk (35–37 weeks + risk factors[a])	15	16	17	18	19
Medium risk (≥38 weeks + risk factors or 35–37 weeks and well)	16.5	18	19	20	22
Low risk (>38 weeks and well)	19	21	22	24	25

[a] Risk factors are defined as isoimmune hemolytic disease, G6PD deficiency, asphyxia, significant lethargy, temperature instability, sepsis, acidosis.

Data from the American Academy of Pediatrics Clinical Practice Guidelines Subcommittee on Hyperbilirubinemia. Management of hyperbilirubinemia in the newborn infant 35 or more weeks of gestation. Pediatrics 2004;114:297–316.

level below 17.5 to 23.4 mg/dL, or for any neonate showing signs of kernicterus [70]. Newman and colleagues [94] found that when high TSB levels were treated with phototherapy or exchange transfusion, there was not an association with adverse neurodevelopment. An exchange transfusion will reduce the bilirubin concentration by approximately 50% and should be used with concurrent phototherapy.

Pharmacologic therapy may also be considered in conjunction with a neonatologist. Phenobarbital and ursodeoxycholic acid have been used to improve biliary flow and lower bilirubin levels [35]. Tin mesoporphyrin decreases bilirubin production by inhibiting heme oxygenase and is awaiting US Food and Drug Administration approval [35].

Admission is indicated for all ill-appearing neonates, for those found to be anemic, for bilirubin levels in the range of phototherapy or exchange requirements, and for pathologic or conjugated hyperbilirubinemia [1]. The latter condition always conceals serious underlying disease. Although conjugated bilirubin lacks the neurotoxicity of the unconjugated form, steps should immediately be taken to identify and treat the precipitating disorder. Jaundice is an early indicator of sepsis or urinary tract infection, and if such an infectious etiology is found, antibiotics should be started immediately. The anatomic causes of biliary atresia or obstruction due to a choledochal cyst must be identified early, and surgical evaluation should be prompt [2].

Prognosis

For the majority of cases, when treated early and appropriately, the prognosis is favorable. This success is evidenced by an investigation by Newman and colleagues [94] who determined that when high TSB levels were treated with phototherapy or exchange transfusion, there was not an association with adverse neurodevelopment.

Summary

Neonatal hyperbilirubinemia is estimated to occur in the majority of term infants in the first week of life, and approximately 2% reach a TSB greater than 20 mg/dL [1–4]. Secondary to early hospital discharge, neonatal jaundice has been transformed from an inpatient issue to an outpatient one that is often dealt with by the emergency physician. Consequently, the emergency physician should be comfortable with the presentation, evaluation, and management of the jaundiced newborn. Kernicterus, a rare but catastrophic complication of neonatal hyperbilirubinemia, is preventable and until recently was thought to be extinct. The role of the emergency physician is to balance the risks and benefits of diagnostic evaluation and management in the care of the jaundiced neonate.

Acknowledgment

The authors thank Jeahan R. Hanna, MD, and Elshaday Messele for their support and contributions to this manuscript.

References

[1] American Academy of Pediatrics, Subcommittee on Neonatal Hyperbilirubinemia. Practice parameter: management of hyperbilirubinemia in the healthy term newborn. Pediatrics 1994; 94:558–5.

[2] Claudius I, Fluharty C, Boles R. The emergency department approach to newborn and childhood metabolic crisis. Emerg Med Clin North Am 2005;23:843–83.

[3] Newman TB, Escobar GJ, Gonzales VM, et al. Frequency of neonatal bilirubin testing and hyperbilirubinemia in a large health maintenance organization. Pediatrics 1999;104(5): 1198–203.

[4] Chou S-C, Palmer RH, Ezhuthachan S, et al. Management of hyperbilirubinemia in newborns: measuring performance by using a benchmarking model. Pediatrics 2003;112(6): 1264–73.

[5] Bhutani VK, Johnson L, Sivieri EM. Predictive ability of a predischarge hour-specific serum bilirubin for subsequent significant hyperbilirubinemia in healthy term and near-term newborns. Pediatrics 1999;103:6–14.

[6] Bhutani VK, Donn SM, Johnson LH. Risk management of severe neonatal hyperbilirubinemia to prevent kernicterus. Clin Perinatol 2005;32(1):125–39.

[7] Eggert LD, Wiedmeiser SE, Willson J, et al. The effect on instituting a prehospital-discharge newborn bilirubin screening program in an 18-hospital health system. Pediatrics 2006;117: 855–62.

[8] Johnson L, Brown AK. A pilot registry for acute and chronic kernicterus in term and near-term infants. Pediatrics 1999;104(Suppl 3):736.

[9] Johnson L, Bhutani VK, Brown AK. System-based approach to management of neonatal jaundice and prevention of kernicterus. J Pediatr 2002;140(4):396–403.

[10] Bhutani VK, Johnson LH, Maisels MJ, et al. Kernicterus: epidemiological strategies for its prevention through systems based approaches. J Perinatol 2004;24:650–62.

[11] Shapiro SM. Bilirubin toxicity in the developing nervous system. Pediatr Neurol 2003;29(5): 410–21.

[12] Tiker F, Gulcan H, Kilicdag H, et al. Extreme hyperbilirubinemia in newborn infants. Clin Pediatr (Phila) 2006;45(3):257–61.

[13] Dennery PA, Seidman DS, Stevenson DK. Neonatal hyperbilirubinemia. N Engl J Med 2001;344(8):581–90.

[14] Gartner LM, Catz CS, Yaffe SJ. Neonatal Bilirubin Workshop. Pediatrics 1994;94(4): 537–40.

[15] Newman TB, Xiong B, Gonzales VM, et al. Prediction and prevention of extreme hyperbilirubinemia in a mature health maintenance organization. Arch Pediatr Adolesc Med 2000; 154:1140–7.

[16] Seidman DS, Stevenson DK, Ergaz Z, et al. Hospital readmission due to neonatal hyperbilirubinemia. Pediatrics 1995;96:727–9.

[17] Maisels MJ, Kring E. Length of stay, jaundice, and hospital readmission. Pediatrics 1998; 101:995–8.

[18] Bhutani VK, Johnson LH, Keren R. Diagnosis and management of hyperbilirubinemia in the term neonate: for a safer first week. Pediatr Clin North Am 2004;51:843–61.

[19] Vales T. Problems with prediction of neonatal hyperbilirubinemia. Pediatrics 2001;108: 175–7.

[20] Maisels M. Jaundice in the newborn. Pediatr Rev 1982;10:305–19.

[21] American Academy of Pediatrics Subcommittee on Hyperbilirubinemia. Management of hyperbilirubinemia in the new born infant 35 or more weeks of gestation. Pediatrics 2004; 114:297–316.

[22] Porter LM, Dennis BL. Hyperbilirubinemia in the term newborn. Am Fam Physician 2002; 65(4):599–605.

[23] Kaplan M, Hammerman C. Understanding and preventing severe neonatal hyperbilirubinemia: is bilirubin neurotoxicity really a concern in the developed world. Clin Perinatol 2004; 31(3):555–75.

[24] Khoury MJ, Calle EE, Joesoef RM. Recurrence risk of neonatal hyperbilirubinemia in siblings. Am J Dis Child 1988;142(10):1065–9.

[25] Knudsen A, Ebbesen F. Cephalocaudal progression of jaundice in newborns admitted to neonatal intensive care units. Biol Neonate 1997;71:357–61.

[26] Bhutani VK, Gourley GR, Adler S, et al. Noninvasive measurement of total serum bilirubin in a multiracial predischarge newborn population to assess the risk of severe hyperbilirubinemia. Pediatrics 2000;106(2):e17.

[27] Davidson LT, Merritt KK, Weech AA. Hyperbilirubinemia in the newborn. Am J Dis Child 1941;61:958–80.

[28] Moyer VA, Ahn C, Sneed S. Accuracy of clinical judgment in neonatal jaundice. Arch Pediatr Adolesc Med 2000;154:391–4.

[29] Tenovuo A. Neonatal complications in small-for-gestational age neonates. J Perinat Med 1988;16:197–201.

[30] Keren R, Bhutani VK, Luan X, et al. Identifying newborns at risk of significant hyperbilirubinemia: a comparison of two recommended approaches. Arch Dis Child 2005;90: 415–21.

[31] Thacker KE, Lim T, Drew JH. Cephalhematoma: a 10 year review. Aust N Z J Obstet Gynecol 1987;27(3):210–2.

[32] Perlow JH, Wigton T, Hart J, et al. Birth trauma: a five-year review of incidence and associated perinatal factors. J Reprod Med 1996;41(10):754–60.

[33] Davies DP, Gomersall R, Robertson R, et al. Neonatal jaundice and maternal oxytocin infusion. Br Med J 1973;3:476–7.

[34] Chung MA. Galactosemia in infancy: diagnosis, management, and prognosis. Pediatr Nurs 1997;23(6):563–8.

[35] Maisels M. Neonatal jaundice. Pediatr Rev 2006;27(12):443–54.

[36] Waldron P, De Alarcon P. ABO hemolytic disease of the newborn: a unique constellation of findings in siblings and review of protective mechanisms in the fetal-maternal system. Am J Perinatol 1999;16(8):391–8.

[37] Zawodnik SA, Bonnard GD, Gautier E. Antibody-dependent cell-mediated destruction of human erythrocytes sensitized in ABO and rhesus fetal-maternal incompatibilities. Pediatr Res 1976;10:791–6.

[38] Kaplan M, Hammerman C. Severe neonatal hyperbilirubinemia: a potential complication of glucose-6-phosphate dehydrogenase deficiency. Clin Perinatol 1998;25(3):575–90.

[39] Iranpour R, Akbar MR, Haghshenas I. Glucose-6-phosphate dehydrogenase deficiency in neonates. Indian J Pediatr 2003;70(11):855–7.

[40] Huang MJ, Kua KE, Teng HC, et al. Risk factors for severe hyperbilirubinemia in neonates. Pediatr Res 2004;56(5):682–9.

[41] Atay E, Bozaykut A, Ipek IO. Glucose-6-phosphate dehydrogenase deficiency in neonatal indirect hyperbilirubinemia. J Trop Pediatr 2006;52(1):56–8.

[42] Hammer SG, Lewan RB. Neonatal hyperbilirubinemia caused by pyruvate kinase deficiency. J Am Board Fam Med 1988;1(4):288–90.

[43] Kedar PS, Warang P, Colah RB, et al. Red cell pyruvate kinase deficiency in neonatal jaundice cases in India. Indian J Pediatr 2006;73(11):985–8.

[44] Trucco JI, Brown AK. Neonatal manifestations of hereditary spherocytosis. Am J Dis Child 1967;113:263–70.

[45] Passi GR, Saran S. Neonatal hyperbilirubinemia due to hereditary spherocytosis. Indian Pediatr 2004;41:199.

[46] Schroter W, Kahsnitz E. Diagnosis of hereditary spherocytosis in newborn infants. J Pediatr 1983;103:460–3.

[47] Laosombat V, Dissaneevate S, Peerapittayamongkol C, et al. Neonatal hyperbilirubinemia associated with southeast Asian ovalocytosis. Am J Hematol 1999;60:136–9.

[48] Austin RF, Desforges JF. Hereditary elliptocytosis: an unusual presentation of hemolysis in the newborn associated with transient morphologic abnormalities. Pediatrics 1969;44(2):196–200.

[49] Gartner LM, Herschel M. Jaundice and breastfeeding. Pediatr Clin North Am 2001;48(2):389–99.

[50] Jansen PLM. Diagnosis and management of Crigler-Najjar syndrome. Eur J Pediatr 1999;158(Suppl 2):S89–94.

[51] Strauss KA, Robinson DL, Vreman HJ, et al. Management of hyperbilirubinemia and prevention of kernicterus in 20 patients with Crigler-Najjar disease. Eur J Pediatr 2006;165(5):306–19.

[52] LaFranchi SH, Murphey WH, Foley TP, et al. Neonatal hypothyroidism detected by the northwest regional screening program. Pediatrics 1979;63(2):180–91.

[53] Schneider AP. Breast milk jaundice in the newborn: a real entity. JAMA 1986;255(23):3270–4.

[54] Kivlahan C, James EJ. The natural history of neonatal jaundice. Pediatrics 1984;74(3):364–70.

[55] Brown LP, Arnold A, Allison D, et al. Incidence and pattern of jaundice in healthy breast-fed infants during the first month of life. Nurs Res 1993;42(2):106–10.

[56] Osborn LM, Reiff MI, Bolus R. Jaundice in the full-term neonate. Pediatrics 1984;73(4):520–5.

[57] Poland RL. Breast-milk jaundice. J Pediatr 1981;99(1):86–8.

[58] Gerardi M. Neonatal emergencies: fever, jaundice, respiratory distress, cyanotic heart disease, and behavioral complaints. Pediatric Emergency Medicine Reports 1996;1(12):113–24.

[59] Brown AK. Neonatal jaundice. Pediatr Clin North Am 1962;9(3):575–603.

[60] Bernstein J, Brown AK. Sepsis and jaundice in early infancy. Pediatrics 1962;29:873–82.

[61] Hamilton JR, Sass-Kortsak A. Jaundice associated with severe bacterial infection in young infants. J Pediatr 1963;63:121–32.

[62] Arthur AB, Wilson BR. Urinary infection presenting with jaundice. Br Med J 1967;1:539–40.

[63] Rooney JC, Hill DJ, Danks DM. Jaundice associated with bacterial infection in the newborn. Am J Dis Child 1971;122(1):39–41.

[64] Littlewood JM. 66 Infants with urinary tract infections in first month of life. Arch Dis Child 1972;47:218–26.

[65] Seeler RA. Urosepsis with jaundice due to hemolytic *Escherichia coli*. Am J Dis Child 1973;126:414.

[66] Linder N, Yatsiv I, Tsur M, et al. Unexplained neonatal jaundice as an early diagnostic sign of septicemia in the newborn. J Perinatol 1988;8(4):325–7.

[67] Escobedo MB, Barton LL, Marshall RE, et al. The frequency of jaundice in neonatal bacterial infection. Clin Pediatr 1974;13(8):656–7.

[68] Chavalitdhamrong PO, Escobedo MB, Barton LL, et al. Hyperbilirubinemia and bacterial infection in the newborn. Arch Dis Child 1975;50(8):652–4.

[69] Maisels MJ, Kring E. Risk of sepsis in newborns with severe hyperbilirubinemia. Pediatrics 1992;90(5):741–3.

[70] Newman TB, Maisels JM. Evaluation and treatment of jaundice in the term newborn: a kinder, gentler approach. Pediatrics 1992;89:809–18.

[71] Schreiner RL, Glick MR. Interlaboratory bilirubin variability. Pediatrics 1982;69:277–81.

[72] Watkinison LR, St John A, Penberthy LA. Investigation into paediatric bilirubin analyses in Australia and New Zealand. J Clin Pathol 1982;35:52–8.

[73] Chan KM, Scott MG, Wu TW, et al. Inaccurate values for direct bilirubin with some commonly used direct bilirubin procedures. Clin Chem 1985;31:1560–3.

[74] Rosenthal P. The laboratory method as a variable in the diagnosis of hyperbilirubinemia. Am J Dis Child 1987;141(10):1066–8.

[75] Newman TB, Hope S, Stevenson D. Direct bilirubin measurements in jaundiced term newborns: a re-evaluation. Am J Dis Child 1991;145:1305–9.

[76] LO SF, Doumas TB, Ashwood ER. Performance of bilirubin determinations in US laboratories–revisited. Clin Chem 2004;51(1):190–4.

[77] Newman TB, Liljestrand PJ, Escobar GJ. Hyperbilirubinemia benchmarking. Pediatrics 2004;114(1):323.

[78] Vreman HJ, Verter J, Oh W, et al. Interlaboratory variability of bilirubin measurements. Clin Chem 1995;42:869–73.

[79] Seeler RA, Hahn K. Jaundice in urinary tract infection in infancy. Am J Dis Child 1969;18:553–8.

[80] Ng SH, Rawstrong JR. Urinary tract infections presenting with jaundice. Arch Dis Child 1971;46:173–6.

[81] Seeler R. Hemolysis due to gram-negative urinary tract infection. Birth Defects Orig Artic Ser 1977;13:425–31.

[82] Garcia FJ, Nager AL. Jaundice as an early sign of urinary tract infection in infancy. Pediatrics 2002;109(5):846–51.

[83] MacDonald MG. Hidden risks: early discharge and bilirubin toxicity due to glucose 6-phosphate dehydrogenase deficiency. Pediatrics 1995;96(4):734–8.

[84] Van Praagh R. Diagnosis of kernicterus in the neonatal period. Pediatrics 1961;28:870–6.

[85] Connolly AM, Volpe JJ. Clinical feature of bilirubin encephalopathy. Clin Perinatal 1990;17:371–9.

[86] Mollison Pl, Cutbush M. Haemolytic disease of the newborn. Recent Advances in Pediatrics 1954;110.

[87] Hsia Dy-Y, Allen FH, Gellits SS, et al. Erythroblastosis fetalis. VIII. Studies of serum bilirubin in relation to kernicterus. N Engl J Med 1952;247:668–71.

[88] Volpe J. Bilirubin and brain injury. Neurology of the newborn. 4th edition. Philadelphia: WB Saunders; 2001. p. 521–46.

[89] American Academy of Pediatrics Subcommittee on Neonatal Hyperbilirubinemia. Neonatal jaundice and kernicterus. Pediatrics 2001;108:763–5.

[90] Maisels MJ, Newman TB. Predicting hyperbilirubinemia in newborns: the importance of timing. Pediatrics 1999;103:493–4.

[91] Sarici SU, Serdar MA, Korkmaz A, et al. Incidence, course and prediction of hyperbilirubinemia in near-term and term newborns. Pediatrics 2004;113(4):775–80.

[92] Mollison PL, Walker W. Controlled trials of the treatment of haemolytic disease of the newborn. Lancet 1952;1:429–33.

[93] Ellis MI, Hey EN, Walker W. Neonatal death in babies with rhesus isoimmunization. Q J Med 1979;48:211–25.

[94] Newman, Thomas B, Liljestrand P, et al. The Jaundice and Infant Feeding Study Team. Outcomes among newborns with total serum bilirubin levels of 25 mg per deciliter or more. N Engl J Med 2006;354(18):1889–900.

ELSEVIER
SAUNDERS

Emerg Med Clin N Am
25 (2007) 1137–1159

EMERGENCY
MEDICINE
CLINICS OF
NORTH AMERICA

The Crying Infant

Martin Herman, MD[a,b,*], Audrey Le, MD[a]

[a]University of Tennessee Health Sciences Center, College of Medicine,
Memphis, TN 38103, USA
[b]Division of Pediatric Emergency Medicine, LeBonheur Children's Medical Center,
50 N. Dunlap Street, Memphis, TN 38104, USA

Crying is a part of normal human behavior. Infants cry for a variety of reasons including the need for attention, hunger, discomfort, or pain. However, when the amount of crying is perceived to be excessive or without discernable cause, it can be the cause of much parental as well as physician anxiety. During the first 4 months of an infant's life, excessive crying has been one of the problems most commonly reported by mothers [1–3]. The prevalence of excessive crying in infants has been estimated to be between 1.5% and 40% [4–7]. Among those 1 to 6 months of age, 1-month-old infants appear to have the highest prevalence [5].

Crying in infants can have a strong impact on both the families and the medical system that supports them. Crying and irritability are among the most common reasons that families seek medical attention during a child's first months of life and therefore it is a frequent presenting complaint for pediatricians and emergency physicians. A study from the United Kingdom has estimated an annual cost of $108 million to the national health system related to the care of infants with crying and difficulty sleeping in the first 12 weeks of life alone [8]. It is an important cause of maternal anxiety and stress, and is strongly associated with maternal depression [9–13]. Infant crying has also contributed to the discontinuation of breast-feeding [2]. Moreover, not only is the relationship between a mother and infant often subjected to stress in such situations, the entire family dynamic including interactions between the infant and father and that between the two parents can be negatively affected [10,14]. In the worst of cases, it has been implicated as one of the inciting factors in physical violence and even infant death [9,15,16].

One of the challenges for every physician presented with a crying or irritable infant lies in discriminating between benign and organic causes for

* Corresponding author. c/o Pediatric Emergency Specialists, P.C., PO Box 637, Ellendale, TN 38029.
E-mail address: martinherman@comcast.net (M. Herman).

0733-8627/07/$ - see front matter © 2007 Elsevier Inc. All rights reserved.
doi:10.1016/j.emc.2007.07.008   *emed.theclinics.com*

crying. Because of the commonality and seeming banality of the problem, the chief complaint of "crying" is at times greeted by the physician with disdain. While it may be tempting to dismiss these patients and assign a preemptory diagnosis of colic after a cursory history and physical exam, they are better served when each case is looked upon as a clinical challenge rather than as an annoyance. It is also an opportunity to educate and counsel parents in regard to the care of their infant. Conversely, excessive caution or fear of "missing" a diagnosis may result in unnecessary and overly invasive tests. Therefore, caring for such patients requires a fine balance.

Crying: how much is normal?

The literature on excessive crying is considerable. For the larger part, the term has been used to describe crying behavior in infants resulting from nonorganic disease. It may denote duration, frequency, and intensity of crying, and has been used interchangeably with "persistent crying," "infantile colic," and "paroxysmal fussing." Before discussing excessive crying in infants, however, it is helpful to understand their usual crying behavior. Fortunately, this has been previously illustrated in a number of studies.

In 1962 Brazelton [17] delineated the crying pattern in infants based on prospective data from 80 infants from birth through 12 weeks of age. He found that infants in their second week of life cried and fussed for a median of 1.75 hours (30 minutes in the upper quartile and 20 minutes in the lower quartile). From there, it increased gradually to a peak median of 2.75 hours at 6 weeks of age, after which there was a decline in the amount of crying. At 3 weeks of age the majority of crying was concentrated in the hours between 6 and 11 PM with smaller concentrations between 4 to 7 AM and 9 to 11 AM. At 6 weeks of age crying occurred more at the end of the day between 3 PM and 12 AM with a smaller peak in the early morning. By 10 weeks of age infants were crying to a lesser extent and mostly between the hours of 6 AM to 12 PM and 5 PM to 11 PM.

Subsequent studies that described crying beyond 12 weeks of age have supported and supplemented Brazelton's original work. Crying in infants has often been described using a behavioral or crying curve characterized by a peak at 2 months of age and a decline thereafter until about 4 months after which it remains relatively steady [17–20]. There appears to be a circadian pattern in which crying is concentrated most in the late afternoon and evening. This decreases by the middle of the first year, and after 9 months of age crying at night becomes more common [18,19]. It is important to note that despite observed trends, there does exist considerable variability of crying between infants as well as day-to-day fluctuations of crying in each infant [18,21].

Perhaps one of the earliest studies that addressed excessive crying was that by Illingworth [22] in 1954 in which he described 50 infants in the first

3 months of life with "rhythmic attacks of screaming." In finely illustrative terms, he described the child thus: "his face flushes, his brow furrows, and then he draws his legs up, clenches his fists and emits piercing, high-pitched screams, which do not stop when he is picked up, continuing unabated in his mother's arms." Such episodes lasted 5 or more minutes, occurred predominately in the evenings, and had no clear inciting cause. Illingworth called this phenomenon "three months' colic" because it improved by the time a child reached 3 months of age.

Contemporaries of Illingworth, Wessel and colleagues [23] used the phrase "paroxysmal fussing" to describe a similar phenomenon in 98 infants. In what has come to be known as the "rule of threes," they defined a fussy infant as one who cried or fussed for a total of more than 3 hours a day occurring on more than 3 days a week. The infants were, furthermore, divided into one of three groups: (1) contented, (2) paroxysmal fussers, and (3) seriously fussy. Contented infants were those who did not meet the criteria outlined above. Seriously fussy infants were those whose paroxysmal fussing episodes continued for more than 3 weeks. As with Illingworth, Wessel's group found that the episodes, in most cases, subsided by the end of the second month of life.

While Wessel's designation of the amount of crying that constitutes excessive has become the most commonly accepted standard, the literature on crying has not always been consistent. Numerous studies have used variations on that definition, which has made it somewhat problematic to interpret the data as a whole. Different definitions have resulted in study groups composed of dissimilar infants between and among studies; this makes it difficult to compare estimations of prevalence as well as the cause and treatment of excessive crying [5]. Similarly, it may be difficult to consistently identify characteristics of at-risk infants [24].

When confronted with a crying infant in the emergency department, while it is helpful to understand the common pattern and distribution of crying, it is important to consider each child individually. Bouts of crying of several weeks' or months' duration with relatively stable frequency may be more reassuring than that which started much more recently even if the latter conforms better to the "normal" infant crying pattern. One may more comfortably attribute the former to benign crying, while the latter may require more in-depth investigation. While the crying curve is helpful in the understanding of infant development, it is meant be applied within the context of a case.

Colic

Colic is a well-known syndrome of excessive crying. Beyond that, the exact definition encompassing etiology as well as possible treatments varies considerably. The term colic itself is perhaps a misnomer. It is a derivation of the

Greek word for colon, and, as such, implies gastrointestinal (GI) dysfunction as the underlying cause. In fact, GI dysfunction is only one of several theories that have been presented over the years to explain the colic syndrome. These theories span physiological, psychological, and behavioral foundations.

Some of the earliest and more popular explanations for colic involve cow's milk protein allergy, malabsorption, and gastrointestinal dysmotility. In 1901 Zahorsky [25] reported that "proteids" found in breast milk caused violent peristalsis in the gastrointestinal tracts of colicky infants. Unfortunately, studies that have examined gastrointestional dysfunction as the source of colic have often been plagued with inadequate sample numbers and faulty methodology [26,27]. A number of studies have demonstrated that crying decreased in formula-fed infants when cow's milk protein allergy was eliminated from their diets [28–30]. However, as Treen [26] has pointed out, some of these studies were not blinded and lacked adequate controls, while others preselected a subgroup consisting of infants with the most severe degree of crying who had already failed standard counseling and medication trials. The data on elimination of cow's milk from the mothers' diets in breast-fed babies have yielded mixed results [31–33].

Malabsorption has been thought to be a possible cause for colic through the production of excess colonic gas, abdominal cramping, and discomfort. However, this has not borne out in all studies. In one prospective study of 56 infants with colic, stool examinations for pH and reducing substances were normal [34]. In another study, breath hydrogen production was measured in 122 healthy infants after feedings containing lactose [35]. The group of colicky infants had more numbers of positive breath tests compared with the noncolicky infants, and failure to produce hydrogen gas throughout the breath test was more frequent in the latter group. However, there was considerable overlap in the hydrogen excretion values between groups. Ultimately, malabsorption may account only for a small subset of infants with colic.

Gastroesophageal reflux disease (GERD) as a cause for colic is a common conception held by both health care providers and parents [36]. One study with 51 infants admitted to the hospital with crying or irritability found that the most common diagnosis previously assigned to them was gastroesophageal reflux disease [37]. The data on this topic, however, has been mixed. In a study of 26 infants with colic of more than 4 weeks' duration that was considered severe enough to prompt referral to a pediatric gastroenterology clinic, pathological GERD was found in 16 (61.5%) using pH-metry [38]. All of those infants experienced a reduction in crying 2 weeks after institution of treatment. Of note, however, the remaining infants without GERD also experienced a resolution of their colic over a 4- to 6-week period. One may question whether the patients who received treatment might have improved even without intervention. In addition, because the median age of the infants in the group was 4.8 months, a number of them had crying that persisted beyond the time when the average infant's crying has abated. Thus, this was a group preselected for the most severe patients, and may not be an accurate reflection of the population of colicky infants as a whole. A review of the relationship between colic and GERD found that there was little evidence to support the connection, and furthermore, that there was poor correlation between irritability and episodes of reflux on pH probe studies [36].

Although gastrointestinal disturbances cannot fully account for the colicky behavior in many infants, they might explain crying and irritability in at least a subgroup of patients. The diagnosis can be considered when the history or physical examination is suggestive, as for example, when there are feeding difficulties, excessive emesis, diarrhea, constipation, or mucous or blood in the stools [26,36,39]. Excessive crying beyond 3 months of age or worsening of crying, although this has been shown to persist into the fifth month of life in otherwise healthy infants, should also raise suspicion of gastrointestinal or other causes of irritability [4,26].

An extensive body of literature has examined infant crying in terms of development and temperament. Barr described four distinct clinical crying syndromes in the first year of life, namely: (1) colic, (2) persistent mother-infant distress syndrome, (3) the temperamentally difficult infant, and (4) the dysregulated infant [40]. Colic, in this view, should be regarded as a manifestation of normal development. Furthermore, if crying syndromes were viewed in terms of responsivity (positive or negative), reactivity (the intensity, threshold, and timing of the response), and regulation (inhibition of the response), colic could be described by increased responsivity and reactivity, and decreased regulation. The persistent mother-infant distress syndrome refers to infants whose crying peaks at 2 months and worsens or fails to decline thereafter. These infants may have additional characteristics including feeding and sleeping disturbances, and familial discord [14,40]. The temperamentally difficult infant has been described as having a predisposition to negative responsivity (crying), and high intensity and low distractibility on the Early Infancy Temperament Scale [40,41]. Finally, dysregulated infants are thought to have central dysfunction and usually present in the latter part of the first year of life with disturbances in multiple behavioral domains including affect, feeding, and motor activity [40]. Viewed in this manner, one can conclude that the crying syndromes can and do overlap.

In the past, one of the theories offered to explain colic was that of the indifferent or aloof mother [21]. This view serves neither the interests of the mother nor the child and has fortunately been discredited in recent years. St. James-Roberts and colleagues [42] compared the caretaking styles of mothers of 67 persistent criers at 6 weeks of age who cried 3 or more hours a day with 53 moderate criers and 35 evening criers who cried less than 3 hours a day in total. They found that there was no significant difference in maternal sensitivity or affection between the groups. The studies examining the possible effects of maternal care on crying in infants 3 months and older have been mixed [43,44]. However, at that age when colicky crying has started to decline, excessive crying may have different implications.

Colic may best be viewed as a syndrome consisting of common symptoms rather than a specific disease entity. It consists of the timing and duration described above; that is, crying for more than 3 hours a day for 3 days a week for 3 or more weeks, which peaks at about 6 weeks of age and starts to decline at about 3 months of age. These crying bouts are characterized by their failure to abate with the usual soothing methods such as feeding, holding, or rocking. Many parents may feel that their child is in pain because of the inconsolability and characteristic posture adopted by these infants consisting of drawing up their legs, furrowing their brows, and screaming. However, they occur by definition in healthy well-fed infants who are growing and developing appropriately and appear "normal" between the bouts.

Colic treatments

Once the diagnosis of colic has been made, one must contend with prescribing treatment and giving the parents suggestions on ways with which to deal with their infant's crying. This is neither straightforward nor always successful. The methods that have been prescribed to control infantile colic thus far have included both medical treatment and behavioral modifications. No one approach works consistently for every infant. The process of trial and error may be discouraging and frustrating for both the parents and their health care providers. In treating patients with colic, it is perhaps just as important to offer support to the parents as it is to find ways to assuage the infant's crying.

A number of medical treatments have been examined regarding their efficacy in reducing crying in colic. Simethicone is one agent commonly used in the treatment of infantile colic, although its effectiveness has not been fully supported. It is a defoaming agent that is thought to accelerate the passage of gas in the gastrointestinal tract. In one randomized, double-blind, placebo-controlled multicenter trial with 83 infants ranging from 2 to 8 weeks of age, simethicone was no more effective than placebo [45]. A systemic review that included three randomized controlled trials found that only one showed possible benefit, but noted that the authors did not elucidate their definition of colic in that study [46]. A second review found that although the use of simethicone was not supported by good quality trials, it has no reported adverse effects and is widely used based upon common consensus [47].

Dicyclomine and dicycloverine are anticholinergic medications that are thought to relieve crying in colic through their actions as smooth muscle antispasmodics. They have been found to be effective treatments in a number of randomized controlled trials [46,48]. However, because of reported adverse events, the manufacturer has contraindicated their use in infants younger than 6 months and they are no longer indicated as treatments for infantile colic. The most frequently reported adverse events were drowsiness, constipation, and diarrhea. The most serious events, occurring most commonly in infants younger than 7 weeks, included shortness of breath, apnea, syncope, seizures, hypotonia, and coma [49].

Sucrose has been studied in the treatment of infantile colic because it is thought to cause release of endogenous opioids providing an analgesic effect in infants [50]. One double-blind double-crossover study examining the effect of 12% sucrose on 19 infants found that 12 had a positive response, although this only lasted for 30 minutes to an hour [51]. A randomized controlled trial using 48% sucrose with 19 colicky infants similarly showed that the response to sucrose was short-lived; in this case only up to 3 minutes [52].

Several studies in which lactase enzyme was introduced into the milk of infants with colic have not shown significant reductions in crying [53,54]. Miller and colleagues [54] conducted a randomized controlled trial with 15 colicky breast-fed infants and found that lactase did no better than placebo in reducing duration of crying. In a second small double-blind crossover study with 10 infants fed both breast milk and cow's milk formula, the duration and severity of their colic was not significantly different when they received milk treated with lactase [53]. One double-blind randomized placebo-controlled crossover trial with 53 infants did find that crying time was reduced in 26% of infants who received lactase, although the difference was not significant [55]. A recent review that included four randomized controlled trials determined that the evidence was such that one cannot draw firm conclusions [47].

A number of dietary changes with the intent to eliminate cow's milk protein have been proposed as interventions for colic or crying. One of the most prevalent is perhaps the use of soy-based formulas as opposed to cow's milk–based formulas. A survey of 1803 mothers in Israel found that 10.4% of infants were given soy-based formulas at 2 months of age, 20.4% at 4 months of age, and 31.5% of infants at 12 months of age [56]. Colic ranked among the main symptoms that triggered medical personnel and/or the mothers to initiate the change to a soy-based formula. One systemic review with three trials found that the substitution of a soy-based formula for cow's milk formula had a small favorable effect in infantile colic [48]; however, the significance disappeared when results were calculated using only the trials deemed to be methodologically sound. A second systemic review found two randomized controlled trials that examined the efficacy of soy formula in reducing symptoms of colic in bottle-fed infants [46]. Both studies showed a decrease in symptoms, but the methodology was found to be flawed. One study enrolled infants admitted to the hospital for colic, selecting a population much different from the majority seen in the outpatient setting. Both studies were thought to have inadequate blinding. A more recent review that included the same trials concluded that although no harms were reported in either, the evidence was of insufficient quality to determine the benefit of soy-based formula in infantile colic [47].

Some studies have addressed the efficacy of a low allergen diet in mothers of breast-feeding infants in reducing symptoms of colic. In one double-blind randomized placebo-controlled study, Hill and colleagues [57] looked at the 77 breast-fed and 38 bottle-fed infants. Mothers of the breast-fed infants were randomized to a low allergen diet free of milk, egg, wheat, and nut, or to a control diet free of artificial color, preservatives, and additives. Bottle-fed infants received either a hypoallergenic casein hydrolysate formula or a control cow's milk formula. When results of the two groups were combined in analysis, 61% of infants randomized to the low allergen or hypoallergenic feeds experienced more than 25% reduction in distress versus 43% of those on the control diets. In comparing the results between the bottle-fed and breast-fed groups, the investigators did not find a significant difference. Evans and colleagues [32] performed another small placebo-controlled double-blind randomized crossover trial with 20 exclusively breast-fed infants. They determined that eliminating cow's milk from the maternal diet did not ameliorate the distress in colic except in infants whose mothers had a history of atopy. A third more recent randomized controlled trial with 90 colicky infants found a significant absolute risk reduction of 37% in cry/fuss duration in 47 infants whose mothers were randomized to a low-allergen diet free of dairy products, soy, wheat, eggs, peanuts, tree nuts, and fish compared with the 43 infants whose mothers were randomized to the control diet [58]. Although there is some conflicting evidence, overall, the studies suggest that some therapeutic benefit may be derived in colicky breast-fed infants when their mothers maintain a low-allergen diet.

Hypoallergenic formulas including casein hydrolysate and whey hydrolysate formulas are potentially promising treatments for colic [46–48]. In Hill and colleagues' [57] study comparing casein hydrolysate formula to cow's milk formula, the infants randomized to the former group did significantly better in terms of reduction of distress. However, there were only 38 bottle-fed infants in the study, and the results were pooled with those of breast-fed infants. A second double-blind crossover randomized study with 17 infants evaluated the effects of alternating casein hydrolysate and cow's milk formula on colic symptoms [59]. Although symptoms were significantly reduced when the infants were on the casein hydrolysate formula, the effects diminished over time and there was no difference between groups by the third change. In addition, eight infants dropped out of the study before completion. Lucassen and colleagues [60] compared whey hydrolysate formula to cow's milk formula in a double-blind, randomized trial with 43 infants with colic. Infants in the first group were found to have an average in decreased crying time of 63 minutes compared with those receiving cow's milk formula. However, blinding may have been inadequate.

A number of herbal remedies have been used anecdotally in the treatment of colic. One study comparing the effects of a tea containing chamomile, vervain, licorice, fennel, and balm-milk to placebo found that after 7 days of treatment 57% of infants in the active treatment group no longer met

Wessel's criteria for colic versus 27% of those in the placebo group [61]. Long-term effects were not studied. In addition, the average amount of tea consumed by infants in the study was 32 mL/kg/day which leads to concerns about nutritional deficiencies should the amount of milk consumed decrease accordingly. No adverse effects were reported in this study. However, not all herbal remedies may be considered safe. In particular, star anise is a spice used among the Caribbean and Latino populations to make tea for the treatment of colic. Chinese star anise is commonly viewed as safe, although neurological symptoms have been seen with higher doses [62]. The closely related Japanese star anise, however, has been reported to cause both gastrointestinal and neurological toxicities including vomiting, jitteriness, myoclonus or clonus, nystagmus, and seizures [62,63].

Along with medical remedies and dietary changes, parents are oftentimes advised to initiate behavioral interventions for their colicky infants. These include increased infant carrying, car rides, decreasing stimulation, and infant swaddling. Two systemic reviews with two randomized control trials found that there was no reduction in symptoms with increased infant carrying [46,48]. One randomized controlled trial showed that the use of a car ride simulator was no better than counseling and reassurance in reducing the amount of infant crying or maternal anxiety [64]. Two systemic reviews found one randomized controlled trial that addressed the question of whether or not decreasing stimulation effectively reduces the symptoms of colic [46,48]. In this study, 93% of infants in the treatment group showed improvement compared with 50% in the control group [65]. However, the study had methodological weaknesses including a subjective case definition that precludes one from drawing firm conclusions [46–48]. A recent randomized controlled trial evaluated the added effect of swaddling to nurse support and stimuli reduction on excessive infant crying [66]. Swaddling was found to have no added benefit for the group as a whole. However, the subgroup of infants younger than 8 weeks did appear to benefit although the results were modest with a crying time reduction of 12 minutes per 24 hours.

Pathological crying

Organic diseases account for less than 5% of infants presenting with excessive crying [67]; however, the importance of distinguishing crying due to pathologic causes from nonpathological causes cannot be understated. In addition, in the face of an actively wailing infant and his or her strained parent(s), the examination room setting can often be tense. Because the complaint of crying is so nonspecific, the differential diagnosis is extensive and may be somewhat overwhelming. The authors find it helpful to use a systems-based approach.

The importance of a thorough history and physical examination cannot be overemphasized. In a prospective study of 56 infants presenting to the

Emergency Department with ages ranging from 4 days to 24 months (median age 3.5 months), Poole [68] found that 61% had diagnoses that were considered serious. The history provided clues that aided in the diagnoses in 20% of these patients, while the physical examination provided the diagnoses in 41% and provided clues leading to the diagnoses in 13%. The remaining 24% of infants with serious conditions continued to cry excessively after the initial assessment. Of note, patients were excluded from the study when they had fever or history of fever, symptoms of acute illness within the past 72 hours, or history of a previously diagnosed disease that could predispose them to bouts of pain or crying including colic, sickle cell anemia, and ventriculoperitoneal shunt.

In addition to the usual questions concerning onset, duration, and frequency of crying, and associated symptoms, the initial history should include a thorough review of systems, birth history, developmental history, past medical history, medications, and allergies. A history of recent immunizations should be included as well. Persistent crying associated with painful local reactions has been reported following administration the diphtheria-tetanus-pertussis vaccine [69]. The infant should be undressed to allow a complete exam. A thorough history and physical examination will go a long way in helping to sort out the possibilities. Box 1 lists some of the more common causes of crying in infants.

Head, eyes, ears, nose, throat

The head and scalp should be palpated carefully. Soft tissue swelling, tenderness, or skull depression suggest trauma and should prompt radiological testing especially when the injury is unexplained or the history is inconsistent. A bulging fontanelle raises concerns about increased intracranial pressure secondary to intracranial infections or intracranial lesions including hemorrhage or space-occupying masses. A large fontanelle along with widely separated cranial sutures suggests hydrocephalus. Prematurely fused cranial sutures, on the other hand, may be indicative of craniosynostosis.

Examination of the eyes should start with an external examination of the eyelids, conjunctiva, sclera, cornea, and iris. The presence of persistent discharge or tearing is associated with lacrimal duct obstruction, infection, allergy, or glaucoma [70]. Corneal enlargement is the hallmark of pediatric glaucoma, but the edema may be subtle especially if both eyes are involved. It is often preceded by the triad of epiphora, blepharospasm, and photophobia. In the presence of consistent signs and symptoms, an intraocular pressure of greater than 20 mm Hg in a resting infant or an asymmetry of more than 5 mm Hg are suggestive of glaucoma [71]. Suspicion for glaucoma should prompt urgent referral to a pediatric ophthalmologist. Direct ophthalmoscopy may be performed to look for the red reflex both individually and simultaneously. The red reflex should be bright reddish-yellow or light gray in the brown-eyed patients and should be symmetrical in both eyes [72].

A blunted or asymmetric reflex suggests intraocular tumors, vitreous opacities, or retinal detachment. The presence of retinal hemorrhages in the absence of a history of robust mechanism is concerning for shaken baby syndrome [73]. A thorough eye examination with fluorescein stain of the cornea should be performed in every infant with unexplained crying. Corneal abrasions have been reported in infants in the absence of trauma history and corneal redness or edema [68,74]. Similarly the lids may be retracted to look for a foreign body.

External examination of the ears is important. Look for signs of external irritation or injury. Contusions on the ear are highly suggestive of nonaccidental trauma. Otoscopy should be performed on every child to look for otitis media. In Poole's [68] study, otitis media was the most commonly diagnosed condition among infants with unexplained excessive crying.

A history of unilateral nasal discharge is suggestive of a nasal foreign body. Because the history can often be unrevealing, nares should be examined in every infant, ambulatory and nonambulatory alike. Examination of the oropharynx may reveal thrush, pharyngitis, or vesicular lesions indicative of stomatitis. Palatal or uvular burns from ingesting hot food or liquid can also become apparent. These conditions may be accompanied by a history of decreased feeding and/or fever.

Cardiovascular

A history of congenital heart disease (CHD) in a child may change one's approach to the work-up, and should be sought out. Many children with CHD are at increased risk for infective endocarditis. Infants can present with nonspecific symptoms such as fever, malaise, and irritability. They may have a new or changing murmur, splenomegaly, or petechiae on exam. Patients with known CHD and those with undiagnosed CHD can present with symptoms of congestive heart failure. In the most severe case, they can have cyanosis or shock; however, many will have less obvious complaints and signs including fussiness, agitation, and feeding difficulty. A cardiac murmur, tachypnea, diaphoresis, and hepatomegaly may be found on physical examination [75]. Infants with an anomalous left coronary artery can present with myocardial infarction and such nonspecific signs as crying and fussiness.

Patients with supraventricular tachycardia may also present with the chief complaint of fussiness. The diagnosis usually starts in triage, with the nurse reporting that the heart rate is "too fast to count." In general, infants will present with heart rater of greater than 220 beats per minute.

Pulmonary

Any history of previous or chronic pulmonary disease such as recent pneumonia, bronchopulmonary dysplasia, reactive airway disease, or cystic fibrosis may be relevant. Procure a history of respiratory symptoms including

Box 1. Differential diagnosis for excessive crying in infants

Head, eyes, ears, nose, throat
Trauma
Corneal abrasion
Ocular/nasal/ear foreign body
Glaucoma
Otitis media
Oral thrush/stomatitis/pharyngitis
Palatal burns
Panniculitis

Cardiovascular
Congestive heart failure
Supraventricular tachycardia
Endocarditis/myocarditis
Myocardial infarction

Pulmonary
Upper respiratory infection
Foreign body aspiration
Pneumothorax
Pneumonia

Gastrointestional
Constipation
Anal fissure
Hemorrhoids
Bowel obstruction
Intussusception
Malrotation/midgut volvulus
Hirschsprung's disease
Milk protein allergy
GERD/Esophagitis
Celiac disease
Appendicitis
Peritonitis

Genitourinary
Testicular torsion
Incarcerated inguinal hernia
Genital tourniquets
Balanitis/posthitis/balanoposthitis
Hydrocele
Urinary retention
Urinary tract infection

Musculoskeletal
Hair/Synthetic fiber tourniquet
Fracture
Osteomyelitis
Arthritis
Rickets
Vasoocclusive crisis (sickle-cell anemia)
Dactylitis

Neurological
Neonatal drug withdrawal
Increased intracranial pressure
    Hydrocephalus
    Mass
    Intracranial hemorrhage
    Cerebral edema
Meningitis/encephalitis

Dermatologic
Burns
Cellulitis
Insect bites/urticaria
Atopic dermatitis
Mastocytosis

Metabolic/Toxigenic
Inborn errors of metabolism
Hypoglycemia
Electrolyte abnormalities
Hyperthyroidism
Pheochromocytoma
Toxic ingestion
Carbon monoxide poisoning

Other
Hunger
Infantile colic
Immunizations
Abuse

cough, wheezing, dyspnea, or tachypnea. This is not always offered without prompting when the main complaint is crying especially if the event was transient and thus deemed insignificant. The possibility of a foreign body in the airway is present even in the nonambulatory infant especially if they have been around other young children. If the index of suspicion is high, bilateral decubitus chest radiographs may be indicated. Inadequate oxygenation or ventilation resulting in air hunger can manifest outwardly with nonspecific symptoms such as irritability. Note the general work of breathing. Auscultation of the lungs yielding abnormal sounds should prompt a chest radiograph.

Gastrointestinal

A history of vomiting or diarrhea or an abdominal examination revealing tenderness, distention, or a mass could direct the work-up and diagnosis in a child with excessive crying. The rectum should be examined in every case for anal fissures or hemorrhoids. Bright red blood may be seen in the stools but not invariably. Constipation is a common problem that can cause discomfort and irritability and, oftentimes, the diagnosis is made based solely on a history of stooling patterns [68]. Bilious vomiting points to a process occurring distal to the ampulla of vater, whereas nonbilious vomiting suggests that there is a problem proximal to the ampulla. Gastrointestinal symptoms are, however, often more subtle especially in young infants.

Intussusception is a serious condition that has a peak incidence between 3 and 9 months of age. One retrospective chart review of 90 patients diagnosed with intussusception found that 92% of patients were under the age of 1 year [76]. Only 30% of patients had bloody stools, while the combination of vomiting, blood per rectum, and abdominal mass was found in 29%. The triad of vomiting, screaming attacks, and lethargy was found in 38%. Vomiting alone or in combination with other signs or symptoms was the most common clinical manifestation of intussusception, but screaming attacks ranked second with 74% of infants presenting with it. The incidence of intussusception appears to be concentrated during the warmer months. It occurs not uncommonly in conjunction with common viral illnesses including upper respiratory infections. The newly released rotavirus vaccine is currently suspected of causing intussusception in vaccine recipients. Suspicion should also be high when there is unexplained crying with vomiting and/or lethargy. Plain radiographs are diagnostic in less than half of cases. Barium enema can be both diagnostic and therapeutic and has traditionally been the study of choice. More recently, air and saline hydrostatic reductions have also been performed. The use of ultrasound as a diagnostic modality has achieved good results at centers with experienced radiologists [77].

Other causes of bowel obstruction that can present early with nonspecific signs and symptoms include midgut volvulus, and Hirschsprung's disease. Although Hirschsprung's disease presents most commonly in the newborn period with bowel obstruction and bilious emesis, children can present later with irritability and a history of chronic severe constipation. Classically there is a failure to pass stools within the first 24 hours of life. The rectal examination may reveal an empty rectal vault [77]. Midgut volvulus occurs in those that have intestinal malrotation during fetal development. They may present from the newborn period into adulthood, but most become symptomatic during the first year of life with a concentration during the first month of life. Early signs include acute onset of abdominal pain and bilious emesis. Abdominal distension and tenderness, hematemesis, and passage of blood from the rectum develop later [77,78]. Again, a high index of suspicion is required for early diagnosis and management. Chronic intermittent midgut volvulus may have a more subtle presentation including recurrent bouts of abdominal pain and malabsorption, constipation alternating with diarrhea, and intolerance to solid food. The upper GI series is the diagnostic modality of choice in the stable patient [77].

Genitourinary

A careful physical examination of the genitourinary area may suggest testicular torsion or incarcerated inguinal hernias, both surgical emergencies. The incidence of congenital inguinal hernia has been reported to be between 0.8% and 4.0% of live births, and during the first 6 months of life the risk of the hernia becoming incarcerated may be as high as 60.0% [79]. An incarcerated inguinal hernia presents as scrotal swelling that can extend to the inguinal area that may or may not be tender [80]. The incidence of testicular torsion peaks during the perinatal period and the peripubertal period. Patients may present with acute onset of scrotal pain, tenderness, and swelling often accompanied by nausea and vomiting. A Doppler ultrasound is needed to diagnose and differentiate it from other causes of scrotal swelling including orchitis, epididymitis, trauma, and hydrocele. Hydroceles are a common cause of scrotal swelling in infants and, although usually painless, can cause diffuse discomfort. Transillumination can help confirm the presence of a hydrocele, but an ultrasound may be needed for evaluation of possible associated pathology [79,81].

Other causes of discomfort that may be uncovered with physical examination include genital tourniquets, balanitis, posthitis, and balanoposthitis. Genital tourniquets are surgical emergencies that can lead to ischemic injury to the organ if not promptly relieved. Balanitis, posthitis, and balanoposthitis are commonly the result of inadequate hygiene or external irritation [79]. A history of recent urethral catheterization or instrumentation may be significant. Obtaining a urinalysis to screen for urinary tract infections in infants with a normal exam and continued unexplained crying can be helpful [68].

Musculoskeletal

A history of trauma is important. It is vital to obtain a clear and detailed history including time of injury occurrence and mechanism of injury. Fractures are the second most common presentation of abuse, and up to 80% of fractures occurring in infants less than a year of age have been attributed to abuse [82]. Carefully palpate the body and extremities for swelling or tenderness. Oftentimes, the chief complaint is vague consisting only of a fussy or irritable infant, swollen extremity, or refusal to move a limb. In one study with 215 children 3 years of age and younger with sustained fractures, 52 (24%) were determined to be the result of abuse. Abuse was found to be more likely if there was no history of trauma, the extent of injury was greater than expected, there was an extremity fracture in a child less than 1 year of age, or there was a midshaft or metaphyseal humerus fracture [83]. Fractures with high specificity for abuse include classic metaphyseal lesions, posterior rib fractures, scapula fractures, spinous process fractures, and sternal fractures [84].

Examine all bones and joints for warmth, swelling, tenderness, or irritability that may suggest osteomyelitis, or arthritis. Osteomyelitis in infants and especially neonates can have delayed diagnoses because signs and symptoms are often nonspecific. These include irritability, decreased use of the affected limb, and fever. There may be redness or swelling of the soft tissue over the affected area. Neonates with osteomyelitis may show solely pseudoparalysis and tenderness over the site. Septic arthritis can present similarly with acute onset of irritability, fever, limp in the ambulatory child, or joint irritability, redness, and swelling [85,86]. The child may hold the joint in such a position that maximizes intracapsular volume and comfort. Hips may be flexed, abducted, and externally rotated, and knees may be moderately flexed [86]. The differential diagnosis includes inflammatory or reactive arthritis and malignancy. Dactylitis, microinfarcts in the phalanges and metatarsal bones, occurs in individuals with sickle-cell disease, most commonly in infancy, and can mimic osteomyelitis [85,87]. Children with acutely swollen digits should be examined carefully for digital tourniquets.

Neurologic

Many neurological disorders can present with nonspecific signs and symptoms especially in young infants. Birth history should include a history of maternal drug use since neonates in drug withdrawal are often irritable, jittery, and difficult to console. A careful neurological exam should be performed on all patients. Focal neurological findings might raise concern for increased intracranial pressure. Infants with acute intracranial hemorrhage, cerebral edema, or hydrocephalus can initially present with fussiness, irritability, decreased activity or feeding, or lethargy. Those with chronic subdural hematomas, hydrocephalus, intracranial mass, or chiari malformation type I may also have poor weight gain or failure to thrive and developmental delay [88].

An external examination of the head and scalp is important as stated above. However, infants with inflicted traumatic brain injuries commonly present without external signs of trauma and a wide spectrum of signs and symptoms. Many have normal neurological examinations [89–91]. Rubin and colleagues [91] reviewed the records of children younger than 2 years with injuries suspicious for child abuse, a normal neurological exam, normal scalp exam, and at least one high-risk criteria, namely rib fractures, multiple fractures, facial injuries, or an age of less than 6 months. They found that 19 (37%) of 51 had occult head injuries found on computed tomography. Consider imaging the head when there is suspicion for abuse in the young infant.

Meningitis or encephalitis should always be a consideration in the irritable infant. During the early course of systemic infections, young infants may present with crying, irritability, or fussiness without fever [92]. Patients who are ill-appearing, or have unabated crying during the emergency department visit should be observed either in the department or in the hospital and may require further ancillary testing. In Poole's [68] small study, serious illness was found to be unlikely in the face of a normal physical exam and an infant who did not continue to cry beyond the initial assessment.

Dermatologic

The skin should be examined thoroughly for infectious lesions, rashes, abrasions, and bruises. Infants with infectious skin lesions such as cellulitis or mastitis do not necessarily have fever or obvious initial findings [93]. The skin exam may also reveal papular urticaria from insect bites or spider bites. Check the child's interdigital web spaces for lesions that could suggest infestation with *Sarcoptes scabiei*, or scabies.

Diaper dermatitis is a common condition in young infants particularly in those with a recent history of diarrhea. The resulting skin irritation can cause aggravation and restlessness. The papulosquamous lesions of atopic dermatitis may be found on the scalp, face, or extensor surfaces on infants usually sparing the diaper area. It is characterized by intense pruritis and scratching that can lead to excoriations and vesiculations [94].

Bruises are extremely rare in preambulatory infants less than 6 months of age and uncommon in those less than 9 months of age [95–97]. Therefore, when they do occur, they raise suspicion for inflicted injuries. Bruises over the ears and genitourinary and buttocks regions are rarely the results of accidental injury. Accidental bruises from falling characteristically occur over bony prominences at the front of the body [96,97]. Any injury that does not fit with the stated mechanism is a cause for concerns about possible abuse. The developmental capabilities of the infant should be taken into account when determining the plausibility of the mechanism. The same is true of burn injuries [98]. Patterned burns from the imprint of hot objects such as a cigarette or hand iron, or immersion of a body area into hot liquid are suggestive of inflicted injuries. Burns to the bilateral lower extremities and buttocks or perineal regions are seen more frequently in inflicted than accidental injuries [99].

Metabolic/toxigenic

The child with an inborn error of metabolism can present in the newborn period or later in life. The intricacies of various biochemical pathway defects that result in the many possible diseases are discussed in detail elsewhere [100–102]. Many of these disorders have in common enzymatic or protein defects that lead to accumulation of toxic intermediates and neurological dysfunction. This can manifest in the early stages as irritability or lethargy and vomiting, and in later stages with a sepsis-like picture. When the toxic intermediates are acids, as is often the case, metabolic acidosis is present inducing tachypnea. Older infants and toddlers typically present during periods of common viral illnesses. There may be a history of poor weight gain, developmental delay, or recurrent severe illness.

Hypoglycemia is important particularly in the neonatal period. It is relatively common in newborns especially in those who are premature or small for gestational age. In most cases, it is a transient process, a consequence of poor glucose and fat stores and immature glucoregulatory mechanisms that resolves over a matter of days. Newborn infants of diabetic mothers can also have hypoglycemia from transient hyperinsulinemia that usually resolves over 3 to 5 days. Hypoglycemia occurring past the newborn period could suggest pituitary or adrenal dysfunction; inborn errors of glucose synthesis, storage, or breakdown or fatty acid oxidation; or congenital hyperinsulinemia [101–103]. Alternatively, infants may be hypoglycemic simply from inadequate nutritional intake. It can also be one of the many manifestations of serious systemic illness including infection [104]. Hypoglycemia in infants presents with any combination of jitteriness, irritability, abnormal cry, poor feeding, respiratory distress, apnea, cyanosis, temperature instability, myoclonic jerks, and seizures.

Consider the possibility of toxic ingestions especially in ambulatory infants. In the same vein, maternal medications can be significant in breast-feeding infants who may be exposed to medications that are excreted in the breast milk. Environmental exposures can also be a consideration. Carbon monoxide poisoning is the most frequent cause of asphyxiant poisoning in the United States, and occurs more commonly in the winter months [105]. Relevant historical factors include indoor heaters and gas stove use, and household members with similar symptoms. It presents in the acute stages in adults and older children with headache, dizziness, blurred vision, confusion, nausea/vomiting, chest pain, weakness, tachycardia, and/or tachypnea. Young infants can present with irritability or lethargy and vomiting [106,107]. The classic findings of cherry-red lips, cyanosis, and retinal hemorrhages are rare. More severe poisoning can lead to apnea, seizures, dysrhythmias, or cardiopulmonary arrest. Pulse oximetry is often falsely elevated, and diagnosis requires the measurement of carboxyhemoglobin in the blood. The mainstay of treatment is supplemental oxygen [107].

Summary

The crying infant is a common clinical dilemma faced by emergency physicians. Careful consideration should be given to every case. The differential diagnosis must be tailored to the history and clinical presentation. Ordering

---

Box 2. IT CRIES mnemonic for infant crying

I – Infections (herpes stomatitis, urinary tract infection, meningitis, osteomyelitis, and so forth)

T – Trauma (accidental and nonaccidental), testicular torsion

C – Cardiac (congestive heart failure, supraventricular tachycardia, myocardial infarction)

R – Reflux, reactions to medications, reactions to formulas

I – Immunizations, insect bites

E – Eye (corneal abrasions, ocular foreign bodies, glaucoma)

S – Surgical (volvulus, intussusception, inguinal hernia)

(S) – Strangulation (hair/fiber tourniquet)

---

arbitrary tests will likely have low diagnostic yield possibly exposing the child to unneeded pain and radiation and adds to the cost burden of the medical system. Colic is a common condition in young infants. The individual history of crying pattern is necessary in making the diagnosis. The first episode of severe crying should not be easily dismissed as colic. Taking the general appearance of the child into account will guide clinical decision making. Any child who is ill-appearing or displays evidence of poor growth or development deserves further investigation. Any child who has cries inconsolably beyond the time of the initial assessment also requires further consideration. Do not forget the possibility of abuse. Screening and diagnostic testing should ideally be guided by the history and physical examination. The differential diagnosis for pathological causes of crying is considerable. To assist clinicians in recalling some of the more common causes of excessive crying, one of the authors has previously proposed the mnemonic IT CRIES (Box 2) [108].

When the diagnosis of colic is made, it is important to offer support and reassurance and suggest different methods of treatment since not all infants will respond to the same treatments. In addition, reviewing signs of ill appearance will empower the guardians and ensure prompt follow-up should the clinical picture change. A thorough systemic evaluation of the infant with the chief complaint of crying is an important skill for any clinician who works with pediatric patients. When the problem is approached in an open-minded inquisitive manner, the experience can be more satisfying for both the family and the practitioner.

References

[1] Forsyth BW, Leventhal JM, McCarthy PL. Mothers' perceptions of problems of feeding and crying behaviors. Arch Pediatr Adolesc Med 1985;139(3):269–72.
[2] Forsyth BW, McCarthy PL, Leventhal JM. Problems of early infancy, formula changes, and mother's beliefs about their infants. J Pediatr 1985;106(6):1012–7.

[3] St. James-Roberts I, Conroy S, Wilsher K. Bases for maternal perceptions of infant crying and colic behavior. Arch Dis Child 1996;75(5):375–84.

[4] Wake M, Morton-Allen E, Poulakis Z, et al. Prevalence, stability, and outcomes of cry-fuss and sleep problems in the first 2 years of life: prospective community-based study. Pediatrics 2006;117(3):836–42.

[5] Reijneveld SA, Brugman E, Hirasing RA. Excessive infant crying: the impact of varying definitions. Pediatrics 2001;108(4):893–7.

[6] Van der Wal MF, van den Boom DC, Pauw-Plomp H, et al. Mothers' report of infant crying and soothing in a multicultural population. Arch Dis Child 1998;79(4):312–7.

[7] Clifford TJ, Campbell K, Speechley KN, et al. Sequelae of infant colic: evidence of transient infant distress and absence of lasting effects on maternal mental health. Arch Pediatr Adolesc Med 2002;156(12):1183–8.

[8] Morris S, St. James-Roberts I, Sleep J, et al. Economic strategies for managing crying and sleeping problems. Arch Dis Child 2001;84(1):15–9.

[9] Oberklaid F. Persistent crying in infancy: a persistent clinical conundrum. J Paediatr Child Health 2000;36(4):297–8.

[10] Raiha H, Lehtenon L, Huhtala V, et al. Excessively crying infant in the family: mother-infant, father-infant, and mother-father interaction. Child Care Health Dev 2002;28(5): 419–29.

[11] Akman I, Kuscu K, Ozdemir N, et al. Mother's post-partum psychological adjustment and infantile colic. Arch Dis Child 2006;91(5):417–9.

[12] Miller AR, Barr RG, Eaton WO. Crying and motor behavior of six-week-old infants and post-partum maternal mood. Pediatrics 1993;92(4):551–8.

[13] Beebe SA, Casey R, Pinto-Martin J. Association of reported infant crying and maternal parenting stress. Clin Pediatr 1993;32(1):15–9.

[14] Papousek M, von Hofacker N. Persistent crying in early infancy: a non-trivial condition of risk for the developing mother-infant relationship. Child Care Health Dev 1998;24(5): 395–424.

[15] Levitzky S, Cooper R. Infant colic syndrome—maternal fantasies of aggression and infanticide. Clin Pediatr (Phila) 2000;39(7):395–400.

[16] Reijneveld SA, van der Wal MF, Brugman E, et al. Infant crying and abuse. Lancet 2004; 364(9442):1340–2.

[17] Brazelton TB. Crying in infancy. Pediatrics 1962;29:579–88.

[18] Barr RG. The normal crying curve: what do we really know? Dev Med Child Neurol 1990; 32(4):356–62.

[19] St. James-Roberts I. Persistent infant crying. Arch Dis Child 1991;66(5):653–5.

[20] Hunziker UA, Barr RG. Increased carrying reduces infant crying: a randomized controlled trial. Pediatrics 1986;77(5):641–8.

[21] St. James-Roberts I, Plewis I. Individual differences, daily fluctuations, and developmental changes in amounts of infant waking, fussing, crying, feeding, and sleeping. Child Dev 1996;67(5):2527–40.

[22] Illingworth RS. Three months' colic. Arch Dis Child 1984;29(145):165–74.

[23] Wessel MA, Cobb JC, Jackson EB, et al. Paroxysmal fussing in infancy, sometimes called "colic". Pediatrics 1954;14(5):421–34.

[24] Reijneveld SA, Brugman E, Hirasing RA. Excessive crying: definitions determine risk groups. Arch Dis Child 2002;87(1):43–4.

[25] Zahorsky J. Mixed feeding of infants. Pediatrics 1901;11:208–15.

[26] Treen WR. Infant colic: a pediatric gastroenterologist's perspective. Pediatr Clin North Am 1994;41(5):1121–38.

[27] Long T. Excessive infantile crying: a review of the literature. J Child Health Care 2001;5(3): 111–6.

[28] Lothe L, Lindberg T. Cow's milk whey protein elicits symptoms of infantile colic in colicky formula-fed infants: a double-blind crossover study. Pediatrics 1989;83(2):262–6.

[29] Iacono G, Carrocio A, Montalto G, et al. Severe infantile colic and food intolerance: a long-term prospective study. J Pediatr Gastroenterol Nutr 1991;12(3):332–5.

[30] Lothe L, Lindberg T, Jakobsson I. Cow's milk formula as a cause of infantile colic: a double blind study. Pediatrics 1982;70(1):7–10.

[31] Jakobsson D, Lindberg T. Cow's milk as a cause of infantile colic in breast-fed infants. Lancet 1978;2(8087):437–9.

[32] Evans RW, Fergusson DM, Allardyce RA, et al. Maternal diet and infantile colic in breast-fed infants. Lancet 1981;1(8234):1340–2.

[33] Jakobsson I, Lindberg T. Cow's milk proteins cause infantile colic in breast-fed infants: a double-blind crossover study. Pediatrics 1983;71(2):268–71.

[34] Liebman WM. Infantile colic: association with lactose and milk intolerance. JAMA 1981; 245(7):732–3.

[35] Moore DJ, Robb TA, Davidson GP. Breath hydrogen response to milk containing lactose in colicky and noncolicky infants. J Pediatr 1988;113(6):979–84.

[36] Sutphen J. Is it colic or is it gastroesophageal reflux? J Pediatr Gastroenterol Nutr 2001; 33(2):110–1.

[37] Armstrong KL, Previtera N, McCallum RN. Medicalizing normality? Management of irritability in babies. J Paediatr Child Health 2000;36(4):301–5.

[38] Berkowitz D, Yehezkel N, Moshe B. 'Infantile colic' as the sole manifestation of gastro-esophageal reflux. J Pediatr Gastroenterol Nutr 1997;24(2):231–3.

[39] Heine RG, Jordan B, Lubitz L, et al. Clinical predictors of pathological gastro-oesophageal reflux in infants with persistent distress. J Paediatr Child Health 2006;42(3):134–9.

[40] Barr RG. Management of clinical problems and emotional care: colic and crying syndromes in infants. Pediatrics 1998;102(5):1282–6.

[41] Blum NJ, Taubman B, Tretina L, et al. Maternal ratings of infant intensity and distracti-bility. Arch Pediatr Adolesc Med 2002;156(3):286–90.

[42] St. James-Roberts I, Conroy S, Wilsher K. Links between maternal care and persistent infant crying in the early months. Child Care Health Dev 1998;24(5):353–76.

[43] Keller H, Lohaus A, Volker S, et al. Relationships between infant crying, birth complica-tions, and maternal variables. Child Care Health Dev 1998;24(5):377–94.

[44] Keller H, Chasiotis A, Risau-Peters J, et al. Psychobiological aspects of infant crying. Early Development and Parenting 1996;5(1):1–13.

[45] Metcalf TJ, Irons TG, Sher LD, et al. Simethicone in the treatment of infant colic: a ran-domized, placebo-controlled, multicenter trial. Pediatrics 1994;94(1):29–34.

[46] Garrison MM, Christakis DA. A systemic review of treatments for infant colic. Pediatrics 2000;106(1):184–90.

[47] Wade S. Infantile colic. Clin Evid 2006;15:439–47.

[48] Lucassen PL, Assendelft WJ, Gubbels JW, et al. Effectiveness of treatments for infantile colic: systemic review. BMJ 1998;316(7144):1563–9.

[49] Williams J, Watkins-Jones R. Dicyclomine: worrying symptoms associated with its use in some small babies. BMJ 1984;288(6421):901.

[50] Stevens B, Ohlsson A. Sucrose for analgesia in newborn infants undergoing painful proce-dures. Cochrane Database Syst Rev 2004;3:CD001069.

[51] Markestad T. Use of sucrose as treatment for infant colic. Arch Dis Child 1997;76(4): 356–8.

[52] Barr RG, Young SN, Wright JH, et al. Differential calming responses to sucrose taste in crying infants with and without colic. Pediatrics 1999;103(5):e68.

[53] Stahlberg MR, Savilahti E. Infantile colic and feeding. Arch Dis Child 1986;61(12): 1232–3.

[54] Miller JJ, McVeagh P, Fleet GH, et al. Effect of yeast enzyme on 'colic' in infants fed human milk. J Pediatr 1990;117(2 Pt 1):261–3.

[55] Kanabar D, Randhawa M, Clayton P. Improvement of symptoms in infant colic following reduction of lactose load with lactase. J Hum Nutr Diet 2001;14(5):359–63.

[56] Berger-Achituv S, Shohat T, Romano-Zelekha O, et al. Widespread use of soy-based formula without clinical indications. J Pediatr Gastroenterol Nutr 2005;41(5):660–6.

[57] Hill DJ, Hudson IL, Sheffield LJ, et al. A low allergen diet is a significant intervention in infantile colic: results of a community-based study. J Allergy Clin Immunol 1995;96(6): 886–92.

[58] Hill DJ, Roy N, Heine RG, et al. Effect of a low-allergen diet on colic among breastfed infants: a randomized, controlled trial. Pediatrics 2005;116(5):700–15.

[59] Forsyth BW. Colic and the effect of changing formulas: a double-blind, multiple-crossover study. J Pediatr 1989;115(4):521–6.

[60] Lucassen PL, Assendelft WJ, Gubbels JW, et al. Infantile colic: crying time reduction with a whey hydrolysate: a double-blind, randomized, placebo-controlled trial. Pediatrics 2000; 106(6):1349–54.

[61] Weizman Z, Alkrinawi S, Goldfarb D, et al. Efficacy of herbal tea preparation in infantile colic. J Pediatr 1993;122(4):650–2.

[62] Ize-Ludlow D, Ragone S, Bruck IS, et al. Neurotoxicities in infants seen with the consumption star anise tea. Pediatrics 2004;114(5):e653–6.

[63] Ize-Ludlow D, Ragone S, Bruck IS, et al. Chemical composition of chinese star anise (*Illicium verum*) and neurotoxicities in infants. JAMA 2004;291(5):562–3.

[64] Parkin PC, Schwartz CJ, Manuel BA. Randomized controlled trial of three interventions in the management of persistent crying of infancy. Pediatrics 1993;92(2):197–201.

[65] Mckenzie S. Troublesome crying in infants: effect of advice to reduce stimulation. Arch Dis Child 1991;66(12):1416–20.

[66] Van Sleuwen BE, L'Hoir MP, Engelberts AC, et al. Comparison of behavior modification with and without swaddling as interventions for excessive crying. J Pediatr 2006;149(4): 512–7.

[67] Gormally SM, Barr RG. Of clinical pies and clinical clues: proposal for a clinical approach to complaints of early crying and colic. Ambulatory Child Health 1997;3:137–53.

[68] Poole SR. The infant with acute, unexplained, excessive crying. Pediatrics 1991;88(3):450–5.

[69] Blumberg DA, Lewis K, Mink CA. Severe reactions associated with diphtheria-tetanus-pertussis vaccine: detailed study of children with seizures, hypotonic-hyporesponsive episodes, high fevers, and persistent crying. Pediatrics 1993;91(6):1158–65.

[70] Swanson J, Yasuda K, France FL, et al. Committee on Practice and Ambulatory Medicine, Section on Ophthalmology. Eye examination in infants, children, and young adults by pediatricians. Pediatrics 2003;111(4 Pt 1):902–7.

[71] Fierson WM, Eisenbaum AM, Freedman HL, et al. Red reflex examination in infants. Pediatrics 2002;109(5):980–1.

[72] Brandt JD. Congenital glaucoma. In: Yanoff M, Duker JS, Augsburger JJ, editors. Ophthalmology. 2nd edition. St. Louis (MO): Mosby, Inc.,; 2004. p. 1475–80.

[73] Buys YM, Levin AV, Enzenauer RW. Retinal findings after head trauma in infants and young children. Ophthalmology 1992;99(11):1718–23.

[74] Harkness MJ. Corneal abrasion in infancy as a cause of inconsolable crying. Pediatr Emerg Care 1989;5(4):242–4.

[75] Woods WA, McCulloch MA. Cardiovascular emergencies in the pediatric patient. Emerg Med Clin North Am 2005;23(4):1233–49.

[76] Eshel G, Barr J, Heyman E, et al. Intussusception: a nine-year survey (1986–1995). J Pediatr Gastroenterol Nutr 1997;24(3):253–6.

[77] Halter JM, Baesl T, Nicolette L, et al. Common gastrointestinal problems and emergencies in children. Clinics in Family Practice 2004;6(3):731–54.

[78] Gosche JR, Vick L, Boulanger SC, et al. Midgut abnormalities. Surg Clin North Am 2006; 86(2):285–99.

[79] Haynes JH. Inguinal and scrotal disorders. Surg Clin North Am 2006;86(2):371–81.

[80] Leslie JA, Cain MP. Pediatric urological emergencies and urgencies. Pediatr Clin North Am 2006;53(3):513–27.

[81] Coley BD. The acute pediatric scrotum. Ultrasound Clinics 2006;1(3):485–96.

[82] Pierce MH, Bertocci G. Fractures resulting from inflicted trauma: assessing injury and history compatibility. Clinical Pediatric Emergency Medicine 2006;7:143–8.

[83] Leventhal JM, Thomas SA, Rosenfield NS, et al. Distinguishing child abuse from unintentional injuries. Am J Dis Child 1993;147(1):87–92.

[84] Kleinman PK. Diagnostic imaging of child abuse. 2nd edition. St. Louis (MO): Mosby; 1998. p. 9.

[85] Gutierrez K. Bone and joint infections in children. Pediatr Clin North Am 2005;52(3):779–94.

[86] Frank G, Mahoney HM, Eppes SC. Musculoskeletal infections in children. Pediatr Clin North Am 2005;52(4):1083–106.

[87] Aguilar C, Vichinsky E, Neumayr L. Bone and joint disease in sickle cell disease. Hematol Oncol Clin North Am 2005;19(5):929–41.

[88] Piatt JH. Recognizing neurosurgical conditions in the pediatrician's office. Pediatr Clin North Am 2004;51(2):237–70.

[89] Bechtel K, Berger R. Inflicted traumatic brain injury: making the diagnosis in the emergency department. Clinical Pediatric Emergency Medicine 2006;7(3):138–42.

[90] Greenes DS, Schutzman SA. Occult intracranial injury in infants. Ann Emerg Med 1998; 32(6):680–6.

[91] Rubin D, Christian CW, Bilaniuk LT, et al. Occult head injury in high-risk abused children. Pediatrics 2003;111(6 Pt 1):1382–6.

[92] Ruiz-Contreras J, Urquia L, Bastero R. Persistent crying as predominant manifestation of sepsis in infants and newborns. Pediatr Emerg Care 1999;15(2):113–5.

[93] Brown L, Hicks M. Subclinical mastitis presenting as acute, unexplained, excessive crying in an afebrile 31-day-old female. Pediatr Emerg Care 2001;17(3):189–90.

[94] Boguniewicz M, Leung DY. Atopic dermatitis. In: Adkinson NF, Yunginger JW, Busse WW, et al, editors. Middleton's allergy: principles and practice, vol. 2. 6th edition. St. Louis (MO): Mosby-Year Book Inc; 2003. p. 1559–75.

[95] Kaczor K, Pierce MC, Makoroff K, et al. Bruising and physical child abuse. Clinical Pediatric Emergency Medicine 2006;7:153–60.

[96] Sugar NF, Taylor JA, Feldman KW. Bruises in infants and toddlers: those that don't cruise rarely bruise. Arch Pediatr Adolesc Med 1999;153(4):399–403.

[97] Carpenter RF. The prevalence and distribution of bruising in babies. Arch Dis Child 1999; 80(4):363–6.

[98] Allasio D, Fischer H. Immersion scald burns and the ability of young children to climb into a bathtub. Pediatrics 2005;115(5):1419–21.

[99] Daria S, Sugar NF, Feldman KF, et al. Into hot water head first: distribution of intentional and unintentional immersion burns. Pediatr Emerg Care 2004;20(5):302–10.

[100] Zinn AB. Inborn errors of metabolism. In: Martin RJ, Fanaroff AA, Walsh MC, editors. Fanaroff and Martin's neonatal-perinatal medicine. 8th edition. St. Louis (MO): Mosby; 2006. p. 409–28.

[101] Claudius I, Fluharty C, Boles R. The emergency department approach to newborn and childhood metabolic crisis. Emerg Med Clin North Am 2005;23(3):843–83.

[102] Filiano JJ. Neurometabolic diseases in the newborn. Clin Perinatol 2006;33(2):411–79.

[103] Sperling MA, Menon RK. Differential diagnosis and management of neonatal hypoglycemia. Pediatr Clin North Am 2004;51(3):703–23.

[104] Losek JD. Hypoglycemia and the ABC's (sugar) of pediatric resuscitation. Ann Emerg Med 2000;35(1):43–6.

[105] Kales SN, Christiana DC. Acute chemical emergencies. N Engl J Med 2004;350(8):800–8.

[106] Kao LW, Nañagas KA. Toxicity associated with carbon monoxide. Clin Lab Med 2006; 26(1):99–125.

[107] Ernst A, Zibrak JD. Carbon monoxide poisoning. N Engl J Med 1998;339(22):1603–8.

[108] Herman MI, Nelson RA. Crying infants: what to do when babies wail. Critical Decisions in Emergency Medicine 2006;20(5):2–10.

ELSEVIER
SAUNDERS

Emerg Med Clin N Am
25 (2007) 1161–1165

EMERGENCY
MEDICINE
CLINICS OF
NORTH AMERICA

Index

Note: Page numbers of article titles are in **boldface** type.

Moving?

Make sure your subscription moves with you!

To notify us of your new address, find your **Clinics Account Number** (located on your mailing label above your name), and contact customer service at:

E-mail: elspcs@elsevier.com

800-654-2452 (subscribers in the U.S. & Canada)
407-345-4000 (subscribers outside of the U.S. & Canada)

Fax number: 407-363-9661

Elsevier Periodicals Customer Service
6277 Sea Harbor Drive
Orlando, FL 32887-4800

*To ensure uninterrupted delivery of your subscription, please notify us at least 4 weeks in advance of move.

1. Publication Title	2. Publication Number	3. Filing Date
Emergency Medicine Clinics of North America	0 0 0 - 7 1 1 4	9/14/07

4. Issue Frequency	5. Number of Issues Published Annually	6. Annual Subscription Price
Feb, May, Aug, Nov	4	$193.00

7. Complete Mailing Address of Known Office of Publication (Not printer) (Street, city, county, state, and ZIP+4)

Elsevier Inc.
360 Park Avenue South
New York, NY 10010-1710

Contact Person
Stephen Bushing

Telephone (Include area code)
215-239-3688

8. Complete Mailing Address of Headquarters or General Business Office of Publisher (Not printer)

Elsevier Inc., 360 Park Avenue South, New York, NY 10010-1710

9. Full Names and Complete Mailing Addresses of Publisher, Editor, and Managing Editor (Do not leave blank)

Publisher (Name and complete mailing address)

John Schrefer, Elsevier, Inc., 1600 John F. Kennedy Blvd. Suite 1800, Philadelphia, PA 19103-2899

Editor (Name and complete mailing address)

Patrick Manley, Elsevier, Inc., 1600 John F. Kennedy Blvd. Suite 1800, Philadelphia, PA 19103-2899

Managing Editor (Name and complete mailing address)

Catherine Bewick, Elsevier, Inc., 1600 John F. Kennedy Blvd. Suite 1800, Philadelphia, PA 19103-2899

10. Owner (Do not leave blank. If the publication is owned by a corporation, give the name and address of the corporation immediately followed by the names and addresses of all stockholders owning or holding 1 percent or more of the total amount of stock. If not owned by a corporation, give the names and addresses of the individual owners. If owned by a partnership or other unincorporated firm, give its name and address as well as those of each individual owner. If the publication is published by a nonprofit organization, give its name and address.)

Full Name	Complete Mailing Address
Wholly owned subsidiary of	4520 East-West Highway
Reed/Elsevier, US holdings	Bethesda, MD 20814

11. Known Bondholders, Mortgagees, and Other Security Holders Owning or Holding 1 Percent or More of Total Amount of Bonds, Mortgages, or Other Securities. If none, check box ☐ None

Full Name	Complete Mailing Address
N/A	

12. Tax Status (For completion by nonprofit organizations authorized to mail at nonprofit rates) (Check one)
The purpose, function, and nonprofit status of this organization and the exempt status for federal income tax purposes:
☑ Has Not Changed During Preceding 12 Months
☐ Has Changed During Preceding 12 Months (Publisher must submit explanation of change with this statement)

PS Form 3526, September 2006 (Page 1 of 3 (Instructions Page 3)) PSN 7530-01-000-9931 **PRIVACY NOTICE**: See our Privacy policy in www.usps.com

---

13. Publication Title	14. Issue Date for Circulation Data Below
Emergency Medicine Clinics of North America	May 2007

15. Extent and Nature of Circulation			Average No. Copies Each Issue During Preceding 12 Months	No. Copies of Single Issue Published Nearest to Filing Date
a. Total Number of Copies (Net press run)			2700	2700
b. Paid Circulation (By Mail and Outside the Mail)	(1)	Mailed Outside-County Paid Subscriptions Stated on PS Form 3541. (Include paid distribution above nominal rate, advertiser's proof copies, and exchange copies)	1509	1348
	(2)	Mailed In-County Paid Subscriptions Stated on PS Form 3541 (Include paid distribution above nominal rate, advertiser's proof copies, and exchange copies)		
	(3)	Paid Distribution Outside the Mails Including Sales Through Dealers and Carriers, Street Vendors, Counter Sales, and Other Paid Distribution Outside USPS®	427	415
	(4)	Paid Distribution by Other Classes Mailed Through the USPS (e.g. First-Class Mail®)		
c. Total Paid Distribution (Sum of 15b (1), (2), (3), and (4))			1936	1763
d. Free or Nominal Rate Distribution (By Mail and Outside the Mail)	(1)	Free or Nominal Rate Outside-County Copies Included on PS Form 3541	119	94
	(2)	Free or Nominal Rate In-County Copies Included on PS Form 3541		
	(3)	Free or Nominal Rate Copies Mailed at Other Classes Mailed Through the USPS (e.g. First-Class Mail)		
	(4)	Free or Nominal Rate Distribution Outside the Mail (Carriers or other means)		
e. Total Free or Nominal Rate Distribution (Sum of 15d (1), (2), (3) and (4))			119	94
f. Total Distribution (Sum of 15c and 15e)			2055	1857
g. Copies not Distributed (See instructions to publishers #4 (page #3))			645	843
h. Total (Sum of 15f and g)			2700	2700
i. Percent Paid (15c divided by 15f times 100)			94.21%	94.94%

16. Publication of Statement of Ownership

If the publication is a general publication, publication of this statement is required. Will be printed ☑ Publication not required
in the November 2007 issue of this publication.

17. Signature and Title of Editor, Publisher, Business Manager, or Owner

[signature]
Jan Ranucci – Executive Director of Subscription Services

Date
September 14, 2007

I certify that all information furnished on this form is true and complete. I understand that anyone who furnishes false or misleading information on this form or who omits material or information requested on the form may be subject to criminal sanctions (including fines and imprisonment) and/or civil sanctions (including civil penalties).

PS Form 3526, September 2006 (Page 2 of 3)